Tending
the
Temple

Kevin Vost

Shane Kapler

Peggy Bowes

Published by
Bezalel Books
Waterford, MI
www.BezalelBooks.com

Printed in the United States of America

Scripture quotations contained herein are adapted from the *Douay-Rheims Bible*, copyright © 1971, by Tan Books, the *Ignatius Revised Standard Version, Catholic Edition*, copyright © 1994, by Thomas Nelson Publishers for Ignatius Press, the *Ignatius Revised Standard Version, Second Catholic Edition*, copyright © 2006, and the *New American Bible*, copyright © 1965, 1966 by the National Council of the Churches of Christ in the United States of America.

Images used in *Tending the Temple*:
Francis Vincent
Soleilc | Dreamstime.com
Jim Mills | Dreamstime.com
oleksandr kalyna | Dreamstime.com
Sufi70 | Dreamstime.com
Robodread | Dreamstime.com
Freeskyblue | Dreamstime.com
Lomachevsky | Dreamstime.com

ISBN 978-1-936453-00-9
Library of Congress Control Number 2011900640

Introduction

Do you not know that your body is a temple of the Holy Spirit within you, which you have from God?   *I Corinthians 6:19*

God has called us to be good stewards of all creation, and this includes our own bodies. We are called to tend our temples—not to become obsessed about the body beautiful or to spend our lives worried about counting carbs, but to take moderate, reasonable measures to keep ourselves fit and healthy, and to help our loved ones do the same. Tending our bodily temples can help us to grow in virtues day by day, like the fortitude required to persistently exercise, and the temperance involved in eating sensible portions of food in our daily diets. It can also open up great new opportunities for prayer—before, after, or intertwined right in the midst of our workouts.

Our hope is that this book will inspire you to grow first and foremost in holiness through the glorious models of saintliness personified by the men and women throughout the world and throughout the centuries profiled within this devotional. Our special intention, of course, is that you and your loved ones will grow in bodily fitness as well. We hope this book will help you gain more energy and confidence to get out there and do good works, to fight the good fight, to become "dynamos of charity," spreading God's message of joyful redemption to all you encounter.

A Thought or Two from Kevin

I am very much honored to share these pages with a talented cast of coauthors and special contributors. Peggy Bowes, author of *The Rosary Workout* (Bezalel, 2010), is your typical devout Catholic housewife, mother, fitness expert, and former Air Force pilot, who home-schooled her children while their family traveled around the country in an RV. (So maybe she's not so typical.)

Shane Kapler, author of *The God Who is Love*, (Out of the Box, 2009), had lauded his results with the fitness methods of my *Fit for Eternal Life* (Sophia, 2007) in his blog. I found his writing most engaging, amusing, and abounding in charity. Thankfully, Shane heeded our call and became this book's third author.

Matt Swaim, the dynamic producer of EWTN/Sacred Heart Radio's Son Rise Morning Show, author of *The Rosary and the Eucharist* and *Prayer in the Digital Age* (Liguorian, 2010 & 2011) graciously provided his inimitable entries for April 14: St Peter Gonzalez, April 25: St. Mark the Evangelist, June 15: St. Vitus, Oct 5: Bl. Bartolo Longo, and last (and shortest), but never to be overlooked, Oct 17: St. John the Dwarf. (I can't help but note as well, in a book such as this, that Matt is a former state powerlifting champion and an avid bicyclist.)

Francis Vincent, M.D., is the author of *The Vagaries of Life* (Vin-Ego Books, 2000). He has graced us with five cartoons scattered about herein. ("The skill of the physician lifts up his head, and in the presence of great men he is admired." Sirach 38:3).

A Thought or Two from Shane

That Shane Kapler would contribute to a book on physical well-being has to be a miracle on par with the parting of the Red Sea (well, it seems that way to me). I have always been passionate about growing in my relationship with the God, but my commitment to caring for the body He entrusted to me has been downright pathetic at times. At about the same time Kevin and Peggy began writing this book though, God's grace finally brought me to the point of "conversion," and I started implementing the recommendations Kevin made in *Fit For Eternal Life*. Over an eight month period I shed over 50 pounds, pounds I had been carrying around for over seven years! When Kevin heard the changes God was allowing me to make, he, Peggy, and their publisher Cheryl Dickow, were kind enough to invite me aboard. So while Kevin and Peggy write from the perspective of fitness instructors, I write from the perspective of so many of you—a student.

I know the value of the instruction you will receive between these pages, because I am living it. Do you know what has surprised me the most these past months? It has been the interconnection between physical virtue and spiritual virtue. I can see how increasing my endurance for cardiovascular exercise for example, has translated into less procrastination in getting jobs done around the house. This goes right back to Aquinas: We human beings are body *and soul*, soul *and body*; and the vigilance or laxity we practice in one part of our nature affects the other. So get reading . . .and praying. . .and exercising—you are tending a temple meant for eternity!

A Thought or Two from Peggy

It is an honor and a privilege to work with such virtuous and amiable gentlemen as Kevin Vost and Shane Kapler. Although we have never met in person, I continue to be impressed by Kevin's wit and wisdom. He is "just" your average log-throwing, kilt-wearing, former Atheist psychologist who can rattle off every book of the Bible, in order, while simultaneously quoting Aquinas and Aristotle.

Kevin "virtually introduced" me to Shane, who shares my love for the Blessed Mother and her favorite prayer, the Rosary. Imagine my surprise when I discovered that I had already referenced Shane's eloquent articles several times in my blog on the Rosary (www.rosaryinfo.blogspot.com). I think the Blessed Mother beat Kevin to our introduction!

I invited two of my favorite women authors to contribute their talents to *Tending the Temple*. Theresa Doyle-Nelson (www.TheresaDoyle-Nelson.com), author of *Saints of the Bible* and *More Saints of the Bible,* penned the November 22nd entry on Sts. Philemon and Apphia. Her books on Bible saints were also helpful resources for writing some of my own entries. Lisa Mladnich, author of *Be an Amazing Catechist* (www.AmazingCatechists.com), wrote the entry on St. John Vianney for August 4th.

Note: The Church dedicates each month of the year to a particular devotion, as outlined below. Keep these overall themes in mind while reading the varied saint biographies and daily physical and spiritual exercises. Perhaps you might want to learn more about a particular monthly devotion and include it in your prayer routine.

January: *Holy Name of Jesus;* February: *Holy Family;* March: *St. Joseph;* April: *Blessed Sacrament;* May: *Mary;* June: *Sacred Heart;* July: *Precious Blood;* August: *Immaculate Heart of Mary;* September: *Our Lady of Sorrows;* October: *Rosary;* November: *Holy Souls in Purgatory;* December: *Immaculate Conception*

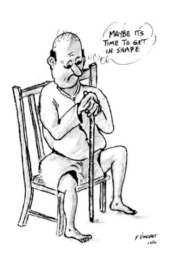

MAYBE ITS
TIME TO GET
IN SHAPE

Cautions:
Temple Building Codes

The things with which prudence is concerned, are contingent matters of action, wherein, even as false is found without true, so is evil mingled with good, on account of the great variety of these matters of action, wherein good is so often hindered by evil, and evil has the appearance of good. Wherefore, prudence needs caution, so that we may have such a grasp of good as to avoid evil.

St. Thomas Aquinas
(Summa Theologica, II-II, Q 60. a.8)

St. Thomas sure has a way of saying things, doesn't he? To translate his Latin into even simpler English that is relevant to our concerns, we will be *prudent* (practically wise) if we exercise *caution* in seeking the good of bodily fitness without encountering the evils of injury or overtraining. While we authors have striven to incorporate information on safe and proper exercise performance throughout our daily entries, we thought it most prudent to start right off the bat (or perhaps right off the couch!) to provide some preliminary cautions, so please note these well:

- The exercises described within this book are intended for healthy men and women. Especially if you are coming to this book straight off the couch and have not been involved in systematic strength or aerobic training, we strongly urge you to seek the advice of our your personal physician before embarking on a training program, lest known or undiagnosed medical problems require that you forgo or modify the training advice within this book.
- The strength training exercises are to be performed in a slow (also see the glossary) and controlled manner with normal breathing patterns (no holding the breath) and without excessively tight gripping of barbells, dumbbells, or machine handles. Holding the breath and tight gripping can elevate the blood pressure to possibly dangerous levels. Fast, sloppy exercise performance can lead to loss of control of the weights and to injuries to the muscles, tendons, ligaments, or bones.
- The pain that comes from lactic acid buildup during strength training exercises should come on gradually and lead to cessation of the set. Sudden pains suggest injury. Stop any exercise in which you feel any sudden, sharp pains. Also, do not do a particular exercise or use a particular machine if it feels like the mechanics

are not right for your body, as if a joint or muscle is placed in an awkward position. If you are training within a fitness center, ask for assistance in learning proper exercise performance.

✦ ✦ Chest pain and dizziness are also serious signs and you should seek medical assistance if you experience such symptoms from your training.

✦ ✦ When walking, running, or biking outside, seek traffic-free paths if possible, and exercise great care if you must share roads with vehicles. Some prefer to walk or run against traffic, to see what is coming. It is usually safer to bike with the flow of traffic, though. Also exercise special caution when approaching curves or hills. And be sure to wear bright clothing and reflective gear like a vest, especially when training at dusk or dawn, in the dark, rain, snow, or fog.

✦ ✦ Also exercise care if using a headset while walking or running. The use of a headset is especially dangerous for biking and *we strongly urge you not to use one while biking.*

✦ ✦ A simple way to gauge that you are not training too intensely in your aerobic/cardiovascular sessions is the simple "talk test." If you are unable to carry on a conversation during your session (unless you are advanced and are performing a brief, intense interval), you may need to slow down a bit.

✦ ✦ For your aerobic/cardiovascular training sessions, always spend a few minutes of gentle warm-up as you increase your speed or resistance, and always end with a few minutes of gentler activity as well. For example, you might spend your first five minutes on an exercise bike gradually increasing the level of resistance and the last five minutes gradually decreasing it. If you are running, you might start by walking or jogging slowly for the first few minutes, and conclude your run with several minutes (maybe five or more) of walking.

Along with the words of caution, the authors wanted you to know the sites and references they used in this tome as they may enrich you further in your temple tending journey. They include:
www.americancatholic.org/Features/Saints/bydate.aspx;
www.catholictradition.org/Saints/feast-days.htm;
www.newadvent.org/cathen/; www.saints.sqpn.com/;
www.wikipedia.org/ (always cross-checked with other sources);
www.NewAdvent.org; www.CatholicOnline.com;
www.HolySpiritInteractive.net; www.CatholicCulture.org;
www.CatholicFire.blogspot.com; www.ewtn.com;
Delaney, John J. Dictionary of Saints. New York: Doubleday, 1980;
Ghezzi, Bert. Voices of the Saints. Chicago: Loyola, 2000;
Bernard Bangley, *Butler's Lives of the Saints: Concise Modernized Edition* Brewster, MA: Paraclete Press, 2005; Fr. Alban Butler, *Lives of the Saints for Every Day of the Year* (Rockford, IL: TAN Books, 1995); Doyle-Nelson, Theresa. *Saints of the Bible*. Huntington, IN: Our Sunday Visitor, 2009; Doyle-Nelson, Theresa. *More Saints of the Bible*. Self-published, 2010; Marbach, Ethel. *Once-Upon-a-Time Saints*. Cincinnati, OH: St Anthony Messenger Press, 1977

Solemnity of Mary, Mother of God

Behold, from henceforth all generations will call me blessed. *Luke 1:48*

The Blessed Virgin's womb remains forever fruitful. Mary leads us to Christ, but Christ leads us back to his Mother, for without Mary's maternity, Jesus would become a mere abstraction to us. The Lord wills to "let his face shine upon" us through the face of the Mother of God. We serve a Mother who seems to grow more beautiful as new generations rise up and call her blessed. *G.K. Chesterton*

Happy New Year! It is fitting that we begin every calendar year by honoring the Blessed Mother. One of Mary's many titles is the Greek word *Theotokos*, or "God bearer." She is truly the Mother of God and not merely the mother of Jesus' human nature. In fact, we honor Mary's role as Mother of God each time we pray the Hail Mary.

From eternity, God chose Mary as the pure vessel who would bring His Son into the world to redeem us. She freely and humbly gave her consent to God's plan at the Annunciation. At the foot of the cross, Jesus declared her to be the mother of all generations to come, "Behold, your mother!" (John 19:27) Mary leads us to Christ and ultimately to the Father.

Exercise: Today let us not sigh and say, "We must go to Mass again since this is a Holy Day of Obligation." Instead, we should rejoice and declare it a Holy Day of *Celebration*, a perfect opportunity to receive the Bread of Life and the Cup of Eternal Salvation. The Blessed Mother will be greatly pleased when we receive her Divine Son's body and blood with joy and reverence.

We also please God when we take good care of the earthly body He has created for us. Take a few minutes today to set realistic goals for healthy eating and exercise. Approach this task with joy rather than trepidation, and pray for the Blessed Mother's assistance in achieving your goals.

St. Basil the Great (329-379)
& St. Gregory Naziazen (329-390)

Iron sharpens iron, and one man sharpens another.   *Proverbs 27:17*

The acts of charity that you do not perform are so many injustices that you commit.   *St. Basil the Great*

There is nothing unusual about two brilliant young students learning abroad becoming fast friends, but for both to later become monks, bishops, theologians, orators, saints, and Doctors of the Church, that we don't see every day. This is why January 2nd is a very special date, a feast in honor of two great and holy friends of the East. Both saints battled against the Arian heresy that denied the full divinity of Christ, despite the fact that the Roman Emperor Valens' own Arianism put their lives in peril. Through their shared holy zeal they helped forge each other's characters sharp and strong.

The mutual support and strengthening that friends can afford each other applies to women as well as men of course, and it applies to the realm of fitness as well as of that of faith. There is even a special term for such fitness-based friendships: "training partners." You can do your body a world of good, and glorify God with it, by exercising on your own. But you might also consider teaming up with a friend for at least a part of your training. I (Kevin) have a Saturday lifting partner of 27 years, a weekend running partner of three years, another of one year, a Tuesday morning (5:30 am mind you) running partner of one year, and a Wednesday lifting and cardio partner of 27 years (and I'm married to her!).

Exercise: Is there a friend, co-worker, spouse, sibling, parent, child or someone you can invite to join you for a regular or occasional workout, run, bike, or even a walk around the neighborhood? Can you invite him, her, or them *today*? Sharing the joys of vigorous fitness can indeed be a charitable act. Let's thank God for our bodies—and for our friends, as we sharpen each other—like iron!

St. Genevieve (422-512) Patron of Paris

...If my people who are called by my name humble themselves, and pray and seek my face, and turn from their wicked ways, then I will hear them from heaven, and will forgive their sin and heal their land.
2 Chronicles 7:14

Saint Genevieve, you who by the days before, penance and prayer, ensured the protection of Paris, intercede near God for us, for our country, for the devoted Christian hearts. From The St. Genevieve Prayer

Born in a small village outside Paris, St. Genevieve exuded holiness even as a young girl. When St. Germanus passed through her village on his way to England, he was captivated by young Genevieve's holy face and stopped to speak to the child. She expressed her intense love for Jesus, and Germanus consecrated her as a virgin and bride of Christ. At the age of 15, Genevieve entered the religious life and devoted her time to fasting, prayer and works of charity. St. Genevieve is honored as the patron of Paris because she helped to save the city from an attack by Attila the Hun. The Parisians wanted to evacuate their beloved city when they discovered that the Huns planned to lay siege to Paris. St. Genevieve urged them not to leave but to pray and fast to spare Paris from attack. Miraculously, the Huns bypassed Paris and changed the course of their attack.

Exercise: Pray daily for our nation's leaders and for our country through the intercession of the patron of the United States of America, Mary in her Immaculate Conception. Every country has a patron saint, and we are certainly blessed to have such a powerful intercessor. If you have the opportunity to travel to Washington, D.C., take the time to visit the Basilica of the National Shrine of the Immaculate Conception. To improve your health, take a cue from St. Genevieve, who is often shown holding a loaf of bread, symbolizing her generosity to the poor. If you haven't already, switch to whole grain breads instead of white or "faux wheat" bread. To tell the difference, check the label and look for "whole wheat flour" as the first ingredient. Avoid breads whose labels read "enriched flour." For something different, try rye or pumpernickel. Breads made with whole grain are high in fiber and contain beneficial nutrients, such as selenium, potassium and magnesium.

St. Elizabeth Ann Seton (1774 - 1821)

We must pray literally without ceasing—without ceasing—in every occurrence and employment of our lives . . . that prayer of the heart which is independent of place or situation, or which is rather a habit of lifting up the heart to God as in a constant communication with Him.

St. Elizabeth Ann Seton

St. Elizabeth Ann Seton was raised in the Episcopalian Church. She would marry and have five children. With her sister-in-law and spiritual friend Rebecca Seton, she went about New York doing charitable deeds. They were called the "Protestant Sisters of Charity." Hers would be a relatively short life of great upheavals and accomplishments. St. Elizabeth would convert to the Catholic Church at age 29, suffer the deaths of her husband, of Rebecca, and of two of her children; ultimately succumbing to tuberculosis at the age of 46. But in those few decades of her adulthood she would found in Baltimore the first American non-cloistered religious order, the Sisters of Charity of St. Joseph, as well as the first free Catholic school in the United States. She would become the first native-born American saint, when canonized by Pope Paul VI on September 14, 1975.

St. Elizabeth was a "dynamo of charity." Can you imagine having the energy and fortitude to found a religious order and a school while still raising your children as a single mother? We can also see the sufferings she endured due to fatal illnesses in her loved ones and finally in herself. Blessed as we are today with comparative freedom from disease, what can we do to foster the spiritual and physical fitness of our own family and friends? How, like St. Elizabeth, can we "pray always" despite the hardships we endure?

Exercise: Have you invited a loved one to share in exercise with you? Have you yet tried praying the rosary or other prayers while you walk, or run, or bike? Let today, the feast of St. Elizabeth Ann Seton, be a day of thanks and prayer, hopefully during a formal exercise session of at least 12 minutes, and also a day of ceaseless prayer, regardless of places that we'll find ourselves in or the situations that we'll face.

St. John Neumann (1811-1860)
Bishop of Philadelphia

Whatever your task, work heartily, as serving the Lord and not men, knowing that from the Lord will receive the inheritance as your reward; you are serving the Lord Christ." Colossians 3:23-24

Everyone who breathes, high and low, educated and ignorant, young and old, man and woman, has a mission, has a work. We are not sent into this world for nothing. St. John Neumann

St. John Neumann was born in Bohemia (now part of the Czech Republic) but had a calling to become an American missionary. He was ordained a priest in 1836 and sent to a remote parish in upstate New York. Since the parish was 900 square miles in size, St. John frequently traveled in harsh conditions to minister to his scattered congregation. It was fortunate that he spoke eight different languages as the area was home to many diverse ethnic groups. St. John built 100 churches and 80 schools and was consecrated as the fourth bishop of Philadelphia in 1852. He established a diocesan system of Catholic schools which is still in use today.

St. John Neumann had a wonderful sense of humor. As bishop, he visited a rural parish whose only available mode of transportation was a manure wagon. Taking his seat on a plank stretched over the wagon's contents, he joked, "Have you ever seen such an entourage for a bishop!"

Exercise: What is your unique vocation? Spend some time today pondering the life that God has called you to live. Are you working with God or against Him? Consider that your physical fitness affects your ability to carry out your vocation. St. John Neumann needed stamina to travel his far-flung parish. Regular exercise will give you more energy to carry out your daily tasks and to do God's work on earth. Get out your calendar (or whatever device you use to schedule appointments), and find three days this week to devote to exercise.

January 6

St. Andre Bessette (1835-1937)

Do not hate toilsome labor, or farm work, which were created by the most high.
                                                                    Sirach 7:15

When I joined this community, the superiors showed me the door, and I remained 40 years.
                                                                    St. Andre Bessette

Andre Bessette was one of those simple, humble, hardworking souls whom God puts to use for surprisingly great things. After failed attempts at occupations including farming, baking, and candlestick making, (sorry, shoemaking actually), this sickly youth was admitted at age 25 to the Congregation of the Holy Cross. He was assigned jobs including doorman and laundry worker at the Notre Dame Cathedral in Montreal. He exercised there a special devotion to St. Joseph, as well as a penchant for visiting the sick and anointing them with oil from a lamp in the chapel.

Could Brother Andre's superiors have foreseen the multitudes who would report healing in body and soul through his caring ministrations? (He attributed the cures to St. Joseph.) Would they have been surprised to see him live to 92 and be canonized by Pope Benedict XVI in 2010?

Exercise: Many of the early scientific studies on the benefits of exercise focused not on formal fitness activities, but on the exercise afforded by occupations that require a good deal of walking or other physical exertion. Even the sedentary desk worker can take advantage of the health benefits of plain old physical work by taking walks on breaks or walking up and down the stairs. If the floor you work on is too many flights up, just climb a few flights, and add a few more over time. You can also still burn about 40% of the calories of walking up those stairs, just by walking down them. Think of some ways you can burn a few calories at work and give your heart, lungs, and skeletal muscles a little something to think about. Do not hate toilsome labor, it could be your doorway to physical and spiritual health!

St. Raymond of Penafort (1175-1275) Patron of Lawyers

Any one whom you forgive, I also forgive. What I have forgiven, if I have forgiven anything, has been for your sake in the presence of Christ, to keep Satan from gaining the advantage over us, for we are not ignorant of his designs.   *2 Corinthians 2:10*

Look then on Jesus, the author and preserver of faith: in complete sinlessness He suffered, and at the hands of those who were His own, and was numbered among the wicked. As you drink the cup of the Lord Jesus (how glorious it is!), give thanks to the Lord, the giver of all blessings.   *St. Raymond of Penafort*

St. Raymond of Penafort was a brilliant Spanish Dominican priest, both a professor of philosophy and a canon lawyer. He wrote a comprehensive guide on the sacrament of Confession titled *The Summa of Penitential Cases.* This work was so well received that he was appointed confessor to Pope Gregory IX. St Raymond was also asked to organize and condense the canon laws (legal system) of the Church. He apparently completed this task well as his code of canon law endured from 1234 to 1917!

An interesting story is told about St. Raymond: He was exiled to the island of Majorca because he refused to turn a blind eye to King James' adulterous affairs. Undaunted, he spread his cloak on the Mediterranean Sea, tied one end to his walking stick as a sail, stepped upon the improvised craft and made the sign of the cross. He briskly sailed to Barcelona, and the astonished king quickly repented.

Exercise: To honor this great saint on his feast day, resolve to go to Confession this week. If necessary, call your parish office to make an appointment. Be sure to examine your conscience beforehand using one of the many helpful guides found online or in Catholic bookstores. While you're in the frame of mind to make appointments, call your doctor and dentist to schedule annual or semi-annual examinations or check-ups for yourself and your family if you've gotten off a schedule—or never started one. "An ounce of prevention is worth a pound of cure," as they say, and regular check-ups are an excellent way to prevent health problems down the road.

Blessed Angela of Foligno (1248-1309)

Put off your former nature which belongs to your former manner of life and is corrupt through deceitful lusts, and be renewed in the spirit of your minds, and put on the new nature, created after the likeness of God in true righteousness and holiness. *Ephesians 4:22-24*

The more perfect a man is, the more earnestly doth he endeavor to do that which is desired, ordained, and counseled of God.
Blessed Angela of Foligno

This wife and mother of thirteenth century Italy has much to teach us today. Absorbed in pursuit of social status, accumulation of wealth, and illicit pleasures of the flesh, it was not until around the age of 40, and shortly before the deaths of her husband and children, that she cast off her old nature and sought to live as a true child of God.

Under the spiritual direction of the early Franciscans, Angela sold her property, formed a religious community and cared for the poor. Her heart and mind devoted now to God, at the advice of her spiritual director, this spiritual late-bloomer recorded her visions and meditations, becoming known as "The Teacher of Theologians." Her writings include *The Book of Visions and Instructions* and *The Book of Divine Consolation of the Blessed Angela of Foligno.*

Exercise: Ask yourself today, am I glorifying God or only myself in my body? Does my clothing adorn my body with modesty and grace, or does it invite others to see me only as an object? Am I seeking status in the eyes of men, or in the eyes of God? Am I sufficiently grateful for the gift of my own family? What little thing can I do today to show them how I love them, to instruct and encourage them to overcome worldly temptations, to honor their own bodies in the right way, to become holy, perfecting their minds and wills as sons and daughters of God?

St. Julian and St. Basilissa (c. 3ʳᵈ Century) Martyrs

Is any among you sick? Let him call for the elders of the Church, and let them pray over him, anointing him with oil in the name of the Lord; and the prayer of faith will save the sick man, and the Lord will raise him up; and if he has committed sins he will be forgiven.   James 3:14-15

Then the king will say to those on his right, 'Come, you who are blessed by my Father. Inherit the kingdom prepared for you from the foundation of the world. For I was... ill and you cared for me.'
Matthew 25:34, 36

St. Julian and St. Basilissa were in a bit of a predicament. They had both taken a vow of chastity but had been forced to marry. On their wedding night, they agreed to live a chaste marriage and to devoutly practice works of charity. They converted their large home into a hospital to care for the poor and sick. Amazingly, they housed up to 1000 people at once! St. Basilissa served as mother superior for the convent she founded and cared for the women in the hospital. St. Julian gathered a group of monks together to care for the men.

Since this holy couple lived during the reign of the Emperor Diocletian, it was inevitable that their Christian hospital would be discovered and its founders persecuted. St. Basilissa managed to survive seven persecutions before dying peacefully. She is honored as a martyr for her willingness to die for her faith. St. Julian was arrested several years later, tortured and died a martyr's death by beheading. The saintly pair's example of holiness and charity resulted in many conversions in their mostly pagan land of Egypt.

Exercise: Call your local hospital and ask permission to visit a patient who does not receive any visitors. You might also drop off flowers at the administration office and request that they be delivered to a patient who is lonely. At the very least, pray for the sick. Take action to improve your own health (and stay out of the hospital!) by eating at least five servings of fruits and vegetables today.

St. Gregory of Nyssa (330-395)

For this very reason make every effort to supplement your faith with virtue, and virtue with knowledge, and knowledge with self-control, and self-control with steadfastness, and steadfastness with godliness, and godliness with brotherly affection, and brotherly affection with love.
2 Peter 1: 5-7

A greedy appetite for food is terminated by satiety and the pleasure of drinking ends when our thirst is quenched. And so it is with the other things... But the possession of virtue, once it is solidly achieved, cannot be measured by time nor limited by satiety. Rather, to those who are its disciples it always appears as something ever new and fresh.
St. Gregory of Nyssa

St. Gregory of Nyssa shared brotherly affection and love with St. Basil the Great (Jan. 2), his own big brother. Along with St. Gregory, these three bishops from what is modern-day Turkey, formed the great "Cappadocian Fathers" of the Church, all fighting the Arian heresy that denied Christ's full nature as God and man, and all defending the doctrine of the Trinity.

St. Gregory, echoing the admonition of St. Peter, also wrote much on man's God-given responsibility to perfect his own human nature (with the assistance of God's grace). Inspired by St. Paul's words "forgetting what lies behind and pressing to what lies ahead, I prize the upward call of God in Christ Jesus," (Philippians 2:13-14), St. Gregory wrote that humans are called to engage in a process of επεκτασισ, *epektasis*, of "constant progress" in godly virtue leading us upward towards Christ.

Exercise: Still early in our march through the calendar of another temporal year, in what ways are you seeking out constant progress in virtue and holiness, in body and soul, in preparation for eternity? Will you commit to God that this is the year you will develop the virtues of fitness within your soul? Will your knowledge of fitness grow, and along with it your affection and love for all around you? What about today? What thoughts and deeds might foster your own spiritual growth and share its bounty with those around you? Let's think about that—and act upon it!

St. Alexander of Comana (died c. 251)
Martyr and Patron of Philosophers

Is not my word like fire, says the Lord, and like a hammer which breaks the rock in pieces?
Jeremiah 23:29

They said to each other, "Did not our hearts burn within us while he talked to us on the road, while he opened us to the Scriptures?"
Luke 24:32

Today is my (Peggy's) birthday and I chose St. Alexander from a list of rather obscure saints because both my beloved husband and son share a middle name of Alexander. St. Alexander is known as the "Charcoal Burner," because out of humility, he took on the job of burning charcoal. Since he was also considered a great philosopher, he no doubt made use of the calm, hypnotic state that comes from staring into a fire to pray and meditate.

The story of how the lowly charcoal burner was chosen as Bishop of Comana (in Asia Minor) reminds me of the story of David's selection as King of Israel. Like David, St. Alexander was brought forward almost as a joke. Dirty and dressed in rags, Alexander was certainly the last man who would be considered as a future bishop, just as the young shepherd boy could hardly be a future king. Yet wisdom prevailed and when Alexander was cleaned up, he was not only handsome and resplendent in his episcopal robes but he astonished the assembly with the wisdom and eloquence of his first sermon. Sadly, but somehow fittingly, the Charcoal Burner became a martyr when he chose to be burned alive rather than to denounce his faith.

Exercise: Your own heart will burn within you if you prayerfully study the Scriptures. *The Ignatius Study Bible: New Testament* is an inexpensive and excellent resource to begin a study of the gospels. Physically strengthen your heart today with a cardio (aerobic) workout. Try adding a few short intervals (bursts of increased intensity, followed by a slower recovery period) to spice up your workout and improve your fitness.

St. Aelred of Rievaulx (1110-1167)

The ideas I had gathered from Cicero's treatise on friendship kept recurring to my mind, and I was astonished that they no longer had for me their wonted savor. For now nothing which had not been sweetened by the honey of the most sweet name of Jesus, nothing which had not been seasoned with the salt of Sacred Scripture, drew my affection so entirely to itself.   St. Aelred of Rievaulx

So much to say and so little space! I (Kevin) first learned about St. Aelred from a book by one of my own friends in Christ, Bert Ghezzi's *The Heart of a Saint*. St. Aelred, you see, literally wrote the book on *Spiritual Friendship*! He also wrote *The Mirror of Charity*. I share St. Aelred's appreciation for the most noble of the pagan moral philosophers who lived before Christ, men like the great Roman Marcus Tullius Cicero, who influenced the likes of Sts. Augustine, Albert the Great, and Thomas Aquinas as well.

But even the sweetest natural wisdom of the greatest and noblest sages fails to satisfy when one has tasted of Christ. St. Aelred knew that Christ had called us to be his friends—that Christ lives in each of us; so we are to also develop spiritual friendships with each other here on earth. Indeed, Christ lives in our own hearts, so we must show concern for our own health and well-being, as we would for a friend.

Exercise: Speaking of that "most sweet name" of our truest friend Jesus, are you familiar with "the Jesus prayer?" Building on the text of Luke 18:13, this simple prayer, "Lord Jesus Christ, Son of God, have mercy on me, a sinner," has been prayed for centuries, especially in the East. Here is a very simple suggestion for making this prayer a habit. In your next strength training workout, say this prayer on the "negative" portion of each of your repetitions. Unless you are doing a super-slow variant of training, you should take about 4 seconds to lower the weight to the starting point of each repetition—fairly close to the time it takes to say this prayer at a natural rate of speech. What a simple way to pace your workout and honor Christ, especially in January, the month of the Holy Name of Jesus.

St. Kentigern (c.518 -614) Patron of Glasgow, Scotland, and the Salmon Industry

---

And [Jesus] said to them, "Follow me, and I will make you fishers of men."
Matthew 4:19

Let the will of the Lord concerning all of us be done. And let him arrange for us as he knows best and as it is pleasing to him.
From "The Life of Kentigern"

S t. Kentigern was born amidst scandal and adventure. His mother, the future St. Thaney, was a Scottish princess who was seduced by a dashing young man and became pregnant. Her irate father hurled her off a cliff, but she miraculously survived. She was then put on a small boat set adrift at sea. The boat eventually landed in another Scottish town where mother and infant were rescued by St. Serf. St. Serf decided to raise Kentigern and affectionately called him Mungo, meaning "darling" or "dear one." (Harry Potter fans will recognize this name.) Under St. Serf's guidance, St. Kentigern became a hermit and missionary renowned for his holiness. He is considered to be the first bishop of Scotland and the patron of Glasgow. His four alleged miracles are represented on Glasgow's coat of arms: a bird, a fish, a tree, and a bell. The bird represents St. Serf's dead pet robin which St. Kentigern brought back to life. The fish, a salmon, was caught by the saint and contained the ring thought to be stolen by a queen who begged him for help, thus exonerating her. The tree represents a miracle from the Kenigern's youth when he fell asleep while tending the fire at St. Serf's monastery. The fire went out, but he used some nearby frozen branches to miraculously rekindle it. The bell was given to the saint by Pope Gregory and placed in a Glasgow church where it rang for daily Mass and for the deceased.

Exercise: To improve your health and honor St. Mungo, include salmon in one of your meals. Fresh wild salmon is hard to find this time of year, but try frozen or canned salmon to make patties with a little egg, bread crumbs and herbs. Salmon contains heart-healthy Omega 3 oils (as do walnuts, tuna and flaxseed) which should be part of a healthy diet.

St. Hilary of Poitiers (315-367)

And when Jesus had crossed again in the boat to the other side, a great crowd gathered about him; and he was beside the sea. Mark 5:21

The Church is the Ship outside which it is impossible to understand the Divine Word, for Jesus spoke from the boat to the people gathered on the shore. St. Hilary of Poitiers

St. Hilary was a learned pagan who converted to Christ around age 35. By the time of his death at age 52, his writings on the Trinity and defense of the Church against heresy—Arianism and others—he had earned the respect of such notable contemporaries as Sts. Augustine and Jerome. A bold champion of orthodoxy, he was also known for his kind and loving manner toward the very heretics whose heresies he fought.

Exercise: Speaking of the Ship of the Church, and of fitness, one of our more recent captains, Pope Pius XII, noted in a 1945 speech to sportsmen that the Church is all for "physical culture,"—an older, more elegant term for fitness training—if it is carried out in the proper proportion: in a way that does not distract us from spiritual pursuits or our duties at work and in the home. Now, St. Hilary was a man who could carry both the sword of fortitude and the laurel wreath of kindness when defending the Church.

Here, I (Kevin) have found a parallel in the world of the gym. The system of HIT (high intensity training) helps keep strength training in proper proportion by its brevity and infrequency. However, many weightlifters are unfamiliar with it and may even try to discredit it.

While I'm not calling those who practice other systems heretics(!), over my 35 years in the gym, I've come to avoid arguments with them by inviting them to join in such a workout or to simply witness one—and the results. I invite you to consider the ways in which your exercise routine may need to be modified so that it is in "proper proportion."

St. Paul of Thebes (229-342) The First Hermit

From now on there is laid up for me the crown of righteousness, which the Lord, the righteous judge, will award to me on that Day, and not only to me but also to all who have loved his appearing.   2 Timothy 4:8

I have always longed to be dissolved and to be with Christ; my course is finished, and there remains for me a crown of righteousness.
                                                                St. Paul the Hermit

S t. Paul the Hermit, as he is often called, was such an important figure in the early Church that his biography was written by none other than the influential Doctor of the Church, St. Jerome. Hermits like St. Paul served as heroes to Christians during the difficult years of persecution in the early Church. Their example of asceticism (extreme self-denial and renunciation of material comforts) led to the rise of monasticism and an increase in religious orders. At age 16, St. Paul fled to the desert near his native Thebes to escape persecution after the death of his parents. He took up residence in a small cave near a palm tree and a spring of fresh water. He enjoyed the ascetic life so much that he decided to remain in the desert after the danger of persecution passed. Near the end of his 100-plus years on earth, St. Paul was visited by St. Anthony Abbot, whose feast we celebrate in two days. St. Anthony mistakenly believed that HE was the first to discover the benefits of austere desert living, but an angel guided him to St. Paul, the true original desert hermit. The two were delighted to meet, but their friendship was brief as St. Paul died several days later. St. Anthony buried his new friend, with the assistance of several heaven-sent lions. (Perhaps this is a legend, but consider that St. Anthony was 90 years old when he visited St. Paul!)

Exercise: We don't like to think of our own death, but stop and think about whether you would receive a "crown of righteousness" if you died today. Has your life been an example to others? If not, take action to change the course of your life. Speaking of death, do you have a will and life insurance? This is especially important if you are married or have children who will depend on your life's assets.

St. Honoratus of Arles (350-429)

And do not seek what you are to eat and what you are to drink, nor be of anxious mind. For all the nations of the world seek these things, and your Father knows that you need them. Instead, seek his kingdom, and these things shall be yours as well.   Luke 12:29-31

St. Honoratus and his brother Venantius were born to a Roman family in Gaul. Forsaking the pagan idols and despite their father's protests, they sought holiness as hermits in Greece. After Venantius fell ill and died, Honoratus returned to Gaul and established a monastery on a small island off the coast of Spain, now known as St. Honore Island. He would be called to the office of Archbishop of Arles, France, where he would serve for the last three years of his life.

Exercise: St. Honoratus worried little about food and drink, so fixed were his thoughts upon God. Today, how much of our time is spent not worrying that we will have enough to eat, but worrying that we won't keep ourselves from eating too much! If you seek to develop the virtue of temperance in your soul and to eat in a way that honors your temple, try this:

The next time you are hungry between meals and some chips, cookies, or candy sound appealing, say a prayer instead, and vow to wait a bit, even if it is just 15 minutes or so, before you eat. If your hunger pangs have not gone by then, consider having a piece of fruit or a previously cut and prepared serving of a vegetable or two

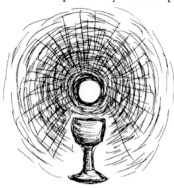

instead. Sometimes when we delay our seeking of less-healthy foods, the real things will taste all the sweeter. We can come to retrain our tastes to the foods that truly feed us. Of course, we can still have the "comfort food" too at times, though not for comfort, but as a small and measured treat. Our true comfort should lie in He Who truly feeds us in body and in soul.

St. Anthony Abbot (c. 250-356) "Father of Monks"

Watch and pray so that you may not enter into temptation; the spirit indeed is willing, but the flesh is weak.   *Matthew 26:41*

Believe me; the devil fears the vigils of pious souls, and their fastings, their voluntary poverty, their loving compassion, their humility, but most of all their ardent love of Christ our Lord. As soon as he sees the sign of the Cross, he flees in terror.   *St. Anthony Abbot*

St. Anthony Abbot received a sizeable inheritance at age 20, but he cared little for material possessions. At Mass one day, he was profoundly affected by the reading of Matthew 19:21: "...*Go, sell what you possess and give to the poor, and you will have treasure in heaven; and come, follow me.*" Young Anthony immediately sold everything he owned and gave all the money to the poor. He felt called to become a hermit and sought a life of solitude in the desert—praying, fasting and doing penance. St. Anthony was frequently tormented by demons, but these attacks only served to strengthen the saint as he grew in virtue. He is considered to be the model of asceticism and the "Father of Monks," greatly influencing successive generations through his belief that the purpose of asceticism is not to destroy the body but to bring it into subjection. St. Anthony built two monasteries on the Nile River and was often sought out for spiritual counseling. He visited St. Paul the Hermit (Jan. 15) and helped bury him after his death.

Exercise: In today's modern secular world, demons and temptations are more apt to be in horror movies than in homilies, but we all experience temptation and must fight our personal demons. Follow St. Anthony's example and practice bringing your body into subjection by fasting from some worldly pleasure today. You might give up your daily cup of coffee, a meal or your favorite TV show. Offer up this small sacrifice as a form of penance. Memorize St. Michael's Prayer and pray it daily to help overcome temptation:

Saint Michael the Archangel, defend us in battle. Be our protection against the wickedness and snares of the devil. May God rebuke him, we humbly pray and do thou, O Prince of the heavenly host, by the power of God, cast into hell Satan and all the evil spirits who prowl about the world seeking the ruin of souls. Amen.

St. Prisca (1ˢᵗ Century)

And do not fear those who can kill the body and not the soul; rather fear him who can destroy both body and soul in hell. Matthew 10:28

St. Prisca was a very early martyr of the Church. Though it is difficult to distinguish historical fact from legend in some of the details of her brief, but glorious, life and her prolonged and painful death, she was said at the mere age of 13 to have refused to worship the god Apollo at the command of Roman Emperor Claudius himself. Her crime was that she was a Christian. The young saint's ordeal would include beating, flogging, the pouring of tallow (boiling animal fat) upon her, being thrown to a lion (who laid down at her feet), the tearing of her flesh with iron hooks, and being thrown upon a burning pyre. When none of these tortures had killed her, she was finally beheaded. Christians buried her in the catacombs and a church was later erected in Rome in her honor. It remains standing today.

Exercise: Fortitude is that natural virtue of *fortis* (strength) that overcomes difficult obstacles to the good. Among the seven gifts of the Holy Spirit is an infused fortitude that enables us to use our strengths as directed not only by our own reason, but according to the stirrings of the Holy Spirit within us. St. Prisca displayed that ultimate fortitude found in the souls of the holy martyrs. It begs us to ask ourselves: Are we working to build the virtue of fortitude within our souls to withstand the immeasurably lesser discomforts involving in exercising our bodies? Do we let the minor muscular pain of completing a set of sit-ups or the respiratory discomfort of those first few minutes of a run or a bike ride prevent us from building our temples to the same Holy Spirit who freely gives us fortitude as a gift? Is there some minor "hard thing" we can do today or in the next few days to tend our bodily temples and build fortitude in our souls? If you are healthy and physically capable, try doing the sets of your next strength training workout to actual "failure," where you try but cannot complete the last repetition (making sure you are doing exercises where this can be safely done – no self-martyrdoms here from getting trapped under a barbell or anything!) Say a brief prayer to God for fortitude and offer up those most minor of pains as you glorify God's temple in your next training session.

St. Canute (c. 1042 -1086) Patron Saint of Denmark

Go therefore and make disciples of all nations, baptizing them in the name of the Father and of the Son and of the Holy Spirit, teaching them to observe all that I have commanded you.   *Matthew 28:19-20*

Show yourself in all respects a model of good deeds.   *Titus 2:7*

St. Canute is the beloved patron saint of Denmark. Not only was he a wise and just king, but he is also the first Dane to be canonized. During his reign, he devoted most of his time, money and effort to spreading the Good News of the Gospel throughout his kingdom. He conquered several neighboring kingdoms, and planted the seeds of Christianity in those pagan lands by building churches and aiding missionaries in their work. Unfortunately, not all of St. Canute's policies were popular with his people. A group of peasants who resented his heavy taxes banded together and conspired to kill the king. St. Canute and his men sought refuge in a nearby church, but the Danish king was slain by a spear while kneeling at the altar just after confessing his sins to the priest.

Exercise: We may not have the money, resources or time to evangelize a kingdom as St. Canute did, but we can make a difference in our own backyards. If you are a godparent, do you take your responsibility to help educate your godchild in matters of the faith seriously? Naturally, you will pray for your godchild, but you can also provide books on the saints, a Rosary blessed by a priest, a study Bible or other helpful aids to lead your godchild closer to Christ. If you are not a godparent, then surely you have a friend or a family member who can benefit from prayer and small gifts to inspire deeper faith.

You can also make a difference in your own backyard by modeling good health habits. When I (Peggy) was an Air Force officer, I discovered firsthand the power of positive example. Every day, I brought my lunch in a cooler, a gym bag and a large bottle of water. It wasn't long before my co-workers started skipping the greasy meals at the nearby bowling alley and joined me in eating lunch at our desks after a workout at the gym. Set a good example, and others will quickly follow.

St. Sebastian (died c. 300) Patron of Athletes and Soldiers

Take your share of sufferings as a good soldier of Christ Jesus. No soldier on service gets entangled in civilian pursuits, since his aim is to satisfy the one who enlisted him. An athlete is not crowned unless he competes according to the rules.   2 Timothy 2:3-5

A favorite subject of Renaissance artists, this holy martyr was portrayed with a most muscular physique as would befit a member of the Roman Emperor Diocletian's elite Praetorian Guard. He has become the patron of soldiers and athletes and was truly a soldier and athlete for Christ. While imprisoned, he gave strength to twin brothers Marcus and Marcellinus, facing death for their Christianity. His message spread outside the prison walls and won more converts to Christ. St. Sebastian was eventually sentenced to death, to be used as a target for the emperor's archers. He is often depicted pierced by arrows. According to legend, however, a widow who came to bury him found that he was alive. When his wounds had healed, this manly solider and athlete of God sought out Diocletian and publicly demanded an end to Christian persecution. For this the Emperor ordered he be clubbed to death, suffering a "double martyrdom." St. Sebastian was a man who had rendered to Caesar what was Caesar's, but had never forgotten that it was ultimately Christ who had enlisted him, and under whose rules he competed.

Exercise: Do you consider yourself a soldier or athlete for Christ? Would those around you know it? Let's ask ourselves how we can play by God's rules, becoming as muscular in spirit as was St. Sebastian in body and in manly fortitude. We are all called at times to suffer—in Shakespeare's Hamlet's words—the "slings and arrows of outrageous fortune," but only metaphorically. And as for physical exercise, in order to be fit to serve those who employ him, rigorous marching is a staple of the soldier's routine. Why not include a vigorously paced walk in your fitness routine today? Decide on the duration, and walk half the time out, before you turn around. See if you can return a little faster than you went out. And while you "march," perhaps with rosary in hand, ask God for the kind of zeal for the Gospel and endurance for suffering he granted to bold St. Sebastian.

St. Agnes (c. 291-304) Patron of Young Girls and Virgins

But I was like a gentle lamb led to the slaughter...   *Jeremiah 11:19*

Do you not know that you are God's temple and that God's Spirit dwells in you? If anyone destroys God's temple, God will destroy him. For God's temple is holy, and that temple you are.   *1 Corinthians 3:16*

St. Agnes, whose name means "lamb" in Latin and "the pure one" in Greek, is one of the most revered virgin martyrs of the early Church. She became a bride of Christ and trusted that He would safeguard her chastity: *"At my side I have a protector of my body, an angel of the Lord."* Agnes' beauty and virtue caught the attention of a Roman prefect, who decided she would make a good wife for his son. When Agnes refused, she was sentenced to death. Since she was a virgin, Roman law protected her from execution so the prefect forced her into a brothel. Various miracles protected her chastity, but she was eventually beheaded at the tender age of 13.

When I (Peggy) was a young girl, one of my most treasured possessions was a beautiful statue of St. Agnes holding a lamb. I have passed this devotion to my daughter, who proudly displays her own St. Agnes statue. She even dressed up as St. Agnes for an All Saints Day pageant, complete with a stuffed animal lamb.

Exercise: Pray to St. Agnes to protect the virtue and purity of your daughters, and ask the same for the future wives of your sons. (Pray to St. John Bosco—see entry for January 31—to protect the virtue and sanctity of your sons and your daughters' future husbands.) St. Agnes will be pleased if you choose the clothing you wear each day with care to safeguard your modesty and create a positive impression. Your body is a gift from God, and you are created in His image. Both men and women should dress with dignity so that others focus on your inner qualities rather than your outward appearance. It's also important to choose your workout attire carefully. Although it should be comfortable and allow you to move freely, it should not be revealing or inappropriate.

St. Vincent Pallotti (1795-1850)

In him we move and breathe and have our being.   *Acts 17:28*

Caritas Christi Urget Nos (The love of Christ impels us)
Motto of the Pallottines, The Society of the Catholic Apostolate

Both a thinker and a doer, though reportedly not the fastest learner, this devout young man, through diligent efforts, would become priest and professor, philosopher and theologian, before devoting his life to spreading the Gospel and tending to the needs of the poor. On a personal level, he was known to give even his own shoes and bed to the needy. He was even willing to risk his own life and dress as a woman to minister to a dying, but pistol-packing man who had vowed to shoot if a priest dared approach him! At age 54 he contracted a cold after giving his cloak to a man on a cold, rainy night. He died soon after on January 22, 1950.

St. Vincent envisioned an apostolate that would spread the Good News to the ends of the earth through its missionary activity, and it exists to this day: The Society of the Catholic Apostolate, also known as the Pallottines and Pious Society of Missions.

Exercise: What is the love of Christ impelling you to do today to tend to the needs of others? Can you train yourself to anticipate their needs before they even ask? And as for yourself and your bodily temple, remember that you move and breathe in Christ. In your strength training exercises, remember then to breathe! Don't hold your breath as you exert as this could give rise to dangerous increases in blood pressure. In your cardiovascular exercises, except for the brief intense intervals of advanced trainees, don't train so hard that you haven't the breath to carry on a conversation. I (Kevin) enjoy conversing with training partners while we run, though they always invite me to tell them a story whenever we start up a steep hill, thus saving their breath (perhaps assuming as well that I'll never run out of hot air.)

St. John the Almsgiver (c. 550-619) Patriarch of Alexandria

And if I should have prophecy and should know all mysteries, and all knowledge, and if I should have all faith, so that I could remove mountains, and have not charity, I am nothing.   *1 Corinthians 13:2*

Those whom you call poor and beggars, these I proclaim my masters and helpers. For they, and they only, are really able to help us and bestow upon us the kingdom of heaven.   *St. John the Almsgiver*

S t. John's life was shaped by a glorious vision he received as a child. A beautiful girl appeared to him who called herself "Charity" saying, "I am the oldest daughter of the King. If you are devoted to me, I will lead you to Jesus. No one is as powerful with Him as I am. Remember, it was for me that he became a baby to redeem humankind." St. John became a priest after his wife and children died of disease. His example of holiness and humility quickly caught the attention of his superiors and he was consecrated as a bishop and later the patriarch of Alexandria, Egypt. As patriarch, he promised to "practice charity without limits," and never strayed from that promise. He inspired the rich to be generous and the poor to trust in God for their needs. A rich man discovered that St. John slept with one threadbare blanket and bought him a luxurious bed covering, begging the patriarch to make use of it. The humble saint obliged, but tossed and turned all night. The next day, he sold the expensive blanket, giving the money to the poor. The rich man recovered his gift and returned it to St. John, who promptly sold it yet again. This little game continued for quite some time, and St. John remarked, "We will see who tires first." I'm sure you can guess who outlasted whom!

Exercise: We often encounter people begging for money on city streets and busy intersections. Often the response is, "Get a job!" or "She doesn't look like she needs any money." Perhaps we recall a TV report on scam artists who disguise themselves as beggars. Consider this anecdote about today's saint: In a long line of the poor begging for alms at the patriarch's palace, a man was discovered who was not particularly needy. When the officers presented this man to St. John, he advised, "Give unto him; he may be Our Lord in disguise."

St. Francis de Sales (1567-1622)

He who does not love does not know God; for God is love.   1 John 4:8

In brief, devotion is nothing other than a spiritual agility and liveliness by which charity acts in us and we act by it promptly and lovingly.
St. Francis de Sales

Have you read St. Francis de Sales' *Introduction to the Devout Life?* If not, we suggest you do so right now! Back already? See what we mean? That book has been called the greatest Catholic spiritual classic for lay people—and rightly so. So bristling with warmth, wisdom, and charity are his lessons that we can give but the most meager of introductions to his own devout life.

A doctor of law, St. Francis became a priest and was later named Bishop of Geneva, Switzerland—the very heart and center of Calvinism. Through his pamphlets on the truths of the Catholic faith and through his own meek and gracious demeanor he converted many souls and earned himself the titles of "Gentleman Saint," and "Patron of the Catholic Press" (so we really like him!) His loving spiritual direction of St. Jane Frances de Chantal (see Aug. 18th) adds yet more depth, relevance, and poignancy to his spiritual writings.

Exercise: Read and meditate upon St. Francis' own writings. (Though absolutely worth buying, his *Introduction to the Devout Life* is even available free online.) For now, let's focus on this theme. Note how devotion produces "agility" and "promptness" in our acts of charity. St. Francis said we can't be *good* unless we practice the Commandments and have charity; but to be *devout*, charity must flow from us in a "lively" and "prompt" manner. So then, the next time you are training your physical body to become quicker and more agile, spend some time in meditating on how you can swiftly and gracefully perform some charitable deeds as soon as you are finished—or even while you're at it. Even a smile and a wave to a stranger you pass while you walk or bike shares a little of that God who is love. So just do it—in a prompt and lively manner!

Conversion of St. Paul

But Saul increased all the more in strength, and confounded the Jews who lived in Damascus by proving that Jesus was the Christ.   *Acts 9:22*

I can do all things in Him who strengthens me.   *Philippians 4:13*

Wouldn't you just love to watch St. Paul's conversion story on EWTN's *The Journey Home*? So much action and drama! Lights flashing from heaven! The booming voice of the Risen Christ! Blindness followed by scales literally falling from Saul's eyes, while the astonished Apostles look on in utter disbelief as the Holy Spirit fills this great persecutor of Christians.

Paul's conversion story teaches us several important lessons. He was literally knocked over by the power and might of God, a lesson that excessive pride in our abilities and accomplishments can lead to a great fall, while submission and humility promote spiritual growth. Paul lost his sight and had to be meekly led into the city, teaching us that only through Christ can we finally see the light of truth. Finally, we learn that a true conversion of heart can lead us to work mighty deeds. Paul went on to become the greatest of missionaries and still speaks to us today through his epistles.

Exercise: Has pride caused you to think that you are responsible for your success or accomplishments? Pride is one of the Seven Deadly Sins and leads us away from God. Your abilities and talents are gifts from God, and it is important to pray for guidance as to how to best to use them in His service.

Carefully ponder the words of St. Paul in the quote above. You can do *all things* through Christ! He will also strengthen you, which means both spiritually and physically. If you struggle with maintaining a regular exercise program, try placing this burden at the feet of the Risen Lord. Trust that He will literally give you strength to build strength, and then take action!

St. Paula (347-404) Patroness of Widows

---

*Then the Lord God said, "It is not good that the man should be alone;
I will make a helper for him."*
Genesis 2:18

*The psalms were her music, the Gospels her conversation; continence
was her luxury, her life a fast.*
St. Jerome

Men and women can bring out the very fullness and best in each other, even among holy celibates. We mentioned the beautiful spiritual friendship between St. Francis de Sales and St. Jane Frances de Chantal just two days (and two pages) ago. About 1200 years before them, another great pair of saints did great things together to spread the news of Christ. We'll address St. Jerome on September 30; for now let's learn of St. Paula.

Paula was a devout Christian widow. She'd been very happily married to Toxotius, a wealthy man who still practiced the pagan religion, and they had five children. After her husband's death, St. Paula embraced a life of devotion to the poor, to learning, and to ascetic self-denial under St. Jerome's spiritual direction. In his *Letter to Asella,* Jerome proclaims his holy friend's graces. She would eventually come to work with Jerome in Bethlehem as his secretary and closest friend. She founded a hospice with her daughter, Eustochium; and she herself headed a convent. She assisted St. Jerome in his great Scriptural and theological works. The death of her children would grieve St. Paula in the last years of her life, though she persevered in her sanctity until she embarked on eternal life.

Exercise: Can we mortify our flesh and build up the capacity for self-denial for the small things that would do us harm? Try this. Though there is nothing contrary to health in having the occasional sweet or crunchy treat, can you forgo them for just today, in honor of St. Paula and other widows?

Four.

You shall love the Lord you[r]
soul, and with all your migh[t]
diligently to your children, and s[h]
house and when you walk by the
when you rise.

Do something! Get moving, be confident, ri[s]
then be ready for BIG SURPRISES!

S t. Angela Merici was an Italian orp[h] firsthand the lack of education among the yo her time, especially in religious matters. As an a[d] was determined to make a difference. She gathered trained a group of like-minded women who taught the girls their homes. This group eventually became the Company of St. Ursula, the first women's teaching order as well as the first secular institute for women. Centuries ago, St. Angela realized that the family was a "Domestic Church" with the father as its head and the mother as its cherished spouse. Both parents have a responsibility to teach their children through word and example how to know, love and serve God. Blessed Pope John Paul II (Oct. 22) revived the concept of the Domestic Church. His Apostolic Exhortation, *Familiaris Consortio – The Role of the Christian Family in the Modern World* emphasizes the role of the family in teaching the fundamentals of our faith. I know St. Angela would be pleased if you read this document, easily available online, as it reflects the values of her life's work.

Exercise: Like St. Angela, resolve to make a difference in the life of a child or teen. Inquire at your parish or local schools to find a child who needs a mentor or a helping hand. You might donate your time, needed supplies or clothing, or financial support. Better yet, follow the advice in the quote from Deuteronomy above and St. Angela's encouragement to "get moving" and talk of the Lord as you walk by the way: Take a child or a friend for a walk or a hike and pray the Rosary together. Afterwards, go out for ice cream and discuss the impact your faith has made in your life.

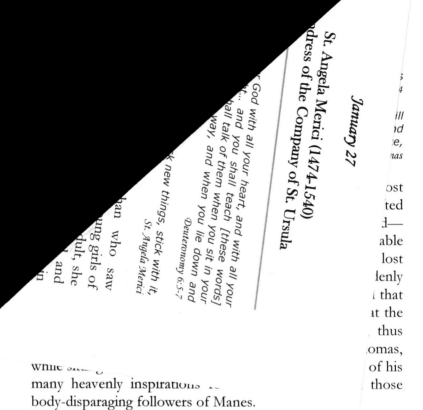

January 27

St. Angela Merici (1474-1540)
...dress of the Company of St. Ursula

God with all your heart, and with all your
... and you shall teach [these words]
...all talk of them when you sit in your
...way, and when you lie down and
(Deuteronomy 6:5-7

...k new things, stick with it.
St. Angela Merici

...an who saw
...ng girls of
...ult, she
...and
...n

while s...
many heavenly inspirations ...
body-disparaging followers of Manes.

What little things can we do today, on the feast of this great saint, to show gratitude to God for the glorious bodies and souls He has given us?

Exercises:

1. Daily bread: Plan your dinner meal tonight as perfect food for your body. Include moderate portions of fruits and whole grain of some sort, a generous portion of vegetables, and a modest portion of some combination of meat, fish, fowl, dairy, or nuts.

2. Words of God: Build virtue within your soul today by reading the 5th chapter of St. Matthew's Gospel. Read of the beatitudes and more in Christ's own words from the Sermon on the Mount. Then meditate upon them for 20-30 minutes while taking a walk or doing the household chores. (If you are doing the chores for exercise, set a timer and do them with gusto!)

St. Angela Merici (1474-1540)
Foundress of the Company of St. Ursula

You shall love the Lord your God with all your heart, and with all your soul, and with all your might... and you shall teach [these words] diligently to your children, and shall talk of them when you sit in your house and when you walk by the way, and when you lie down and when you rise. *Deuteronomy 6:5-7*

Do something! Get moving, be confident, risk new things, stick with it, then be ready for BIG SURPRISES! *St. Angela Merici*

St. Angela Merici was an Italian orphan who saw firsthand the lack of education among the young girls of her time, especially in religious matters. As an adult, she was determined to make a difference. She gathered and trained a group of like-minded women who taught the girls in their homes. This group eventually became the Company of St. Ursula, the first women's teaching order as well as the first secular institute for women. Centuries ago, St. Angela realized that the family was a "Domestic Church" with the father as its head and the mother as its cherished spouse. Both parents have a responsibility to teach their children through word and example how to know, love and serve God. Blessed Pope John Paul II (Oct. 22) revived the concept of the Domestic Church. His Apostolic Exhortation, *Familiaris Consortio – The Role of the Christian Family in the Modern World* emphasizes the role of the family in teaching the fundamentals of our faith. I know St. Angela would be pleased if you read this document, easily available online, as it reflects the values of her life's work.

Exercise: Like St. Angela, resolve to make a difference in the life of a child or teen. Inquire at your parish or local schools to find a child who needs a mentor or a helping hand. You might donate your time, needed supplies or clothing, or financial support. Better yet, follow the advice in the quote from Deuteronomy above and St. Angela's encouragement to "get moving" and talk of the Lord as you walk by the way: Take a child or a friend for a walk or a hike and pray the Rosary together. Afterwards, go out for ice cream and discuss the impact your faith has made in your life.

Feast of St. Thomas Aquinas (1225-1274)
Doctor of the Church and Patron of Scholars

Man shall not live by bread alone, but by every word that proceeds from the mouth of God.   *Matthew 4:4*

But if a man uses exercise, food, and drink in moderation, he will become physically strong and his health shall be improved and preserved. It is the same with the virtues of the soul, for instance, fortitude, temperance, and the other virtues.   *St. Thomas Aquinas*

St. Thomas Aquinas, the Angelic Doctor and the most sublime of intellects, knew so well that God has crafted us as beings of body and soul, and that both are good— very good. The story is told that at the crowded dinner table of the king of France, St. Louis IX (Aug. 25), St. Thomas, lost in deep thought, startled all present when he suddenly slammed his massive fist upon the table, shouting, "And that takes care of the Manichees!" The Manichees taught that the material world, including the human body, was evil, thus denying God's fleshly incarnation in Jesus Christ. Thomas, while sitting down for his daily bread, had received one of his many heavenly inspirations for an argument against those body-disparaging followers of Manes.

What little things can we do today, on the feast of this great saint, to show gratitude to God for the glorious bodies and souls He has given us?

Exercises:
1. Daily bread: Plan your dinner meal tonight as perfect food for your body. Include moderate portions of fruits and whole grain of some sort, a generous portion of vegetables, and a modest portion of some combination of meat, fish, fowl, dairy, or nuts.
2. Words of God: Build virtue within your soul today by reading the 5th chapter of St. Matthew's Gospel. Read of the beatitudes and more in Christ's own words from the Sermon on the Mount. Then meditate upon them for 20-30 minutes while taking a walk or doing the household chores. (If you are doing the chores for exercise, set a timer and do them with gusto!)

St. Gildas the Wise (c. 517-570)
Missionary and Hermit

By rejecting conscience, certain persons have made a shipwreck of their faith. 1 Timothy 1:19

Seeing that you are intoxicated by the habit and dense mass of your sins... seek with all effort of soul the one plank of penance, as if after shipwreck, on which you may escape to the land of the living. In this way the wrath of the Lord may be averted from you, inasmuch as He mercifully says: I wish not the death of the sinner, but that he may be converted and live. St. Gildas, The Ruin of Britain

St. Gildas the Wise lived in Great Britain during a time when the people turned away from God and toward a life of sin, but he worked tirelessly to change their hearts and minds. St. Gildas traveled as a missionary for many years, but he preferred to spend most of his time in isolation, praying and doing penance in reparation for the sins of his people. He wrote a book called *The Ruin of Britain,* calling the British rulers to task for their lax morals and laying direct blame on them for the decline of their society.

St. Gildas plays a part in the legend of King Arthur. According to Carodoc's book, *The Life of Gildas,* the fair Lady Guinevere was kidnapped by King Melwas, and an irate King Arthur planned a siege to rescue his wife. St. Gildas stepped in to negotiate a peaceful settlement between the two monarchs and arranged Guinevere's safe return.

Exercise: We must pray and take action to prevent our country from becoming a shipwreck. You may not agree with those who govern us, but it is important to pray that they are open to God's plan for our country and that we will return to our foundation as "One nation, under God." If you disagree with the direction our country is taking, then do something! Vote in local and national elections. Write or email your Congressman or Senator, sign a petition, volunteer for an organization that supports your beliefs or donate money to it. You can even get in shape for a cause by participating in a Walk for Life event or a bike ride to raise money for a charity you support.

St. Bathildis (c. 630-680) Queen of France

A disciple is not above his teacher, nor a servant above his master.
Matthew 10:24

[Queen Bathildis] ordered that many captives should be ransomed, paying for many of them herself. She established many of the captives she released in monasteries as well as many others of her own people. She could thus care for them. *The Life of Saint Bathildis*

St. Bathildis' story sounds like a Catholic version of Cinderella. As a child, she was kidnapped by pirates and sold as a slave to the French palace. The hard-working, humble and beautiful Bathildis soon caught the attention of King Clovis, who realized the young slave possessed all the qualities he sought in a wife and queen. They married and had three sons, but King Clovis died when the eldest son was just five years old. Since her son was too young to assume the throne, Bathildis ruled France until he came of age. Her experience as a poor slave taught her that each person has value and dignity, and she governed France in the true spirit of Christian charity. She abolished slavery, cared for the poor, and built many hospitals, monasteries, and abbeys. When her son turned 15, St. Bathildis willingly gave up her Queenship and became a nun, continuing her humble and obedient service to God.

Exercise: We can become slaves to things like money, fame, wealth, and material possessions. Such attachments focus our attention on worldly pursuits and away from God. Instead, chain yourself to Christ so that you will always be aware of His presence and the fact that He sees all that you do and knows your innermost thoughts.

It's also possible to become a slave to your workout routine. Repeating the same workout over and over leads to boredom and a lack of progress as your body adapts. Spice things up a bit and try something new. If you usually walk around your neighborhood, go for a hike instead. Try a new cardio machine or aerobics class at the gym. Sign up for lessons in a sport you've always wanted to try or join a recreational league. Exercise should be fun and enjoyable, not a labor to be endured.

St. John Bosco (1815-1888)

Let the children come to me, do not hinder them; for to such belongs the kingdom of God. Truly I say to you, whoever does not receive the kingdom of God like a child shall not enter it. And he took them in his arms and blessed them, laying his hands upon them. Mark 10:14-16

Trust all things to Jesus in the Blessed Sacrament and to Mary Help of Christians and you will see what miracles are. St. John Bosco

I (Kevin) have a special affinity for St. John Bosco, since his feast day falls on my birthday! (and on Thomas Merton's too.) Whenever I think of this great saint, I can't help but picture him surrounded by boys. In these times when the heinous actions of a very small percentage of priests make headline news, we must never forget those legions of holy, priestly men who have helped raise countless young men of character and sanctity throughout the centuries.

Imbued with the practical spirituality of our great saint of January 24 (St. Francis de Sales), John founded the Salesians and opened the Oratory of St. Francis de Sales for boys, which included workshops for the practical arts of shoemaking and tailoring. He imbued his own young charges with the virtues of reason, religion, and loving kindness. Always fond of sports, he loved to play right along with his young charges. Always loving to entertain, he was skilled in acrobats, and was also a magician. Indeed, in 2002 Pope John Paul II (see Oct. 22nd) would call him the patron of magicians.

Exercise: Do you have an ability to spend some time with children at Church or in your neighborhood? Do you have nieces or nephews or grandchildren who could benefit from time with you? This Sunday, why not take them to Mass, pray a rosary with them, and then go out and play or hike together? Who knows what miracles might come from our imitation of such a manly, though nurturing, saint.

February 1

St. Brigid of Kildaire (453-523) Patroness of Ireland

S t. Brigid, like St. Patrick, (March 17) brought the love of Christ to pagan Ireland. As powerful as was St. Patrick's apostolic zeal for evangelization was also St. Brigid's boundless love for living the Gospel in ceaseless acts of generosity, kindness, mercy, and hospitality; earning her the nickname of "The Mary of Ireland." St. Brigid reportedly chose the beatitude of mercy as a motto and guide for her life. She was so generous in tending to the needs of the poor, sick, and unfortunate, that her father felt she was breaking the bank and tried to give her away. Even while he negotiated her transfer, she gave his prize sword to a beggar. Happily for her father, the King of Leinster, so impressed by her deed, replaced it with a resplendent blade with an ivory hilt. Later as a great abbess of convents, her own sisters would chide her at times for her incredible—they thought excessive— generosity. The Catholic Church has long taught seven corporal works of mercy: feeding the hungry, giving drink to the thirsty, sheltering the homeless, clothing the naked, visiting the sick and imprisoned, and burying the dead. The biographies of St. Brigid abound in these acts. Some miracles attributed to St. Brigid involve giving drink to the thirsty (coaxing cows of the convent to provide milk for visitors through a third milking in the same day) to producing from one bag of malt enough beer for seven churches for Holy Thursday and the eight days of Easter!

Exercise: Is there a corporal work of mercy you can perform today, on this feast of St. Brigid? What will it be? Providing some food to a food bank, visiting a sick relative or parishioner? And speaking of milk and the thirsty, have you been tending to the corporal needs of your family and yourself with sufficient intake of dairy products? The USDA, in its food pyramid, recommends 2-3 servings per day of milk, yogurt, or cheese. This supplies your body with nutrients including high quality protein, calcium, and vitamin D. Studies have linked regular, sufficient consumption of various dairy products to benefits including bone health, digestive health, and even weight control. So, let's have a cold one (of milk) for St. Brigid today!

The Feast of the Presentation (Candlemas)

And when the time came for their purification according to the law of Moses, they brought him up to Jerusalem to present him to the Lord.
Luke 2:22

If Candlemas be fair and bright, Come winter, have another flight;
If Candlemas bring clouds and rain, Go winter, and come not again.
Old English Carol

The feast of the Presentation is celebrated 40 days after Christmas based on the Jewish law requiring the redemption of the firstborn male (Ex. 13:11-15) and the ritual purification of a woman after childbirth (Lev. 12). Of course, Jesus, as the Son of God, did not need to be redeemed; nor did Mary, the Immaculate Conception, need to be purified. Yet the Holy Family modeled obedience by submitting to Jewish laws and customs. At the Temple, the Holy Family encountered Simeon, a righteous old man who instantly knew that he held the Messiah when Mary placed her infant Son in his arms. The Holy Spirit had made known to him that he would not die until he beheld the Redeemer. Simeon's prayerful canticle, the *Nunc Dimittis*, is the traditional *Gospel Canticle of Night Prayer* (Compline) in the Liturgy of the Hours. Today's feast is also known as Candlemas, an ancient tradition rich in symbolism which has been recently revived in some parishes. Before Mass, blessed candles are carried to the church in procession to show the arrival of Jesus as the light of the world.

Exercise: Do you have a prayer corner or table in your home? If not, dedicate a space in your home for prayer and meditation. You might include a Bible, a statue of Jesus, the Blessed Mother or a favorite saint and some holy cards or prayer books. In honor of Candlemas, ask a priest to bless some candles to light in your prayer corner. You can honor the Feast of the Presentation in a physical way by following in the footsteps of Jesus and Mary as they walked the five mile journey from Bethlehem to the Temple in Jerusalem. If you're not up to five miles, try to walk for 20 minutes as you pray the Joyful Mysteries of the Rosary, focusing especially on the fourth mystery which we celebrate today.

February 3

St. Blaise (died 316)

Your neck is like the tower of David, built for an arsenal.
Song of Solomon 4:4

May God at the intercession of St. Blasius preserve you from throat troubles and every other evil. Prayer for the Consecration of Throats

Have you ever had your throat blessed with crossed candles on St. Blaise's Day? St. Blaise was a physician before his conversion to Christ. Yet another Cappadocian bishop, he was sentenced to death for his Christian beliefs. On his way to prison, at the entreaties of a distressed mother, his prayer healed a boy who was choking on a fishbone. St. Blaise would face martyrdom through beheading.

Exercise: Strong neck muscles help protect the cervical spine from injury. (Just ask a football player or a wrestler.) The many small muscles of the neck receive indirect training through many standard upper body strength training exercises. But did you know there are many simple exercises to directly strengthen your neck? Various neck muscles are involved in moving the head downward, back, tilting to the right and left, and turning to the right and left. Companies including Nautilus and MedX have designed advanced machines for working these muscles. Simple barbell-plate loading neck harnesses with chains are also available, but you can also gently stretch and strengthen your neck muscles with nothing but your own two hands.

Try this: Place your chin on or near your chest; with hands wrapped behind your head, gently resist while you raise your head to a straight up position. Repeat the process 5 or 6 times with all of these motions. Next, reverse the motion, pressing lightly against your forehead as you move your head down. Then, push against the right side of your head as you bend it toward your right shoulder. Same with the left. Lastly, look to the left and resist a little as you turn to the right, and do the same for the other side.

St. Jane Valois (1464-1505)

In this you rejoice, though now for a little while you may have to suffer various trials, so that the genuineness of your faith, more precious than gold which though perishable is tested by fire, may redound to praise and glory and honor at the revelation of Jesus Christ.
1 Peter 1:6-7

S t. Jane was born in a palace but was never treated like a princess. Since she was deformed and sickly, her father, King Louis XI of France, sent her away to be raised outside the palace. Jane was sweet, gentle, and humble. She was very devoted to the Blessed Mother and the Angelus, which she prayed daily. At the age of nine, St. Jane was forced to marry the Duke of Orleans for political reasons. Her husband loathed her, but she tenderly loved and prayed for him through 22 years of marriage. When the duke became king, he quickly had their marriage annulled. Poor St. Jane was once again humiliated and banished from the palace, but she took this as an opportunity to serve God and others by founding the Order of the Annunciation. The community's goal was to imitate Mary by practicing her 10 Virtues, as described in the Gospels: Most Pure (Mt 1:18, 20, 23; Lk 1:27,34), Most Prudent (Lk 2:19, 51). Most Humble (Lk 1:48), Most Faithful (Lk 1:45; Jn 2:5). Most Devout (Lk 1:46-7; Acts 1:14), Most Obedient (Lk 1:38; 2:21-2, 27), Most Poor (Lk 2:7), Most Patient (Jn 19:25), Most Merciful (Lk 1:39, 56), and Most Sorrowful (Lk 2:35).

Exercise: St. Jane's life embodies the saying, "When life gives you lemons, make lemonade!" She was constantly humiliated but resolved to work even harder to serve God. Follow her example today by looking at life's roadblocks as opportunities to practice virtue. Look at the bright side of things or simply thank God for your blessings—or the ways in which you can grow in virtue because of the roadblocks. In honor of St. Jane's favorite prayer, try an Angelus Abs workout. Lie on your back with your knees bent and gently support your neck. Alternate twisting to the right, then crunching to the center, then twisting to the left, then back to center, repeating the sequence while you pray the Angelus (see glossary).

February 5

St. Philip of Jesus (1572-1597) Patron of Mexico City

Some went down to the sea in ships, doing business on the great waters; they saw the deeds of the LORD, his wondrous works in the deep.

Psalms 107:23

The seven gifts are to a soul what seven sails would be to a boat....In the spiritual order, virtues are oars. Greater speed and comfort follow from favorable winds blowing into the sails.

R. Garrigou-LaGrange, O.P.

St. Philip of Jesus was born in Mexico City. After spending some time in his youth in a Franciscan monastery, his wealthy father sent him to the Philippines with money to start a mercantile shipping business. After a few years of a worldly life, he felt called again to God and to the Franciscans. He entered the order and cared for the sick. On a journey home to Mexico with a few other Franciscans, Augustinians, and a Dominican, his storm-tossed shipped was wrecked on the shores of Japan. Pirates confiscated their possessions and accused them of spying in preparation of a Spanish invasion of Japan. The Japanese Emperor ordered their deaths by crucifixion. St. Philip called his cross the "happy ship" that would take him to God. And in 1862 he would become Mexico's first canonized saint.

Exercise: St. Philip embraced a life of virtue, sailed off in his own direction for a time, and later aligned his sails again with the winds of God. This lesson can serve us well as we strive too for bodily fitness. How common it is to steer off course. If the zeal of your New Year's fitness resolution has begun to fizzle, or life's responsibilities have led to missed workouts, let today be the day you begin anew to follow God's course. Open your Bible to read and pray Psalm 107 in its entirety. Let this renew your spirits and place your sails in the winds of God's gifts and graces. Then pull out that rosary, begin a rosary workout (highlighted on Feb. 11), and get down to getting yourself back into ship shape for God.

St. Dorothy (died c. 311) Virgin Martyr

Let my beloved come into his garden, and eat the fruit of his apple trees.   Song of Solomon 5:1

There are few facts available on the life of St. Dorothy, but a colorful legend has become her lasting legacy. After both her parents were martyred during the Diocletian persecutions, Dorothy was next in line. She was stretched on a rack and offered her freedom if she would consent to marry a pagan or to worship the pagan gods. When she refused, she was tortured and sentenced to beheading. As the young maiden was paraded through town before her execution, a lawyer named Theophilus mockingly asked her to send a basket of roses or apples from the garden of her spouse, Jesus. The ground was hard and frozen, making his request appear impossible to fulfill. St. Dorothy smiled sweetly and promised to do as he asked. As the beautiful virgin turned to face her executioner, a young child appeared by her side bearing a basket of three shiny red apples and three perfect long-stemmed roses. Dorothy instructed the child to give them to Theophilus, and then fearlessly earned her crown of martyrdom. The stunned lawyer answered the knock at his door shortly thereafter and soon realized that the child was an angel in disguise and that the fruit and flowers were not of this earth. He immediately converted to Christianity and joined Dorothy and the saints in heaven when he too was martyred for his faith.

Exercise: Have fun today honoring this saint by making good use of roses and apples. Purchase three red roses and send them anonymously to three people who might need some cheering up. You could also simply leave them on the windshields of random cars in a parking lot or pass them out to three people you encounter. Ask St. Dorothy to pray for the recipients of the roses. At the grocery store, buy one each of three different varieties of apples that you have not tried before. Apples are high in fiber and contain vitamin C and other nutrients. If you are uncertain as to which varieties to try, search online or ask the produce manager to give you some recommendations.

February 7

Blessed Pope Pius IX (1792-1878)

Furthermore, you realize that spiritual exercises contribute greatly to the preservation of the dignity and holiness of ecclesiastical orders. Therefore do not neglect to promote this work of salvation and to advise and exhort all clergy to often retreat to a suitable place for making these exercises. Laying aside external cares and being free to meditate zealously on eternal divine matters, they will be able to wipe away stains caused by the dust of the world and renew their ecclesiastical spirit. And stripping off the old man and his deeds, they will put on the new man who was created in justice and holiness.

Blessed Pope Pius IX

O f the 265 men who have sat in St. Peter's chair at the head of Christ's Church, none have reigned longer the Blessed Pope Pius IX—save St. Peter himself! St. Peter guided the church for approximately 34 years; Blessed Pius IX for 31 years, 7 months and 21 days. So much happened during his reign and as a result of his leadership! However, space allows mention of only a small sample: the convocation of the first Vatican Council, the proclamation of the dogma of Mary's Immaculate Conception and, of national interest, the elevation of the first American to the College of Cardinals. One can simply read the title's of his 38 encyclicals to get a taste of the multitude of the issues he faced as the modern world's philosophies and politics grew in rejection of God and his Church. When church bells rang and prayers were raised for everywhere as his recovery as his death neared, he asked with a smile why everyone wanted to stop him from getting to heaven.

Exercise: Note how St. Peter's longest reigning successor stressed the importance of the interior life—regardless of life's demands! Consider ways in which you allow some of your life's own demands to impede your interior life and examine ways in which you can make changes so that your priorities indicate your commitment to your eternal life. Do you need to eliminate your time online and devote it to Adoration? Is there a television show you watch that should be sacrificed for time in Scripture? Finding time may not be easy; but you want to be willing to follow Pius' example of staying true to your spiritual life.

St. Josephine Bakhita (1868-1947) Patron of Sudan

If I were to meet the slave-traders who kidnapped me and even those who tortured me, I would kneel and kiss their hands, for if that did not happen, I would not be a Christian and Religious today.

St. Josephine Bakhita

St. Josephine was born in Sudan and given a name she could no longer remember after being kidnapped and repeatedly sold by Arab slave traders. She was nicknamed "Bakhita" by her captors (Arabic for "lucky"), an ironic choice as she was often brutally beaten and endured an intensely painful scarring and tattooing ritual by one of her owners. She was eventually sold to an Italian diplomat who was forced to leave Sudan and return to Italy. Bakhita begged the family to take her with them, and they consented. When her new owner had to leave Italy on business, he placed Bakhita in the care of the Canossian Sisters in Venice. When he returned, Bakhita refused to leave the convent. An Italian court declared that she had been illegally enslaved and was now free. She converted to Christianity and joined the order that had cared for and sheltered her. Bakhita took the name of Josephine when she was baptized and devoted her life to serving God and others. Her primary duty was door keeper, giving her frequent contact with members of the Italian community. Josephine's sweet melodious voice and gentle nature charmed everyone who met her. Her holiness and charisma were noticed by the other sisters, and she was asked to write her memoirs about her life, trials and faith. Her last years were marked by pain and suffering, yet she maintained her cheerful attitude and trusted in the will of her true Master.

Exercise: So often we ask, "Why must I suffer?" Suffering can bring us closer to Christ if we unite our sufferings with His. Today, carry your cross with joy and offer it to the Lord while doing an exercise that makes you stronger by bearing a heavy load. Lift two fairly heavy objects (dumbbells, buckets of water, etc), one in each hand, and hold them by your side. Stand straight and tall and carry them a short distance. Turn around and return to the starting point. Repeat 2-5 times, resting if needed.

St. Miguel Cordero (1854-1910)

And his gifts were that some should be apostles, some prophets, some evangelists, some pastors and teachers.   *Ephesians 4:11*

The heart is rich when it is content, and it is always content when its desires are fixed on God.   *St. Miguel Cordero*

Francisco Luis Febres Cordero Muñoz was born with some physical disadvantages. He was unable to stand until 5 years old when he saw a vision of the Virgin Mary. He was also gifted by God with a powerful mind, which he applied to broad and vast learning, and then to teaching others.

At age 13, he joined the Christian Brothers order, taking the name of Brother Miguel. He was a master of languages, translating works for his order in Belgium and in Spain, writing children's textbooks, and teaching school children for more than 30 years. He died of pneumonia in Barcelona on February 9, 1910. This favorite son of Ecuador was canonized by Pope John Paul II on October 21, 1984.

Exercise: Reflect on your own special gifts from God, and thank him for them. Is your heart rich and your mind fixed on God as you work each day in your own vocation? Regardless of your unique gifts though, we all share alike in the gifts of our bodies which are so wondrously made. Think of the ways in which a healthy, more vibrant and energetic body would help you in whatever vocation to which you've been called. Then, build up that temple and get to God's work today!

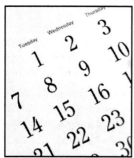

If you made resolutions at the beginning of the year to "tend to your temple" but have fallen away from those resolutions, revisit them—and revise them as necessary.

Remember: Tending to your "temple" allows you to fulfill your unique vocation!

St. Scholastica (c. 480-543)
Patron of Protection from Storms

Imagine being the parents of twin saints! Sadly, the mother of St. Scholastic and St. Benedict (July 11) died in childbirth and never witnessed the heroic virtue of her saintly offspring. Although much has been written about her famous brother, the scant information we have on St. Scholastica comes from Pope St. Gregory's *Second Book of Dialogues*. Scholastica, a consecrated virgin, founded a convent near her brother's abbey, Monte Cassino. The twins could only visit once a year in a house near Monte Cassino. During what was to become their last meeting, Scholastica begged her brother to stay. He refused, as the Rule of his order forbade him to spend the night outside his abbey. Scholastica bowed her head and prayed earnestly, tears flowing from her eyes. At the moment she finished her prayer, the clear sky turned dark, thunder echoed, and a heavy rain fell, making travel impossible. Benedict was initially angry but soon realized that God had honored his sister's request when he could not. They spent the rest of the night in lively conversation on spiritual matters and returned to their respective residences in the morning. Three days later, St. Benedict looked out his window and saw the soul of his sister flying toward heaven under the appearance of a dove. He arranged for her burial in his own tomb in Monte Cassino so that they would be together again after this own death.

Exercise: If you have siblings, pray for them today. Buy each a card or write a heartfelt note. Your words will be a welcome surprise! (Please, no texts, emails or e-cards!) If you don't have siblings, mail a card to your parents, spouse or children. Playing outside games can be a fun. Organize a three-legged race. Gather your family or a group of friends in an open area with soft grass and pair everyone up. Stand side by side and tie the two inner legs together, giving everyone time to practice before staging a race to see which pair of "twins" is the fastest.

February 11

Feast of Our Lady of Lourdes

From this grotto I issue a special call to women. Appearing here, Mary entrusted her message to a young girl, as if to emphasize the special mission of women in our own time, tempted as it is by materialism and secularism: to be in today's society a witness of those essential values which are seen only with the eyes of the heart. To you, women, falls the task of being sentinels of the Invisible!   *Pope John Paul II*

How fortunate we are to have so many ways and so many days to honor Mother Mary. Through her *fiat*—the yes, let it be done—that she answered to God, the omnipotent Lord of the universe took on human flesh to redeem us. Countless great saints and learned theologians, from St. Bernard of Clairvaux to St. Albert the Great to Pope John Paul II in our own time have felt and expressed their powerful and heartfelt devotions to Mary.

When Jesus said to his beloved disciple John, "Behold, your mother!" he was speaking to every one of us. On February 11, 1858, Mary appeared for the first time to a poor, humble, and not particularly devout young girl, Bernadette Soubirous (Feb. 18). On March 25, the beautiful lady announced herself with the words, "I am the Immaculate Conception." Little Bernadette had no idea Pope Pius IX (Feb. 7) had officially proclaimed—four years prior—the dogma of the Mary's Immaculate Conception. The Feast of our Lady of Lourdes was declared by the Church in 1907. Countless pilgrims have journeyed to the healing waters of Lourdes, France in the century since.

Exercise: Our Lady of Lourdes appeared with a rosary draped over her right arm. What better day for a rosary workout? If you have not explored the ways in which The Rosary Workout combines the spiritual with the physical, we invite you today to do just that! Visit www.RosaryWorkout.com to see how caring for yourself spiritually and physically will energize you and will allow you to fulfill your vocation more joyfully!

St. Apollonia (died 249)
Patron of Dentists and Toothaches

You have heard that it was said, "An eye for an eye and tooth for a tooth." But I say to you, "Do not resist the one who is evil. But if any one strikes you on the right cheek, turn to him the other also."
Matthew 4:38-39

St. Apollonia was an elderly deaconess who was seized and tortured during an anti-Christian uprising in Alexandria, Egypt. Her teeth were either forcibly extracted or knocked out of her mouth by beatings. She was about to be burned alive when she hesitated briefly. Her tormenters thought she was about to recant her beliefs, but she actually used this opportunity to fool her captors so that she could leap into the fire of her own accord. In later years, her actions were thought to be suicidal and her martyrdom doubted. St. Augustine of Hippo (Aug. 28) addresses this concern in his work, *The City of God:*

This is a matter on which I dare not pass judgment lightly. For I know not but that the Church was divinely authorized through trustworthy revelations to honour thus the memory of these Christians. It may be that such is the case. May it not be, too, that these acted in such a manner, not through human caprice but on the command of God, not erroneously but through obedience.

Exercise: If you have young children, you can put a Catholic spin on the tooth fairy story by telling them that St. Apollonia is the patron saint of teeth. You might not want to frighten them with the story of her martyrdom, but simply tell them to pray to her when they worry about losing their teeth or going to the dentist. Dental health is very important and the condition of our teeth can have an impact on other parts of the body. Poor dental hygiene can contribute to diabetes, respiratory problems and even heart disease. If you can't remember when you purchased your toothbrush, it's probably time to replace it. A good habit is to replace it with the change of each season, or every three months. Regular flossing is crucial as is scheduling a cleaning appointment every six months.

St. Catherine de Ricci (1522-1589)

Whoever does not bear his cross and come after me cannot be my disciple.
Luke 14:27

St. Catherine de Ricci, a Dominican prioress in Prato, near Florence Italy, was most known for an unusual mystical experience. For a period of 12 years, on every Thursday from noon until 4:00 p.m. on Friday, she would miraculously experience the "ecstasy of the Passion," feeling Christ's sufferings in his last hours.

Exercise: "The Stations of the Cross Workout." St. Catherine's story has been kept brief to allow for elaboration of a strength training workout inspired by her ecstasy. Do you know the fourteen Stations of the Cross? If not, refer to the glossary and other sources and learn them by heart.

Next, choose four strength-training exercises to be performed in super-slow fashion incorporating "a leg, a push, and a pull" (see glossary). A sample routine would be a chest press, row, abdominal machine, and leg press. Choose a weight that will limit you to 4 slow repetitions for the first two exercises and 3 slow repetitions for the last two, yielding a total of 14 repetitions of at least twenty-second duration each. During each repetition meditate upon one station of the cross, imagining the scene through Christ's eyes (or Mary's) as you perform each repetition. On the last repetition of each of the four exercises, lower the weight as slowly as possible taking even more than 10 seconds if possible, while breathing naturally and relaxing the muscles not involved in that movement.

Offer your minor discomfort in honor of St. Catherine de Ricci and her ecstasy, and in loving thanks to the truly unimaginable suffering Christ undertook for us all.

St. Valentine (dates vary)

So faith, hope, love abide, these three; but the greatest of these is love.   *1 Corinthians 13:13*

For this was sent on Seynt Valentyne's day Whan every foul cometh ther to choose his mate.   *Chaucer, "Parliament of Foules"*

I t is important to remember that this highly-commercialized holiday was originally the feast day of St. Valentine. Interestingly, there are 14 St. Valentines, three whose feast days were celebrated on February 14th. One was a priest in Rome who was beaten and beheaded in the late third century. The second was a bishop in central Italy. A third St. Valentine was martyred in Africa. Few verified facts can be found regarding these St. Valentines, but archaeologists did unearth a catacomb and church dedicated to St. Valentine in Rome.

Even more varied are the stories of how Valentine's Day became a holiday for couples in love. My (Peggy's) favorite tradition is from the Middle Ages. It was noted that halfway through February, on St. Valentine's feast, that the birds began to pair (see Chaucer's quote above). It seemed natural to celebrate by sending love letters and tokens of affection.

Exercise: Instead of giving your loved one a card covered in someone else's sentiments or a supermarket bouquet of roses, why not send a spiritual bouquet? A spiritual bouquet is a promise to offer prayers or devotions for the intention of another person. You can offer Masses, Rosaries or any other prayer or good deed. These are usually written on a card and given as a gift. You can make your own or choose from the many spiritual bouquets offered by various Catholic organizations.

Since hearts are everywhere today, use them as a reminder to work your heart muscle through some type of aerobic activity. In fact, celebrate Valentine's Day by asking the person you love most to join you in a walk, hike or trip to the gym.

St. Sigfrid (died 1045) Apostle to the North

So if you are offering your gift at the altar, and there remember that your brother has something against you, leave your gift there before the altar and go; first be reconciled to your brother, and then come and offer your gifts.
                                                                    Matthew 6: 22-24

Gruesome barbarism and sublime Christian love feature in the intriguing life and legends of this English Benedictine monk turned bishop and apostle to Norway and Sweden. Not every saint is depicted carrying three human heads in a bowl. St. Sigfrid was called to help Christianize Northern Europe, baptizing the great pirate turned king, Olaf of Norway, and also evangelizing in Sweden.

The story is told that while off on a mission, pagan marauders beheaded Sigfrid's three nephews. One gruesome legend holds that he retained their three heads and terrified pagans by claiming that they still talked to him. The amazing lesson from these barbarous times is that when Olaf vowed to execute the murderers, St. Sigfrid dissuaded him from using capital punishment. When he then ordered them to pay Sigfrid a large sum, he refused their money as well. Reminiscent of Pope John Paul II's forgiveness of his own attempted assassin, St. Sigfrid's display of Christian forgiveness in action helped bring souls to Christ.

Exercise: Forgiveness and reconciliation are prerequisites for prayer, and this year we are turning our workouts into prayers. Here's a wonderful parallel that I (Kevin) picked up from Peggy's *The Rosary Workout*. Just as we recommend a physical checkup before you would begin an exercise regimen, so to should you do an examination of conscience before every workout, bearing no grudges and forgiving all in your heart. Further, your soul would do well to include a regular visit with your priest to obtain the wonderful healing benefits of the Sacrament of Reconciliation.

St. John de Brito (1647-1693) Jesuit Missionary and Martyr

My friend, I have prayed to God. On my part, I have done what I should do. Now do your part.   *St. John's last words, to his executioner*

St. John de Brito was born to a wealthy Portuguese aristocrat but preferred life as a missionary in India to wealth and power. He was part of the Madura Mission, an attempt to establish a Catholic Church in India that was free from European cultural influence. As a result, St. John dressed in yellow cotton, learned the local language and abstained from every type of animal product and from wine. He studied the Indian caste system and realized that most Christians were of the lowest caste. Knowing that he needed to convert the upper classes to ensure widespread conversion, he became a pandaraswami (Indian ascetic) as they were permitted to approach the members of all castes. He taught the people the Catholic faith using language and concepts that they would understand; he met with much success. Due to his preaching, he was sentenced to death by beheading. His executioner hesitated, not wanting to end the life of this holy man. He is still honored in India as the patron saint of Sakthikulangara Parish, which holds an annual procession in his honor.

Exercise: St. John de Brito was willing to use drastic measures to win converts to Christianity. Sometimes we should do the same, trying to "speak the language" of those we are trying to convert. Approach non-Catholics with respect for their point of view and use that as a starting point for a meaningful dialogue.

Adopting a vegan or vegetarian diet is certainly not for everyone, but we can all benefit from adding more fruits and vegetables to our diet. At least once a week, I (Peggy) make a vegetarian meal for my family. I usually prepare it on Fridays, in honor of the Catholic tradition of meatless Fridays. I might make a bean soup, a strata (baked dish with bread, eggs and cheese) or an interesting meatless ethnic dish. I add a salad with lots of fresh vegetables. I love to share what I am doing and invite you to visit my blog at www.RosaryWorkout.com to get some great cooking ideas and to share yours!

St. Finan of Lindisfarne (died 661)

For just as the body is one and has many members, and all the members of the body, though many, are one body, so it is with Christ.   *1 Corinthians 12:12*

Born in Ireland and educated as a monk in Iona, Scotland, St. Finan served as the second bishop of Lindisfarne on the Northumbrian coast of England. A tireless evangelizer, he founded monasteries and baptized princes. He is also known for rebuilding the cathedral for his See at Lindisfarne (aka Holy Island), which at low tide twice daily, is accessible by foot from the mainland. The church was built of wood in the traditional Celtic fashion and the roof was thatched with a grass they called "bent," which is seaweed.

As Ireland, Scotland, and England converted from paganism to Christianity through the impassioned efforts of so many great saints, the body of Christ multiplied, and new churches sprang up all over the lands. The Irish typically built these churches of wood—and how interesting to think of a cathedral with a roof thatched with seaweed! (Is yours?) The great Catholic basilicas and Gothic cathedrals throughout Europe are the most magnificent architectural wonders on earth, yet how many churches all over the world, though on far less grand scales, can lay claim to a heavenly beauty and majesty of their own—holy structures constructed to glorify God.

Exercise: Our theme in this book, of course, is those wonderful little temples that each and every one of us builds for God—the temples that are our bodies. Recall well that regardless of our size and shape, whether our roofs are of thatch or of gold (or maybe are losing their thatch as the years go by), and regardless of how far along we are on the road to fitness, our bodies are all beautiful and valuable. We are made in the image of God. Recall too that all of us together form that one mystical body in Christ. What will you do today to tend to your temple and to aid in the physical and spiritual well-being of other members of the body of Christ?

St. Bernadette (1844-1879) Patron of Sick People

Whoever drinks of the water that I shall give him will never thirst; the water that I shall give him will become in him a spring of water welling up to eternal life.   *John 4:14*

Holy Mary, pray for me, a poor sinner.   *Last words of St. Bernadette*

Marie-Bernadette Soubirous was a poor, illiterate and sickly child, but she was chosen as a special messenger by the Blessed Mother. At age 14, she received 18 visions of a glorious young woman who stated, "I am the Immaculate Conception." Mary instructed Bernadette to dig up a spring in the mud nearby and to ask that a church be built at the site. Today the miraculous healing waters of Lourdes, France, are visited by over five million people each year.

Bernadette did not become a saint because she was asked to dig up a spring of healing waters. She lived a life of heroic virtue, prayer, and sacrifice which serves as an example for all of us. Interestingly, she never used Lourdes water to cure her own painful illnesses. Instead she calmly declared, "My job is to be ill," knowing that offering up her daily suffering to God was her life's vocation.

Exercise: If you are unable to make a pilgrimage to Lourdes, order a bottle of the healing water online. (The water is free, but you may have to pay for shipping and a container to hold it.) Although it is not holy water or supernatural water, Mary has attached special favors to its use. It is God who cures, of course, and the use of Lourdes water or holy water should be accompanied by prayer and a corresponding faith. While we're on the topic of water, be sure to stay hydrated, especially on days when you are exercising or if the weather is hot and humid. The old adage of drinking eight glasses of water each day still holds true for most people. Keep a water bottle on your desk or the kitchen counter and sip from it throughout the day, refilling as needed. If you don't like the taste of plain water, squeeze a wedge of lemon, lime or orange to add a little flavor.

St. Odran (died 452)

Greater love has no man than this, that a man lay down his life for his friends.

John 15:13

No task was too humble or too dangerous for thee, O Martyr Odran, for in thy station as a servant thou didst render the ultimate service giving thy life for thy master and Ireland's Enlightener. Pray that we may have the courage to hold nothing back, that at the last Christ our God will not withhold His mercy from us.

Troparion of St, Odran, Tone 5

Rumors of an assault on St. Patrick, Patron of Ireland (March 17) had reached the ear of Odran, the great saint's chariot driver. At Odran's request, Patrick switched places in the chariot, leaving Odran in the place of honor. Soon after, they were ambushed by a group of pagans. St. Odran took a lance through his heart becoming the first of the Irish martyrs.

Exercise: Let's ask ourselves, in what ways are we holding back? Are we too proud, afraid, or slothful to subject our bodies to the "assault" of a simple workout? Do we lack the courage to serve as a model for our loved ones that we (and they) can do hard things to build up our temples and glorify God? Think of a way that you, today, or in the next few days, can, like Odran, "switch places with Patrick,"—not to put yourself in harm's way—to do an unpleasant or uncomfortable physical task that will benefit your soul, your body and your neighbor.

At the request of two friends, (quite fittingly, one a Patricia, the other an Erin!), I (Kevin), Mr. Early-Riser, run at 5:30 A.M., fall asleep by 9:00 P.M., ran 6 miles in the dark at 6:30 P.M. last night. I did for them what I wouldn't have done for myself, run at a time so contrary to my natural preferences. No big deal, but better than nothing! So what switch will you make today? Will you work out at an unusual hour, substitute broccoli for fries, or perhaps choose an hour of study or prayer or play with your children instead of your favorite TV show?

Blessed Jacinta (1910-1920)
and Francisco Marto (1908-1919)
The Little Seers of Fatima

Give my greetings to Our Lord and to Our Lady and tell them that I am enduring everything they want for the conversion of sinners.
Blessed Jacinta's words to her brother, Blessed Francisco, on his deathbed

Siblings Jacinta and Francisco Marto are the youngest non-martyr children to be beatified by the Church. They, along with their cousin Lucia Santos, were visited by the Blessed Mother in Fatima, Portugal. During a series of visions in 1917, Mary, calling herself the Lady of the Rosary, encouraged daily recitation of the Rosary and asked the children to make sacrifices for the conversion of sinners. Jacinta and Francisco were poor, illiterate shepherd children and their account of the visions was met with scorn and disbelief by many people. They were even put in jail to prevent them from returning to the place where Mary promised to appear. Undaunted, the sweet children led the inmates in reciting the Rosary. Francisco died peacefully of influenza just two years later at age ten. Jacinta died of the same illness less than a year after her brother. She endured much suffering, including an operation to remove two of her ribs, performed without anesthesia due to the condition of her heart. Jacinta courageously offered up her suffering for the Holy Father, the conversion of sinners and peace in the world.

Exercise: There are many versions of the story of Fatima available on DVD. Purchase a copy to watch with your family, or rent one of several versions available from a wonderful Catholic online DVD rental company, PiusMedia.com. While you're on the website, check out the variety of DVDs available for spiritual enrichment or uplifting entertainment. During the movie, enjoy a healthy snack mix: In a large bowl, combine a bag of prepared low-fat microwave popcorn, a small box of raisins, a handful of mini pretzel twists, a small handful of mixed nuts, a snack-sized bag of cheese crackers and a small package of gummy fruit or M&Ms. Toss to combine, and serve with real fruit juice mixed with soda water for a little fizz.

St. Robert Southwell (1561-1595)

May the Lord direct your hearts to the love of God and to the steadfastness of Christ.   2 Thessalonians 3:5

Passions I allow, and loves I approve, only I would wish that men would alter their object and better their intent.   St. Robert Southwell

St. Robert Southwell had a burning passion from a young age to join the Society of Jesus—the Jesuits— and to bring the word and sacraments of God to the Catholics of England; though it was the law of that land that any English-born subject of Queen Elizabeth who had become a priest since she attained the throne, must leave England within 40 days upon penalty of death. St. Robert Southwell ministered to faithful Catholics in England. He wrote beautiful and inspiring poetry and prose, suffused with religious emotion and expressed with literary finesse. After six years of his self-chosen ministry, he would face that awful legal penalty in the form of imprisonment, torture, hanging, disembowelment, and quartering. He himself had written, *"To him I live, for him I hope to dye."* His reward must be great in heaven.

Exercise: Who or what are the objects of your love? Christ told us to love God, our neighbors, and ourselves. How much do we think about that; pray about it; and act upon it? We, in America, have relative freedom of religion expression compared to late sixteenth century England—so what are we doing to proclaim it? Do we sit by idly when the faith is attacked in our presence, or do we give reasons for our passion for Christ and for the hopes that are in us? Do our facial expressions reveal our joy? Do we plod along our paths, or is there a bounce in our step that bespeaks of our walk with the Lord? How can you fire up your passion today to build your bodily temple, as the Jesuits would say, *"ad majorem gloriam Dei"*? (For the greater glory of God.)

Chair of St. Peter

And I tell you, you are Peter and on this rock I will build my Church, and the gates of Hades shall not prevail against it. I will give you the keys of the kingdom of heaven, and whatever you bind on earth shall be bound in heaven and whatever you loose on earth shall be loosed in heaven.
Matthew 16:18-19

[The Church] has received the keys of the Kingdom of heaven so that, in her, sins may be forgiven through Christ's blood and the Holy Spirit's action. In this Church, the soul dead through sin, comes back to life in order to live with Christ, whose grace has saved us.
Catechism of the Catholic Church, 981

Today we honor the role of the pontiff, initiated when Christ entrusted the keys of the kingdom to St. Peter, which has continued in an unbroken line over 2000 years to our current Holy Father. Do you know that the Chair of St. Peter still exists? A bishop's throne is called a cathedra (Latin for "chair"), and it symbolizes the teaching authority of the person who holds the office. The original cathedra upon which St. Peter and other early popes sat was destroyed by barbarians in the fifth century. The second chair was moved to the baptistery of the Vatican basilica by Pope Damascus in the late fourth century. Newly elected popes were enthroned on St. Peter's Chair until the late 1300's. By that time the chair, which was made primarily from oak, had deteriorated and was carefully restored. In the mid-1600s the Italian artist Bernini designed and built an exquisite reliquary for the chair made from gilded bronze. It is currently on display at St. Peter's Basilica in Rome.

Exercise: It is customary to pray for the pope after you finish the Rosary. The physical exercise today will remind you of the chair of St. Peter. This isometric exercise strengthens the leg muscles. Lean against a wall with your feet shoulder width apart and about two feet in front of you. Slowly sink down as if sitting in an imaginary chair. Your thighs should be parallel to the floor with hips and knees at a 90-degree angle, and your back should be straight. Hold the position for 30-60 seconds. If your legs begin to shake, stand up and relax. Repeat 2-3 times. If the full sit is too difficult, then modify with a partial sit, sinking until the legs are at a 45-degree angle, or hold the position for a shorter period.

St. Polycarp of Smyrna (69-155)

My fruit is better than gold, fine gold, and my yield than choice silver.
Proverbs 8:19

Pray also for kings and magistrates and rulers, as well as for those who persecute and hate you and for the enemies of the cross, that your fruit may be manifest to all and you may be made perfect in him.
St. Polycarp

A disciple of the St. John the Evangelist himself, St. Polycarp is part of that special group known as the Apostolic Fathers, formed in their faith by the very apostles of Jesus Christ. Furthermore, we are blessed to have ancient written texts by him, (*Letter to the Phillipians*), to him (from St. Ignatius of Antoich), and about him (*The Martyrdom of Polycarp*). A bold bishop who declared the faith for many decades, this brave man, 86 years old, defied a Roman proconsul's attempts to have him renounce Christ, despite the threat of lions and fire. A fire built around him did not consume him, but enclosed him as if in a vault. A guard was then ordered to stab him. The story is told that so much blood gushed forth from his side that the fire was completely quenched.

Exercise: St. Polycarp, an early martyr, lived long for God, before he died for him. We benefit from the fruit of his example, his writings, and his intercession, even to our day. That fruit of the book of Proverbs, so much better than gold, is the fruit of wisdom. Fruit, as a metaphor, implies an end result that is ever so good and healthy, so sweet and succulent, so refreshing and rewarding, like the literal fruit of the vine and the branch. We are wise when we include fruit in our diets—at least two servings a day. They provide a variety of vitamins, minerals, and clean-burning fuel for our bodies. And here is a special tip for weight control. Try having a serving of fruit a few minutes to a half-hour before your lunch and dinner. The fiber and water content will help fill your stomach, and the natural fructose (fruit sugar) just might render that gooey desert a little less appealing. So, let's make those fruits manifest to help perfect our forms!

St. Matthias (died 80 AD) Apostle and Martyr

We must combat our flesh, set no value upon it, and concede to it nothing that can flatter it, but rather increase the growth of our soul by faith and knowledge.   *Attributed to St. Matthias by Clement of Alexandria*

Many Catholics are not familiar with St. Matthias, the "thirteenth apostle." After Jesus ascended to heaven, the first order of business for the new leader of the Church, St. Peter, was to oversee the selection of an apostle to replace the traitor Judas. Two men were brought forward, Joseph and Matthias. After praying for guidance, the Apostles cast lots and chose Matthias. Not much is known about St. Matthias. Some accounts state that he was a follower of Jesus and was one of the 72 disciples who were sent out in pairs to preach and heal the sick. There are several conflicting stories regarding his death. One states that he was stoned and then beheaded by the Jews. Another tells that he preached the Gospel to the barbarians and cannibals in Ethiopia and died of natural causes. A third account says he was crucified. Despite his relative anonymity on earth, he is certainly immortalized in heaven: *"And the walls of the city had twelve foundations, and on them the twelve names of the twelve apostles of the Lamb."* (Rev 21:14)

Exercise: Like St. Matthias we too can do good works that will not be recorded in history. Today do something nice for a stranger who will never be able to thank you. Pay for the order for the car behind you in the drive-through. Leave coupons by the items they discount in the grocery store. Tuck a $5, $10 or $20 dollar bill some place where a stranger can find it. Leave a bouquet of flowers on someone's door step. Say a prayer for the anonymous stranger who will receive your small gift. While you're in the gift-giving spirit, give yourself a gift that will help improve your health. Buy a new pair of walking or running shoes, a workout journal, an exercise DVD, a gym membership or several sessions with a personal trainer. You don't have to spend a lot of money, but do purchase something that will help motivate you to exercise more frequently.

Blessed Sebastian of Aparicio (1502-1600)
Angel of Mexico

Sell your possessions, give alms; provide yourselves with purses that do not grow old, with a treasure in the heavens that does not fail, where no thief approaches and no moth destroys. For where your treasure is, there will your heart be also. *Luke 12: 33-34*

The son of Spanish peasants, Blessed Sebastian sailed for Mexico at age 31 and started to work as a farmhand. He later spent 10 years building a 466 mile road from Mexico City to Zacatecas that was used for the post and for commerce—providing a boon to the region. He became a very wealthy rancher. At 60 he married a poor young girl at the request of her parents, noting they would live as brother and sister. She died young and Sebastian contracted another virginal marriage under similar circumstances. She too passed away, whereupon, at age 72, he gave away his possessions, became a lay Franciscan brother, and spent decades begging alms for the Franciscans, earning him the nickname of "The Angel of Mexico." Beatified in 1789, his body remains incorrupt. He is a patron of travelers and road builders.

Exercise: Do you ever "hit the road," for bikes, or runs, or walks? What a great service those road-builders have performed for us who would use them to care for our temples. Have you thanked them in your heart for building so many free gymnasiums?! By varying your workout routes you can get a refreshing change of scenery, and also of terrains.

Got hills? A nice, steep hill or two can change a simple walk in the park to a mini-mountain climb if you attack it with gusto. One variant is to do an occasional briefer, more intense cardiovascular "hill workout," consisting of nothing, besides warm-up and cool-down, but ascending and descending a hill. So, on your next outdoor jaunt, why not set your heart on the things of God, and meditate on the example that the angel of Mexico has set for us—to detach our hearts from earthly treasures.

Saint Mechtildis (1240-1298) Abbess

But nothing unclean shall enter [heaven], nor anyone who practices abomination or falsehood, but only those who are written in the Lamb's book of life.
Revelation 21:27

What do you fear? This child most certainly will not die, but she will become a saintly religious in whom God will work many wonders, and she will end her days in a good old age.
Priest who baptized St. Mechtildis, thought to be near death at her birth

St. Mechtildis wanted to devote her life to God from a very young age. When she was just seven years old, she begged her parents to enroll her in the monastery school where her older sister served as abbess. Ten years later, she joined the convent as a Benedictine nun. She was put in charge of the young school children, one of them the future St. Gertrude the Great (the patroness of this book, see Nov. 16). Mechtildis also led the choir and was known for her beautiful voice. Upon learning that some of the sisters had been writing down her words and visions, she became concerned and prayed for guidance. She had a vision of Christ who held her book and reassured her that the work would draw many closer to him. She edited the writings herself and published them under the title, *The Special Book of Grace*. St. Mechtildis was immortalized in Dante's *Purgatorio* as the Donna Matelda in the vision of purgatory as a seven-terraced mountain, similar to what she had described in one of her visions.

Exercise: The *Catechism* says, "*All who die in God's grace and friendship, but still imperfectly purified, are indeed assured of their eternal salvation; but after death they undergo purification, so as to achieve the holiness necessary to enter the joy of heaven.*" (CCC #1030) One of the spiritual works of mercy is to pray for the living and the dead. Since St. Mechtildis described Purgatory as a mountain, the exercise for today will draw on that by doing "mountain climbers." Start in the standard push-up position, with abs drawn in. Bend one leg, bringing your knee up toward your chest with the ball of your bent leg on the floor. Quickly switch legs, bringing the first leg back to the starting position and the opposite leg up toward your chest. Repeat 10-20 times, alternating legs.

St. Gabriel of Our Lady of Sorrows (1838-1862)

Let them praise his name with dancing, making melody to him with timbrel and lyre! For the LORD takes pleasure in his people; he adorns the humble with victory.   *Psalms 149:3-4*

I will attempt day by day to break my will into pieces. I want to do God's Holy Will, not my own!   *St. Gabriel*

Born Francis Possenti, baptized in the same Assisi fountain as St. Francis himself (Oct. 4), and not unlike his namesake, this saint's youthful passions for the music, theatre, and the company of young ladies, earned him the nickname "The Dancer." He soon came to answer the call to a religious life with the Passionist Order, however. With a special devotion to Mary, and to the contemplation of her sorrows at the passion of Christ, he assumed the name Gabriel of Our Lady of Sorrows. Always positive and cheerful, despite recurring illness, he died of tuberculosis just two days short of his 24th birthday. Canonized in 1920 by Pope Benedict XV, he's a patron of youths, of students, of seminarians, and of Abruzzi, Italy.

Exercise: Perhaps dancing and the breaking of one's will, cheerfulness and sorrow, seem an incongruous mix, but these are the stuff of which lives are made, yours and mine, and even the greatest of saints. Note how this young saint's very name proclaims this paradox. It was Gabriel who made the joyful announcement to Mary that she would receive the greatest honor of any human being, to conceive the very Son of God. Yet with that highest of all graces would also come incomparable sorrows, as she observed that Son's passion. Of course, to contemplate these mysteries, we need look no further than the beads of the rosary itself. The next time you contemplate those joyful and sorrowful mysteries in a rosary workout, set aside time for a prayer to young St. Gabriel of Our Sorrowful Mother.

St. Jadwiga (1373-1399) King of Poland

D o you know that a woman can be crowned king? Such was the case with St. Jadwiga. Her father, King Louis I of Hungary, had no male heirs and decreed that upon his death his two daughters would rule his kingdom as monarchs in their own right. Jadwiga was crowned King of Poland at age eleven and her sister Mary as King of Hungary. The young king was fittingly qualified for the crown. Jadwiga was well-educated, spoke six languages, and was known for her piety. Due to political reasons as well as her beauty, many men wished to marry her. She wisely put the needs of her kingdom over her personal preferences and married Duke Jagiello of Lithuania, a pagan man nearly three times her age. Jadwiga insisted that he convert to Christianity as well as his entire nation. There are several colorful legends told about St. Jadwiga. According to one, she often used an apron to smuggle food to the poor through a secret door from the palace. She was observed and thought to be spying, so her husband was informed. He followed her one night and demanded to know what she was doing. She certainly wasn't a spy but smuggling food would have been a death sentence according to the current law. When she opened her apron, the food miraculously turned into fresh flowers.

Exercise: Find some way to help feed the poor today. Call your parish office and ask if there are any needy families in the parish whom you could help with a donation. Or, call your local food bank or homeless shelter, ask what they need, and go buy a few items and drop them off. Since your legs are probably sore from this week's hill workout and mountain climbers, this is a good day to do some gentle stretches. Warm up briefly by going for a short, brisk walk or simply march in place for a few minutes in your living room. Find a mat or a comfortable place on the carpet and stretch your legs using a variety of different stretches. Hold each stretch for at least 30 seconds. The longer you hold the stretch, the more you'll increase your flexibility.

St. Oswald (died 992)

So God created man in his own image, in the image of God he created him; male and female he created them. *Genesis 1:27*

St. Oswald, a Saxon, was said to be blessed with unusual beauty of body and soul. Born into nobility, he was raised by his uncle St. Odo, Archbishop of Canterbury. He was named dean of the secular church canons at a young age, and when his attempts to reform lax practices failed, he became a religious monk of the Benedictine order. Soon after St. Odo's death, St. Dunstan nominated Oswald to the See of Worcester. Here St. Oswald worked many reforms, established seven religious houses, and helped effect the monastic revival of tenth century. In an ingenious move to reform the secular canons without removing them, he had his monastic brethren construct a church dedicated in honor of the Mother of God, adjoining the secular cathedral. He himself assisted in the Divine Offices at this church and the people, moved by his and his monk's holy example, deserted the cathedral. The canons had but little choice to abandon their worldly ways. In the leap year of 992, this highly gifted, yet piously humble man resumed his Lenten tradition of washing the feet of 12 poor men each day. On February 29, after kissing the feet of the 12th man and delivering a blessing, St. Oswald would die, spreading grief throughout the diocese.

Exercise: Some pious souls fear that physical exercise might lead to an impious vanity, that too much focus on the body will take away focus from the things of the soul. With our fallen natures, this is a legitimate concern. But take particular notice how St. Oswald, graced with great physical beauty, focused on things of the soul and humbled himself before the feet of beggars. We can thank God for the natural beauty of our bodies while making the effects of training on the beauty of our bodies, a mere side effect, not a goal. Especially in the case of young women today, the focus of fitness training needs to be more on function than on form, more on the good we can do with fit bodies than on how they look; always remembering that God wants us to image him foremost in love.

St. David of Wales (died c. 589) Patron Saint of Wales

Count it all joy, my brethren, when you meet various trials, for you know that the testing of your faith produces steadfastness. James 1:2-3

Be joyful, brothers and sisters. Keep your faith, and do the little things that you have seen and heard with me.   *Last words of St. David*

Many of us would find it odd that St. David found joy in his difficult life as a monk and missionary. He and his Welsh monks worked in silence and ate only bread, vegetables and water. They did not use animals to farm but pulled the plow with their own strength, finding joy in living out their vocations in the service of God. St. David must have also experienced great joy as he converted countless pagans to Christianity and built and founded many monasteries in Wales.

St. David is often pictured with a dove on his shoulder based on a Welsh legend. He was preaching to a large crowd, and the people began to complain that they could not see or hear him. A dove suddenly appeared and rested on his shoulder. At that moment, the earth on which he was standing rose up to elevate him above the people so that all could hear his inspiring words.

Exercise: Follow in St. David's footsteps today and eat only bread, water and vegetables—and do it with great joy! Thank God for the food He has provided and offer up your hunger for someone who has no joy in his or her life.

Continue to imitate St. David by using your own strength to do most of your work today. If possible, walk or bike to work or at least park at the back of the parking lot. Take the stairs instead of the elevator and avoid automatic doors. Walk to a co-worker's office rather than use the phone, text or email. Put away the remote control and get up and change the channel. Most importantly, do not grumble about these minor sacrifices but joyfully thank God for the many blessings He has given you.

Blessed Charles the Good (1083-1127)

The good man out of his good treasure brings forth good, and the evil man out of his evil treasure brings forth evil.   *Matthew 12:35*

The object of our inquiry is not to know what virtue is but how to become good.   *Aristotle, Nichomachean Ethics*

Charles I, Count of Flanders—now Belgium—this son of King Canute of Denmark is often depicted with a money purse and a sword. A brave knight and crusader, he turned down the title of King of Jerusalem, and later even that of Emperor. A man of thought and devotion, as well as of action, he preferred to spend his evenings at court discoursing on the Scriptures with three learned theologians. A great defender of the poor, he took forceful action against a prominent family that was hoarding grain to sell later at exorbitant prices. For this action, after one of his daily barefooted walks to the Church of St. Donatian, while kneeling in prayer before a statue of Mary, he was attacked and beheaded by a group of knights in the employ of the family of hoarders. The nobles and commoners of the land soon brought those evil knights to justice.

Exercise: Blessed Charles was such a good man that "the good" would become his nickname. A wealthy and powerful governor, he gave even his life so the poor could share in the treasures of their land. And what an interesting spiritual exercise and penance: to walk barefoot to daily mass. While going barefoot is probably not practical in our day of cement and pavement, is your own church of a reasonable distance for you to occasionally walk there as a special penance? If not, make your own room a shrine of prayer. Today or tomorrow, walk from your house for 10 to 30 minutes, rosary in hand. Come back and pray awhile, before a statue of Mary, a crucifix, or both, and thank Blessed Charles for setting such a good example.

St. Katherine Drexel (1858-1955)
Patron Saint of Racial Justice

There is neither Jew nor Greek, there is neither slave nor free person, there is not male and female; for you are all one in Christ Jesus.
Galatians 3:28

St. Katherine gives us a wonderful example of how to be a saint in modern-day America. She was born in Philadelphia to a wealthy family who believed in sharing their good fortune with others, opening the doors of their home to the poor several days each week. When her parents died, she inherited a vast fortune and was determined to use the money to help the Indian people, having been profoundly moved by Helen Hunt Jackson's book, *A Century of Dishonor.* While traveling in Europe, Katherine met Pope Leo XIII and asked him to send more missionaries to minister to the tribes in America. The pontiff surprised her by suggesting that she become a missionary herself! She did just that and met with the Sioux leader in the Dakotas to determine the needs of his people. St. Katherine established schools, recruited priests to lead the missions, and provided food, clothing and other needed essentials. Years later, she moved to Santa Fe, became a nun and started the Sisters of the Blessed Sacrament for Indians and Colored (now simply called Sisters of the Blessed Sacrament). She founded Xavier University in New Orleans, the first black Catholic university in America. In her lifetime, St. Katherine established 50 Indian missions and a system of black Catholic schools in 13 states.

Exercise: Are you prejudiced against any group of people? We are all equal in the eyes of God. Pray for the grace to see the presence of Christ in everyone. In your exercise time today, open your heart with joy by doing an interval workout. After a 5-10 minute warm-up period, increase your exercise intensity for 15-30 seconds while you pray a joyful prayer of your own choosing, memorized or spontaneous. Slow your pace until you catch your breath, then repeat the increased-intensity interval 3-5 times. Cool down for at least 5 minutes.

St. Casimir of Poland (1460-1484)
Patron of Poland, Lithuania, and of Youths

Blessed are you among women, and blessed is the fruit of your womb.
Luke 1:42

O blessed shoot of Jesse's root, that bears the flower of hope divine; the world's clear light, its glory bright, God's temple, yea, his inner shrine, Hail Mary.
From "St. Casimir's Hymn"

Son of King Casimir of Poland and Queen Elizabeth of Hungary, Crown Prince Casimir would live only a brief time; remarkable for his responsibilities (briefly serving as King of Hungary as a teen, and ruling Poland in his father's absence in his early twenties), as well as for his piety (such as kneeling in prayer before the locked doors of churches in the hours before or after they opened.) He was loved for his charming character and chose the celibate life even though his father had pressed for a political marriage with young Casimir and the daughter of Emperor Frederic III. Casimir died of tuberculosis at age 23. His special devotion to Mary is evidenced by his desire to be buried with a copy of his favorite hymn, *Omni die dic Mariae* (Daily, Daily Sing to Mary), now believed to have been penned by St. Bernard of Clairvaux (Aug. 20), but often referred to as "St. Casimir's Hymn."

Exercise: In your next cardiovascular workout, why not sing a hymn to Mary? If that is not appropriate for the setting, or if you're not too fond of your own voice, why not pop in a CD or turn on your iPod and listen to hymns in her honor by some modern Catholic singers. A few of these wonderful musicians that I (Kevin) have had the honor to meet and would gladly recommend include Dana, Katrina Rae, and Annie Karto. So, why not listen, sing, workout, and pray to Mary, she who was God's temple in the most uniquely possible way?

St. John Joseph of the Cross (1654-1734)
Patron of the Island of Ischia, Italy

Even though I walk through the valley of the shadow of death, I fear no evil; for you are with me.   *(Psalms 23:4*

Whoever walks always in God's presence, will never commit sin, but will preserve his innocence and become a great saint.
St. John Joseph of the Cross

Despite the fact that he was a wealthy young Italian nobleman, Charles Cajetan (the saint's name at Baptism) dressed in humble clothing, slept on a hard, narrow bed and dedicated his life to practicing virtue. He was very devoted to the Blessed Mother and to Jesus' sufferings on the cross. At age 16, he entered the Franciscan Order of the Strictest Observance and took the name John Joseph of the Cross. While still a teenager and not yet ordained a priest, he was asked to found a new monastery. Always humble and hardworking, John Joseph helped with its construction and willingly took on tasks that the other brothers avoided. He was later ordained a priest and named as the superior of Santa Lucia in Naples where he lived the rest of his life.

St. John Joseph worked several miracles and had the gift of prophecy. He was also one of very few saints known to levitate (float above the ground) and bi-locate (be at two places at the same time).

Exercise: Catholics are the only Christians who display the crucifix (rather than an empty cross) as a reminder that Jesus redeemed us through His suffering and death. In imitation of St. John Joseph's dedication to the cross, spend 15 minutes today praying and meditating in front of a crucifix. Or reread today's quotes and spend 10-20 minutes walking either outside or indoors. As you walk, place yourself in God's presence. Pray that you may always keep God by your side as you work toward avoiding sin and becoming a saint.

St. Colette (1381-1477)

May you be strengthened with all power, according to his glorious might, for all endurance and patience with joy, giving thanks to the Father, who has qualified us to share in the inheritance of the saints in light.   *1 Colossians 1:11-12*

If there be a true way that leads to the Everlasting Kingdom, it is most certainly that of suffering, patiently endured.   *St. Colette*

Born in Picardy France, St. Colette was orphaned at 17 and left to the care of a Benedictine abbot. After brief attempts as a religious in the orders of the Beguines and Benedictines, she eventually became a Third Order Franciscan and lived several years as a hermit. St. Francis appeared to her in a vision and instructed her to restore the vigor of the barefoot St. Clare's. She would go on to establish multiple convents and even help heal, with the assistance of St. Vincent Ferrier, a Church schism in which three men laid claim to the papacy. She suffered much abuse from tormenting visions, as well as from those who thought she was a sorceress because of those mystical visions and ecstasies.

Exercise: I (Kevin) had been pondering this idea early yesterday and then, quite fortuitously, the topic was brought up later at dinner by Rick and Karen, my weightlifting friends since the mid-1980s. If you train at a gym, patience is a virtue you'll definitely need to develop! There are unspoken rules of gym etiquette, of sharing equipment ("working in"), of putting your weights away when you're finished, and of checking to see if others have finished before you unload their bars or change their equipment adjustments. We need to be patient if we suffer these minor transgressions, and maintain enough flexibility in our routines so that we can change the order of our exercises if our time is limited and our equipment is in use. We also need to use good gym etiquette ourselves. This way we can all share in the joy of training our temples—without trying each other's patience!

March 7

Saints Perpetua (181-203)
and St. Felicity (died 203) Martyrs

Where you go I will go, and where you lodge I will lodge; your people shall be my people and your God my God; where you die I will die, and there will be buried.   *Ruth 1:16-17*

It shall happen as God shall choose, for assuredly we depend not on our own power but on the power of God.   *St. Perpetua*

St. Perpetua was a beautiful, well-educated young wife and mother living in Carthage, North Africa. She, her beloved African slave named Felicity, and several other catechumens (Christian converts studying the faith) were imprisoned and sentenced to death. While in prison, the two women received some measure of comfort and consolation from their children. Felicity gave birth to a daughter and Perpetua was able to nurse her own infant several times. The two women, joyful at the prospect of martyrdom for their new faith, were brought to a crowded amphitheater and attacked by a wild cow. Both were severely gored but helped each other to get up and face the final deadly assault. The crowd called out that it was enough, and Perpetua and Felicity were brought forward to be beheaded.

We have many details regarding the martyrdom of these two brave women as St. Perpetua recorded the events leading up to her death in a diary. An eyewitness finished the account. Perpetua's diary is the oldest preserved written text by a Christian woman. Both saints are honored in the Roman Canon of the Mass during Eucharistic Prayer I.

Exercise: In the final weeks before Easter, many catechumens are preparing to enter the Catholic faith at the Easter Vigil Mass. Please pray for all catechumens, especially those in your own parish, through the intercession of St. Perpetua and St. Felicity. Make an effort to introduce yourself and welcome them to your parish. Exercise is so much more enjoyable if done with a partner. Ask a friend or family member to join you in a workout or a walk today. If you can't find anyone to join you, then talk to your Guardian Angel who is always with you.

March 8

St. John of God (1495-1550)

Those who are well have no need of a physician, but those who are sick; I came to call not the righteous, but sinners. Mark 2:17

I don't know of any bad person in my hospital other than myself. St. John of God

This Portuguese soldier and pleasure-seeker had a conversion when nearing the age of 40. He first sought to ransom Christian slaves in Africa, then, having received great joy and instruction from reading spiritual books, he became a religious bookseller in Spain. Upon hearing a moving sermon by St. John of Avila (May 10), he experienced a deeper conversion, cast off his books and other possessions, and scourged himself publicly in penance. Indeed, he was considered insane and placed in a hospital. St. John of Avila visited him and convinced him his call was to care for others. John of God opened a hospital himself and worked tirelessly for the sick and the poor. The quotation above is his response to critics for caring for the likes of prostitutes, tramps, and criminals. He is the patron of firefighters because he charged in and saved many people when his hospital caught fire. He died not long after saving a boy who was drowning in a river.

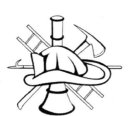

Exercise: No matter how badly or how long we may have abused our bodily temples, the time is always right for repentance and reform. Imagine the joy in heaven when any one of us decides to truly start tending them as they were intended to be tended! Note well too, for certain ailments, physical exercise itself can be effective medicine. For example, exercise can be good therapy for depression. It works chemically through the release of endorphins; and, when combined with prayer, it works psychologically and spiritually by shifting the focus from one's own woes to the wonders of God. When acutely physically ill, during a bout with the flu, for example, rest and not training is in order. After you've healed, the gym or the road will still be there waiting for you.

St. Frances of Rome (1384-1440)
Patron Saint of Motorists and Widows

Are you crying because you want to do God's will or because you want God to do your will? Advice to St. Frances from her confessor

Young Frances was 13 years old, living a life that most girls would envy. She had just married a wealthy nobleman who adored her, she had a closet full of beautiful clothes, and her only responsibility in life was to attend parties and banquets. Frances was completely miserable. She wanted to devote her life to Christ as a nun, but her father insisted that she marry. Her family was baffled by her despondency and told her to act more like her sister-in-law Vannozza, a cheerful and charming hostess. One day Frances was crying bitterly in the garden when Vannozza walked by and stopped to comfort her. Frances poured out her heart and told Vannozza how much she wanted to live a simple life devoted to God. To Frances' astonishment, Vannozza confessed that she felt exactly the same way! The two girls became great friends and went to Mass together, visited prisoners, and volunteered in hospitals. When the plague swept through Rome, Frances gave her own family's food to the poor and turned her house into a makeshift hospital. St. Frances is the patron saint of motorists based on a legend that her guardian angel used to light the road in front of her with a lantern when she travelled, keeping her safe from hazards.

Exercise: Like the young St. Frances, we might wish that God would choose another course for our lives. It is important to spend time in prayer for discernment and acceptance of our vocations and to live our lives in service to God and neighbor. God has a unique plan for each of us. We are all called to be saints, even if our stories will not be told in books and legends. In honor of St. Frances, be especially attentive when you drive today (and every day!). Obey the speed limit and be courteous to other drivers. If another driver is too slow or indecisive, cuts you off, or acts in an inconsiderate manner, just ignore it and pray for that person.

St. John Ogilvie (1580-1615)

Jesus said to them, "Render to Caesar the things that are Caesar's, and to God the things that are God's."   *Mark 12:17*

In all that concerns the king, I will be slavishly obedient; if any attack his temporal power, I will shed my last drop of blood for him. But in the things of spiritual jurisdiction which a king unjustly seizes I cannot and must not obey.   *St. John Ogilvie*

Like St. Robert Southwell, (Feb. 21), St. John Ogilvie chose to minister to the Catholics of the British Isles when this was an illegal and most deadly profession. Raised Calvinist, John joined the Catholic Church at age 17. After many years of study, he was ordained a Jesuit priest and requested to be sent back to Scotland. His identity as a priest was betrayed in Glasgow. During many days of torture, his legs were crushed, he was deprived of sleep for nine days and night by pricks from needles, but he resolutely refused to recant his faith or betray other Catholics. He suffered death as a traitor by hanging, but not before winning the respect of even the Protestant Archbishop by his courage and equanimity during his ordeal.

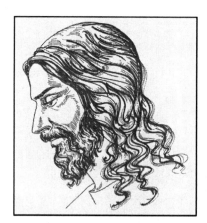

Exercise: What inspiration can we draw from such bold martyrs for Christ? How little we are asked in comparison. The next time you are tempted to skip that morning workout, Mass, prayer time, or spiritual study session because you've missed a few hours of sleep, think of St. John Ogilive, pray for his intercession, and then just do it. We need to train ourselves so that minor discomforts or inconveniences will not deter us from rendering what's due to the King of Kings.

St. Eulogius of Spain (died 859) Martyr

He has sent me to proclaim release to the captives... to set at liberty those who are oppressed.   *Luke 4:18*

The sacrifice most pleasing to God is contrition of heart, and that you can no longer draw back or renounce the truth you have confessed.
                                                                  St. Eulogius

St. Eulogius, the son of a Spanish senator, became a priest during a time when the Muslims controlled Spain. Christians were frequently persecuted for their faith, and Eulogius was captured and imprisoned with many others who refused to renounce their beliefs. In the jail cell, he calmly read the Bible to his fellow prisoners and encouraged them to die bravely for their faith. Eulogius was so successful at calming the fears of the future martyrs that he was encouraged to write a book to inspire other Christians. When he was unexpectedly released from prison, he published a book called *Exhortation to Martyrdom*. Eulogius continued to preach against the persecutions and converted many Muslims to Christianity. He was arrested once again but this time would not escape martyrdom. After earnestly preaching to the judge and council in an attempt to win more conversions, he was beheaded.

Exercise: Sadly, Catholics are still persecuted in many parts of the world. It is important that we not only know our faith but that we can also respond to challenges against it. Apologetics is a branch of theology that teaches us to defend our faith. If you have not heard of this term or have not studied apologetics, spend some time today researching a good book or website to help you better defend your Catholic beliefs. You might start with Shane's book, *The God Who is Love: Explaining Christianity From Its Center*, available at www.explainingchristianity.com!

While you're working to defend your faith, it's also important to defend your house and your family from emergencies. Everyone in your home should know what to do in case of a fire, earthquake, tornado, hurricane or other tragedy. Keep extra food, flashlights, a fire extinguisher, candles and batteries in a safe place where everyone can access them.

March 12

St. Luigi Orione (1872-1940)

Pray constantly...   *1 Thessalonians 5:17*

Without prayer nothing good is done. God's works are done with our hands joined, and on our knees. Even when we run, we must remain spiritually kneeling before Him.   St. Luigi Orione

St. Luigi Orione knew from the age of 10 that he wanted to be a priest, but in the intervening years before his ordination at 23, he would work with his father paving streets and serve as custodian for a Church in Tortona. He joined the Franciscans for a time, but left due to poor health. He would later study with the Salesians and St. John Bosco himself (Jan. 31). Like that great saint, he would impact the world for the good. St. Luigi had special concern for the poor, the sick, orphans, the developmentally disabled and the elderly. He would found the Little Work of Divine Providence with male and female active religious and contemplative orders. He began a first mission in Brazil in 1913. Today the Little Work is involved with over 300 foundations including schools, hospitals, day cares, and parishes found in England, Ireland, North and South America, the Philippines, Kenya, Jordan, India and elsewhere throughout the globe. His body lies incorrupt in the shrine of La Madonna della Guardia in Tortona, Italy, a church that he himself had established in 1931.

Exercise: The next time you run, walk, or bike, remain spiritually kneeling. Before you head out the door, kneel in prayer for a few minutes. As you run, whether doing a rosary workout, listening to spiritual music, or even if conversing with a running partner, take time to visualize yourself still kneeling in prayer to God, asking for the tireless energy and loving goodness of St. Luigi Orione. That way, the workout you get done will be good!

St. Leander (c. 534-600) Bishop of Seville

[The Son] reflects the glory of God and bears the very stamp of his nature, upholding the universe by his word of power.
Hebrews 1:3 (often cited against the Arian heresy)

This man of suave eloquence and eminent talent shone as brightly by his virtues as by his doctrine. By his faith and zeal the Gothic people have been converted from Arianism to the Catholic faith.
St. Isidore writing about his brother, St. Leander

The next time you recite the Nicene Creed at Mass, think of St. Leander. He instituted the practice of praying this summary of our faith as part of the Sunday liturgy in order to defeat several heresies that were popular at the time. As bishop of Seville in Spain, St. Leander worked tirelessly to combat one of these heresies—Arianism, a false belief that Jesus was created by God the Father and therefore inferior to Him. His efforts were so successful that he was banished for several years by the Arian king of the Visigoths who ruled Seville. Eventually the king died and Leander returned to lead the Third Council of Toledo, during which the new king converted to Christianity. The Filioque ("and from the Son") was also added as part of the Nicene Creed, stating that the Holy Spirit proceeds from both the Father and the Son.

St. Leander was part of a very holy family! His brothers are St. Isidore of Seville (April 4) and St. Fulgentius, both bishops, and his sister is St. Florentine.

Exercise: Sometime today, find time to carefully and prayerfully read the Nicene Creed. If you don't fully understand each statement of our faith, reference Part I of the *Catechism of the Catholic Church* (which can be found online if you don't own a copy).

St. Leander was known for his boundless energy. You'll find more energy too if you get a good night's sleep. Most adults need a minimum of 7-8 hours of restful sleep each night. Avoid caffeine and heavy meals in the evenings and try to go to bed early and read for half an hour or so.

St. Maud (aka Matilda) (895-968)

A foolish son is a grief to his father and bitterness to her who bore him.

Proverbs 17:25

St. Maud was raised in a monastery. In 909 she would marry Henry I, the man who would make her the Queen of Germany. Her own children would come to include an archbishop, a duke, and an emperor. Two of those sons, Emperor Otto I, and Duke Henry of Bavaria, would accuse her of impoverishing the realm by her excessive almsgiving (recall February 1 and St. Brigid's similar holy fault). The queen mother responded by relinquishing the property she'd inherited from Henry I and retiring to her villa. Later, when hard times befell those proud sons, in dire need of her advice and her pardon, they welcomed her back to the palace. Generations benefitted from St. Maud's humane counsel to royal rulers and her establishment and support of several German monasteries.

Exercise: St. Maud's boys got carried away by their exercise of power. Too many boys of our day sit away with no physical exercise whatsoever! Childhood obesity and related disorders such as diabetes are becoming a modern plague. We need to set our children examples through our own physical endeavors. We need, as well, to exercise our royal authority within our own households to set time limits on sedentary pursuits (yes, for computers, televisions, cell phones, video games—for the sundry, shimmering, seducers toward sloth of all sorts.) In psychology it's called the Premack Principle or "grandma's law:" first you work, and then you play. Let some limited session of sedentary play (perhaps an hour or so) follow the outdoor, physical play that will build sturdy temples, not mini-basilicas! Better yet, incorporate at least one day per week where you play (or at least walk) with them. In fact, God crafted such a day for leisure pursuits in his honor, and there are plenty of hours left after Mass.

St. Longinus (1ˢᵗ Century) Martyr

When the centurion, who stood facing him, saw that he thus breathed his last, he said, "Truly this man was the Son of God."

Mark 15:39

O Blood and Water, which gushed forth from the Heart of Jesus as a fountain of mercy for us, I trust in you.

From the diary of St. Faustina, Apostle of Divine Mercy

The Roman centurion who testified that Jesus was truly the Son of God is certainly a real person but is unnamed in the Gospels. The name Longinus (derived from the Greek word for spear) is attached to his legend, along with the assertion that he was the soldier who pierced the side of Christ with a lance. According to many accounts, Longinus was nearly blind, perhaps due to an accident in battle. When he pierced the side of Jesus, the precious blood fell on his eyes and restored his sight. He converted to Christianity, left the army and became a monk in Cappadocia. Ironically, a blind governor sentenced him to death by beheading. During Longinus' execution, some of his blood fell upon the governor's eyes, miraculously restoring his sight. He too converted to Christianity. St. Longinus is immortalized in the Basilica of St. Peter in Rome where his statue stands guard over the relics of his lance, now encased in a column that supports the dome over the papal altar.

Exercise: If you have not yet prayed the Chaplet of Divine Mercy, St. Longinus is the perfect inspiration to learn more about this powerful prayer for the conversion of sinners. The Divine Mercy image depicts the blood and water which flowed from the pierced heart of Jesus as rays of light. There are many books and websites devoted to the Divine Mercy devotion. The chaplet and associated prayers are usually said at 3:00 pm, the hour we honor Jesus' death on the cross. St. Longinus' story should also inspire you to schedule an appointment for an eye exam. If you wear glasses or contact lenses, it's important to get an updated prescription. Even if your vision does not require correction, your optometrist will check for serious eye diseases, many of which have no symptoms.

March 16

Blessed Torello of Poppi (1202-1282) Hermit

And Peter remembered the saying of Jesus, "Before the cock crows you will deny me three times." And he went out and wept bitterly.
Matthew 26:75

[Torello] spend all the days of this life, serving God with fasts, vigils, discipline, and prayers, and bitterly lamenting his past sins and evil life.   From "The Life of Beatro Torello da Poppi" by Torello of Casentino

Torello was a happy young Italian boy until his father died. For a time, he continued to practice his faith but then befriended a group of young men who drank and caused trouble. Torello decided it was more fun to hang out with his new friends than to work, pray, and go to Mass. One day, while he was outside playing sports with his companions, a rooster suddenly landed on his shoulder and crowed three times before flying back to its perch. Torello immediately understood that he had just been given the same warning that St. Peter received after denying Jesus three times. He immediately left his friends and spent eight days in fervent prayer for guidance to reform his life. He felt a calling to become a hermit and had a small cell built in the wilderness. He planted a garden and subsisted on the food he grew with water from a nearby stream.

There are several legends about Blessed Torello and his friendship with the wolves of the wilderness. A friend of the hermit sent his steward to Torello with a basket of delicious food. The astonished steward watched with amazement as a wolf came to the door of the cell, ate from Torello's hand and then curled up by the saint like a pet dog.

Exercise: Are your friends leading you toward heaven or away from it? Certainly you can positively influence friends, but if your companions are leading you down the wrong path, it might be time to part ways. Also, if you don't have your own garden, visit a farmer's market and buy some local fruits and vegetables.

St. Patrick (387–461) Patron of Ireland

Arise, shine; for your light has come, and the glory of the Lord has risen upon you.   *Isaiah 60:1*

Christ with me, Christ before me, Christ behind me, Christ in me, Christ beneath me, Christ above me, Christ on my right, Christ on my left, Christ when I lie down, Christ when I sit down, Christ when I arise, Christ in the heart of every man who thinks of me, Christ in the mouth of everyone who speaks of me, Christ in every eye that sees me, Christ in every ear that hears me. I arise today through a mighty strength, The invocation of the Trinity, Through belief in the threeness, Through confession of the oneness Of the Creator of Creation.   *Patricus Magonus Succatus (St. Patrick)*

A rise today and thank God you're Irish! But you're not? Blarney! "Everybody's Irish on St. Patrick's Day!" Even St. Patrick himself wasn't born in Ireland. God guided him to the emerald isle of Erin to bring the good news of Christ there, a place that at the time seemed the very end of the earth. And as we can see in the brief excerpt above from the magnificent prayer known as "St. Patrick's Breastplate," St. Patrick sought to armor himself with Christ, and to honor the Father and Holy Spirit as well.

Exercise: When you literally arise today, in the wee hours of the morning, do one smooth, intense, and focused set of sit-ups or abdominal crunches, reciting one phrase from St. Patrick's Breastplate as you arise with each repetition. Meditate on its meaning as you lower yourself back to the floor. Which of your acts today will help others see Christ in you? Do this daily and perhaps you'll add your own "abs of steel" to St. Patrick's breastplate.

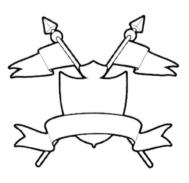

St. Cyril of Jerusalem (315-386) Doctor of the Church

Give me understanding that I may keep your law and observe it with my whole heart.
Psalms 119:34

Children of justice, follow John's exhortation: "Make straight the way of the Lord." Remove all obstacles and stumbling blocks so that you will be able to go straight along the road to eternal life.
Saint Cyril of Jerusalem

St. Cyril was born the same year the Emperor Constantine ended the persecution against Christians. Despite the newfound freedom to practice their faith, many Christians disagreed and several heresies (false teachings) became popular. As Archbishop of Jerusalem, St. Cyril worked hard to defeat the heresies and to teach the truths of Christianity. He was exiled three times and spent over 16 years away from Jerusalem. Cyril refused to give up and was always welcomed back by the people who appreciated his holiness and charity. St. Cyril was something of a rebel and didn't always follow the rules. He often disagreed with his superiors, and he secretly sold Church property. When caught, he argued that his intentions were honorable as he used the money to provide food to those starving in his city. St. Cyril is honored as a Doctor of the Church. His teachings for converts preparing to receive the sacraments are especially inspiring.

Exercise: Do you disagree with any Church teachings? Have you studied the teaching thoroughly or do you just not like a certain restriction on your lifestyle? Pray for guidance and do some research so that it will no longer be a stumbling block. The *Catechism of the Catholic Church* is a good place to start, and Shane's *The God Who is Love* may prove a helpful next step. Ask St. Cyril to help you. Don't let a heavy stumbling block hurt your back! If you must lift a heavy object, start with your feet shoulder-width apart. Bend your knees and keep your back straight while lifting with your legs. Tighten your abdominal muscles to protect your back, and keep the object close to your body rather than at arm's length. Never bend your back or twist your body. If the object is too heavy or you start to strain, ask for help. These suggestions also apply when picking up weights, even if they're fairly light.

St. Joseph (1ˢᵗ Century) Patron of the Universal Church

An angel of the Lord appeared to him in a dream, saying, "Joseph, son of David, do not fear to take Mary for your wife, for that which is conceived in her is of the Holy Spirit; she will bear a son, and you shall call his name Jesus, for he will save his people from their sins."
Matthew 1:20-21

Glorious St. Joseph, pattern of all who are devoted to toil, obtain for me the grace to toil, in the spirit of penance, in order to thereby atone for my many sins... *Pope Pius X*

St. Joseph, the foster-father of Jesus, is a glorious model for all fathers. A man more of actions than words, scripture recounts for us his brave and honorable deeds. He took Mary for his wife, though she was with child through the Holy Spirit. He protected the infant Jesus in their flight to Egypt during King Herod's terrible reign of infanticide. Though he had apparently passed from this earth by the time of Christ's adult ministry, his vital role in salvation history has become increasingly manifest in the Church throughout the centuries. In the nineteenth century, Pope Pius IX (Feb. 7) proclaimed him the patron and protector of the Catholic Church as well. In 1989, Pope John Paul's Apostolic Exhortation *Redemptoris Custos* (Guardian of the Redeemer) sparked new interest in the theological discipline of Josephology.

Exercise: Let's apply a little Josephology in our own homes today. A question for fathers: What can you do today to guide and protect the physical and spiritual health of your family? Are you brave enough to counter the cultural messages telling your loved ones their bodies are not holy? A reminder for all of us: Joseph toiled hard with his hands in the carpenter's shop. Surely his bodily temple was hardened through his labors. Why not do some chore in the house or yard today with prayers in St. Joseph's honor?

St. Maria Josefa (1842-1912)

Beloved, I pray that all may go well with you and that you may be in health; I know that all is well with your soul. 3 John 2

Do not believe, sisters, that caring for the sick consists only in giving them medicine and food. There is another kind of care you should never forget – that of the heart which seeks to adapt to the suffering person, going to meet his needs. St. Maria Josefa

When Maria Josefa joined the Servants of Mary in Madrid, taking the name Sister Maria of Health, she had realized her vocation of ministering to the sick in the hospital and in their homes. She realized, however, an essential element missing in her calling that would strengthen her, her religious sisters, and those they served – devout communal life. St. Maria left with a few sisters and strove to attract the five members required to found a new communal order devoted to the care of the sick. In 1886, Pope Leo XIII would declare approval of the Servants of Jesus. St. Maria would serve as its mother superior for the next four decades until her death. Today, her order has grown to over 1,000 members in 43 houses throughout the globe.

Exercise: St. Maria Josefa was fired by devotion to bringing health to her neighbors in body and soul. Indeed in the third article of her order's institutes she makes clear that tending to physical and material needs of the sick, of children, and the needy, is actually a means to their spiritual sanctification. When St. John addressed Gaius in his third letter quoted above, he wished him physical health, but he knew his soul to be healthy because brethren had told him Gaius "followed the truth." Think now of some small thing we can do today to follow the truth by attending to some physical or spiritual need of the sick, of the family and friends of our own community, or of ourselves?

St. Nicholas of Flue (1417-1487)
Patron Saint of Switzerland

I am the bread of life, he who comes to me shall not hunger, and he who believes in me shall never thirst. John 6:35

Each state of life has its special duties; by their accomplishments one may find happiness. St. Nicholas of Flue

Unlike many male saints, St. Nicholas of Flue was not only married but also fathered ten children. At around age 50 and just after the birth of his tenth child, he felt called to live the life of a hermit. (It was a calling from heaven, not a desire to leave the daily uproar that must be involved in a house with ten children!) With the blessing of his wife and children, he relocated to a hermitage a few miles away. Word of his holiness quickly spread, and he was often called upon for spiritual advice. In fact, Nicholas was so wise that he was consulted when the delegates of his native Switzerland disagreed and civil war seemed imminent. The illiterate saint drafted a proposal that was accepted by everyone, thus uniting Switzerland and preventing war. Six years later, he died of a painful sickness in the arms of his wife and children.

Nicholas is quite a fascinating saint. He was a soldier by profession before becoming a hermit, and was said to fight with a sword in one hand and a Rosary in the other. He received many symbolic visions, and his only sustenance for 19 years was the Eucharist.

Exercise: Although most of us would not be able to live on the Eucharist alone, we can make our reception of it more devout. The next time you go to Mass, try to fast for several hours before Communion (the Church currently requires a one-hour fast, per Canon 919). Let your hunger remind you that you are receiving the true Bread of Life. Focus deeply on your prayers before Communion and your prayers of thanksgiving afterward. Imitate St. Nicholas in battle by praying the Rosary as you perform a repetitive but rigorous chore such as vacuuming, mowing the lawn, or washing the car.

St. Nicholas Owen (1550-1606)

For he will hide me in his shelter in the day of trouble.   *Psalms 27:5*

I verily think no man can be said to have done more good of all those who laboured in the English vineyard. He was the immediate occasion of saving the lives of many hundreds of persons, both ecclesiastical and secular.   *Fr. John Gerard*

Like St. Joseph, (March 19), St. Nicholas Owen was another holy carpenter, and like St. Robert Southwell, (Feb. 21), he was a Jesuit who gave his live for his faith. St. Nicholas was best known as a masterful craftsman of "priest holes," hiding places for priests built in floors and walls of the homes and mansions of faithful Catholics who would house them during the time of great persecution in Britain and Wales from 1535-1679. Nicholas was later captured and tortured in hopes he would reveal the locations of many priests, but his lips were sealed unto his death.

Exercise: A torture that St. Nicholas bore with equanimity until his death was to be hung from his shackled hands with heavy weights attached to his feet. Ironically, when done in the proper manner, hanging from the hands with moderate weights attached can build tremendous strength, and here I mean simply chin-ups. In my 20's, I (Kevin), would perform 22 full chins with a 20 lbs. dumbbell attached to a belt harness and 6 repetitions with a dangling 100 lbs. barbell plate.

Now I'm not recommending such stunts to you (or to myself anymore), but be aware that good old fashioned chin-ups are still a top notch way to strengthen the muscles of the back, shoulders, biceps, and forearms. There are also machines and special bands on the market that will assist you in doing chins if your own bodyweight is too much for you. Various overhead pull-down machines also make a fine substitute. The discomfort from either is negligible, of course, compared to that which St. Nicholas Owen endured.

St. Turibius of Mongrovejo (1538-1606)
Patron Saint of Peru

The harvest is abundant but the laborers are few; so ask the master of the harvest to send out laborers for his harvest.   *Matthew 9:37-38*

Time is not our own, and we must give a strict account of it.
St. Turibius of Mongrovejo

S t. Turibius was a Spanish nobleman, lawyer and chief judge on the Court of the Inquisition. His comfortable life was turned upside down when he was asked to become the archbishop of Lima, Peru. This was a very unusual request as he was not even a priest! His objections were overruled, and Turibius was quickly ordained a priest and bishop and sent to Peru. There he found horrible abuses and oppression of the native people by both the Spanish settlers and the clergy. Turibius learned the language of the people so that they could hear Mass and confess their sins in their native tongue. He built roads, schools, churches and hospitals and established the first seminary in the western hemisphere. St. Turibius possessed incredible stamina. Three times he traveled the 18,000 miles in his diocese, often on foot, baptizing and confirming over half a million people. St. Rose of Lima (Aug. 23) was one of the Peruvian natives he confirmed.

Exercise: St. Turibius made very good use of his time, knowing that he was accountable to God. Today, use your time as wisely as possible. It's perfectly fine to relax by watching TV or surfing the internet, but set a timer so that you keep track of time. Better yet, set aside some time to read the Bible or a book about your favorite saint.

Since you're being extra careful with your time today, you should be able to improve your stamina by doing a long, fairly slow-paced workout. If you're fit, try to exercise for 45-60 minutes or at least 15 minutes longer than your usual routine. If you don't exercise regularly, try a 25-30 minute easy-paced walk or hike. Make your workout even more productive by praying the Rosary, meditating on the Jesus' Passion and Crucifixion or examining your conscience.

St. Gabriel the Archangel, "The Strength of God"

"Oh Daniel, I have now come out to give you wisdom and understanding."   *Daniel 9:22*

St. Gabriel, God's special messenger, first appears in the Bible when he interprets a vision for the prophet Daniel. In the New Testament he brings good news and indeed, the greatest of all news, in announcing to Zechariah, and soon after to the Virgin Mary, the births of John the Baptist and of Jesus Christ. Quite fittingly, Gabriel greets both Zechariah and Mary with the words, "Do not be afraid." Surely, the sudden appearance of an archangel could probably startle anyone! But notice as well that unwarranted fear is opposed to the virtue of fortitude, and fortitude derives from the Latin word *fortis*, for strength. St. Gabriel brings God's special messages and inspires with God's strength.

Exercise: In St. Gabriel the Archangel we have found our ideal patron for strength training, since the very name of Gabriel, means in the Hebrew, "the strength of God." So, have you been keeping up with your physical strength training? Recall that high intensity (HIT) methods can take as little as one 20-minute workout per week. Also, to grow in your strength, you will need to strive to gradually progress, using slightly heavier weights, doing more repetitions with a given weight, and perfecting your form to eliminate cheating or momentum. Be not afraid though! God has enabled us to find methods for building our physical strength in a very safe and controlled manner. As for our spiritual strength, let's always add prayer to our workouts, today with a prayer to the St. Gabriel the Archangel.

Feast of the Annunciation of the Lord

And Behold, you will conceive in your womb and bear a son, and you shall call his name Jesus.   _Luke 1:31_

Without God's Son, nothing could exist; without Mary's Son, nothing could be redeemed.   _St. Anselm of Canterbury_

The details of the Annunciation are related in just one small paragraph in the Gospel of Luke, yet it is one of the most pivotal events in human and salvation history. Mary's obedient fiat ("yes") to the Angel Gabriel's request to become the mother of the Savior reverses Eve's disobedience in the Garden of Eden and paves the way for mankind's redemption through the Word Incarnate. Interesting, several early Christian writers believed that March 25th (as translated from the Jewish lunar calendar) was a very historical date. It was believed to mark the day that God created the world, the day that Adam and Eve fell from grace, the date of Jesus' conception and finally, the date that He suffered and died on the cross. Further testimony of the importance of this date can be found in the original Anno Domini (AD) calendar. When it was first introduced in 525 AD, March 25th marked the first day of the New Year to commemorate the beginning of the era of grace at the Incarnation. Note that as of today, there are exactly nine months until Christmas.

Exercise: This feast often falls during the season of Lent but is to be observed as a celebration. It would be a fun family tradition to buy or bake an angel food cake to celebrate the Annunciation. Angel food cake is a low-fat treat, and its circular shape reminds us of the Blessed Trinity. At the Annunciation, Mary is forever united to the Trinity. She is the daughter of God the Father, the mother of God the Son and the spouse of God the Holy Spirit. You can add more symbolism to your special dessert, as well as some disease-fighting antioxidants and bone-building calcium, by topping with blueberries (blue is Mary's color), strawberries (red for the Precious Blood of Christ), and low-fat whipped cream (white symbolizes Mary's perpetual virginity). Before serving dessert, read the Biblical account of the Annunciation (Luke 1:26-38).

St. Ludger (743-809)

But when you pray, go into your room and shut the door and pray to your Father who is in secret; and your Father who sees in secret will reward you.   *Matthew 6:6*

St. Ludger was born in Holland, studied in England, and became a bishop in Munster, Germany. He was a student of the learned Blessed Alcuin of York and a missionary for the conversion of the Saxons. The Emperor Charlemagne himself gave him charge of the spiritual direction of five provinces. St. Ludger was once accused of mismanagement of his diocese and called by a chamberlain before the presence of Charlemagne. He had reached St. Ludger, however, in the midst of his morning prayers. The saint told him he'd come when he had finished. After two more summons that day, he finally appeared. Advisors had told the emperor that the bishop's delay displayed his contempt for his majesty. When St. Ludger explained that he held the highest earthly respect for the emperor, but was delayed only by the duties he owed to a Majesty of infinitely higher authority, Charlemagne was well pleased, honored the bishop, and dismissed the charges against him.

Exercise: When St. Ludger had shut the door of his mind to outward distractions and raised his prayers to God, not even the summons of the most powerful ruler on earth could distract him from those prayers and budge him from that room. When we have set aside time for prayer, for physical exercise, or time for both combined, how effective are we at keeping the doors of our minds and hearts closed to distractions from outside and from within ourselves? Are we led away by the lure of a warm bed, a glowing television, a stream of daydreams? Alright then, the next time you are tempted to skip a session of prayer or exercise, to cut it short, or to let your attention wander, think of St. Ludger, of Emperor Charles the Great, and of the Father who will reward your perseverance.

Blessed Francis Faa di Bruno (1825-1888)
Priest and Scholar

The heavens are telling the glory of God; and the firmament proclaims his handiwork. *Psalms 19:1*

Science and technology are ordered to man, from whom they take their origin and development; hence they find in the person and in his moral values both evidence of their purpose and awareness of their limits. *Catechism of the Catholic Church, section 2293*

Blessed Francis was a wealthy nobleman who served as an officer in the Italian army before resigning to study mathematics and astronomy in Paris. One of his astronomy professors helped to discover the planet Neptune. He returned to Turin, Italy, as a Professor of Mathematics at the university but devoted much of his free time to charity. He established hostels for the poor and elderly, built a church to honor fallen Italian soldiers, and established the Society of St. Zita (April 27) for domestic servants. At the age of 51 he was ordained a priest and continued his works of charity until his death in 1888.

Blessed Francis is also famous in the secular world. He invented several scientific apparatus and made many important contributions to the field of mathematics. An advanced mathematical formula he derived is named after him.

Exercise: If you really want to see the glory of God's creation and discover Blessed Francis' love for astronomy, take a good look at the night sky. On a moonless night, find a place that is very dark with few lights nearby. Lie on your back and just enjoy the spectacular display of stars and planets. (Make your stargazing night an opportunity to exercise by hiking to a remote location and camping for the night.) Notice how the stars rise and set in a predictable pattern. Imagine the power and might of a God who could create such beauty and order!

St. Tutilo (850-915)

May you be strengthened with all power, according to his glorious might, for all endurance and patience with joy, giving thanks to the Father, who has qualified us to share in the inheritance of the saints in light.
                                                                 Colossians 1:11

This Irish-born Benedictine monk of the abbey of St. Gall in Switzerland, was described as a large, handsome, quick-witted and powerfully built man who excelled in music, painting, sculpture, poetry, mechanics, metalworking, teaching, and public speaking. An incredibly well-rounded "Renaissance Man" many centuries before the Renaissance, this pillar of mind and body prefigures for me both that nearly all-knowing saint "with the shoulders of a giant," St. Albert the Great (Nov. 15) and his most famous student, the "dumb ox of Sicily," that massive man with the mind and the heart of an angel, St. Thomas Aquinas (Jan. 28). And like those two remarkable saints, St. Tutilo's gifts were matched only by his humility. He was known to have a special devotion to the virtue of obedience and preferred to live in the relative seclusion of the monastery.

Exercise: What wonderful inspiration St. Tutilo provides for all who would make the most of the gifts God has given us in mind, body, and soul. Let's focus today on strengthening the glorious might of our own God-given skeletal muscles. To make our muscles large and strong (with women bearing in mind that their lower testosterone levels will not produce the lumpy bulging muscles of a man—thank God!), we would do well to focus our energies on the true "core" of physical strength, by emphasizing the "big three," exercises: "a leg, a push, and a pull." By performing a squat or leg press ("a leg"), a chest press or overhead press ("a push"), and a chin-up, pull-down, or rowing motion, ("a pull"), you will stimulate virtually every major muscle group in the body. The classic three power-lifting exercises: squat, bench press, and dead-lift, have been building powerful bodily temples for generations. Other movements are but icing on the cake. Like St. Tutilo then, let's do some sculpting, and let's use our own muscles serve as our clay.

St. Joseph of Arimathea (1ˢᵗ Century) Patron Saint of Funeral Directors, Undertakers and Pallbearers

---

Joseph of Arimathea... went to Pilate and asked for the body of Jesus... And he bought a linen shroud and taking him down, wrapped him in the linen shroud, and laid him in a tomb.   *Mark 15:43, 46*

The story of Joseph of Arimathea, the man who buried Jesus in his own tomb, is a mixture of fact and legend. The Gospels give us several facts regarding his life, character and actions. Joseph was a just and wealthy man who was a member of the council (probably the Sanhedrin). He followed Jesus in secret due to fear of the Jews, but he found the courage to ask Pontius Pilate for Jesus' lifeless body. Joseph purchased fine linen and spices for burial and laid Jesus in his own, unused tomb. It was hewn from rock and was located in a garden near Calvary.

According to legend, Joseph was Jesus' uncle and amassed his wealth in tin trading. He occasionally traveled to England and might have taken Jesus with him on a trip, where they were shipwrecked on the coast. After Jesus' death, Joseph returned to England and settled in Glastonbury. There he built what is believed to be the first above-ground church in Western Europe. He placed a great treasure in this church—the cup from the Last Supper, which is often called the Holy Grail. When Joseph left to spread Christianity to other nations, he buried the Holy Grail and marked it with his staff. It miraculously took root and turned into a beautiful flowering tree, but no one has yet found the elusive Holy Grail.

Exercise: Today is my (Peggy's) daughter Rebecca's birthday, one of the most important dates of my life. I'm glad she shares a celebration with someone who was so close to Jesus. From the time she was little, Rebecca always blessed every morsel of food that went into her mouth. We sometimes feel awkward about blessing our food in public, but it provides an opportunity to witness to our faith. Make it a habit to bless every meal, even if it's in a fancy restaurant or eaten with friends who don't share your beliefs.

St. John Climacus (579-649)

If I ascend to heaven, though art there!   *Psalms 139:8*

The man who pets a lion may tame it, but the man who coddles the body makes it ravenous.   *St. John Climacus*

This great Church Father, esteemed in the East and the West, became a novice at a monastery at age 16, spent twenty years in isolation studying the lives of the saints, and ended his life as abbot of the monastery at Mt. Sinai. His most notable book is a superb and enduring spiritual classic called *The Ladder of Divine Ascent*. Here, the reader is guided through thirty chapters called "steps," each devoted toward building higher levels of physical and spiritual ascetic virtues. Among the highest of special value to monks are prayer, stillness, and dispassion. The highest step of the ladder (echoing St. Paul's appraisal of the virtues in 1 Cor.13:13) is *agape*, or love. An Eastern icon depicting monks ascending the ladder shows Jesus at the top, welcoming the climbers to heaven.

Exercise: To ascend the spiritual ladder we must bring the body under the sway of the will. This is the stuff of the virtues, like the temperance that brings our appetites in line with the body's needs, not gluttony's wants, and the fortitude we that enables us to do hard things, like regular strength-training and cardiovascular exercise. And speaking of strength and ladders, at my 18-year-old son Kyle's recent leadership retreat for his college's honors group, one task involved ascending a 50-foot rope ladder with a harness attached for safety. No one in the camp's history had ever climbed to the top using their arms alone—and then came Kyle! He had never climbed a rope ladder before, but had trained in a HIT fashion twice weekly for ½ hour for the last 3 years. Virtues, like physical strength, once built in one domain, can be used in many others. (And the stronger the climbers we become, the easier it becomes to extend a hand to help raise up others.)

Blessed Joan of Toulouse (died 1286)
Foundress of the Carmelite Third Order

Fear not, for I have redeemed you; I have called you by name; you are mine.   *Isaiah 43:1*

When you look at the Crucifix, you understand how much Jesus loved you then. When you look at the Sacred Host you understand how much Jesus loves you now.   *Blessed Mother Teresa of Calcutta*

Most Catholics are not aware that it is possible to join a religious order as a lay person. A tertiary (third order) can join a religious community while living in his or her own home rather than a convent or monastery. Tertiaries can wear the habit of the order and participate in works of charity with the nuns or monks. Many follow the Rule of the order. Blessed Joan was fascinated by the Carmelites at the monastery in her hometown of Toulouse, France. When St. Simon Stock (July 16), a well-known Carmelite reformer, passed through Toulouse, Joan approached him and asked to be allowed to enter the order. He agreed, and she became the first Carmelite tertiary. She took a vow of perpetual virginity and followed the Carmelite Rule, performing many acts of charity and doing penance daily. Her most important role in the community was training the young boys of the town as altar servers and helping them discern a possible vocation as a Carmelite. Blessed Joan was very devoted to the Blessed Mother and her Divine Son. It's said that she always carried a picture of Jesus on the cross in her pocket and would frequently pull it out to gaze lovingly on the face of Christ.

Exercise: Blessed Joan would be pleased today if you prayed for more vocations to the priesthood and religious life. Part of the Carmelite Rule that Blessed Joan followed states, *"The Apostle would have us keep silence, for in silence he tells us to work. As the Prophet also makes known to us: Silence is the way to foster holiness."* Follow that simple rule for a time today and work or exercise in silence. (You might need to find some ear plugs!) Use this time to meditate and pray or simply put yourself in God's presence.

April 1

St. Hugh of Grenoble (1052-1132)

The saying is sure: If anyone aspires to the office of bishop, he desires a noble task. Now a bishop must be above reproach...

1 Timothy 3:1-2

St. Hugh aspired to be a priest, a monk, a holy man, a saint, but not necessarily a bishop, despite his 52 years in episcopal office. The son of the former soldier Odilo, St. Hugh would have the rare honor of administering the sacraments of extreme unction and viaticum to his father, who was by then a Carthusian monk, before his death at age 100. St. Hugh desired the contemplative life of a monk himself. Two years after he became bishop, he even resigned and became a novice at the monastery of Casa-Dei in Auvergne France. Soon after, Pope Gregory VII ordered St. Hugh to return to his bishopric to continue the rigorous reforms of the clergy and laity that he had begun. St. Hugh had underestimated his own prior success in this regard. Though he would help St. Bruno found the Carthusian order, and would later petition Pope Innocent II to retire to the monastic life, St. Hugh would serve the remainder of his life, until nearly age 80, as shepherd of a diocese. St. Hugh sought solitude and contemplation. He was able to attain it even at times as a bishop by brief visits to monasteries. Because of his talents as a learned an able administrator and reformer though, he would lead the majority of his life as a man of action and great responsibility for others.

Exercise: It's time for one of my (Kevin's) simple recipes to nourish the body and soul. Here's a simple, austere meal for when you are eating alone: Prepare a low sodium tomato soup, reconstituting it with water. Toast a whole grain bagel. Crumble the bagel into the soup and eat with a side salad of greens, vegetables, and a little vinegar or lemon juice. When feeding a family some heartier fare, reconstitute the soup with skim or 1% milk, add some shredded cheese and turkey bacon pieces to the bagel and toast in the oven before adding to the soup. Have the dressing of your choice on the salad and throw in a few nuts and olives. There you go; two meals fit for a monk – or a bishop.

April 2

St. Richard of Chichester (1197-1253)

If you love me, you will keep my commandments.   *John 14:15*

May I know thee more clearly, love thee more dearly, and follow thee more nearly, day by day.   *St. Richard of Chichester*

St. Richard was young when he and his older brother were orphaned. He was so successful in helping his brother manage his estate that he was offered management of all his lands and marriage to an excellent woman. St. Richard chose instead the priesthood, and would later be named bishop. Perhaps hinting at the rift between the papacy and the British crown to come in the centuries ahead, King Henry III, resenting Pope Innocent IV's appointment of Richard over his own unworthy nominee, confiscated all of Richard's property. Undaunted, Richard fed the poor, held the sick, passed just judgment on even knightly transgressors, and restored the income to his diocese in only two years.

Exercise: Today's entry provided a most pleasant surprise for me (Kevin). Are you familiar with the incredibly beautiful song, "Day by Day," made famous in the 1973 musical *Godspell?* If not, give it a listen. Growing up in the 70s, I was quite moved by some of the music of *Godspell* and *Jesus Christ Superstar* as well (e.g., "I Don't Know How to Love Him.") Do you see where the classic lines from "Day by Day" first came from? 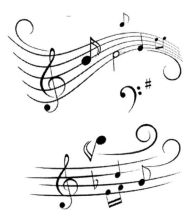 They ended one of St. Richard's beautiful prayers. Here's a suggestion for a change of pace for your next cardio workout, walk, or bout of good old-fashioned, high intensity house or yard work. Turn on the stereo or pop in the MP3 player earplugs and do your workout listening to the stirring tunes of one of those movies. The theme, "day by day," by the way, works perfectly well for this book, wouldn't you say?

St. Ulpianus (died 306) Martyr

---

*Thou art my refuge from the trouble which hath encompassed me:
my joy, deliver me from them that surround me.*   *Psalms 32:7*

*Glorious the northern lights astream; Glorious the song, when God's
the theme; Glorious the thunder's roar; Glorious hosanna from the
den; Glorious the catholic amen; Glorious the martyr's gore.*

Christopher Smart

I (Peggy) came across this obscure saint while reading my beloved *Magnificat* magazine. I have read and researched many martyrs who died in horrible ways, but the chilling story of St. Ulpianus' death has particularly affected me. I hope that this holy teenager's suffering was brief and that his glory in heaven is great. Ulpianus was a devout and zealous Christian who lived in Tyre (now part of Lebanon). At that time, the Roman Emperor Maximinus Daia decreed that Christians were to be arrested and killed. Ulpianus was brought before the cruel judge Urbanus and asked to renounce his faith. The young man refused and courageously confessed Christ before the judge. Something he said must have particularly aroused Urbanus' ire because a horrible series of tortures was devised. After severely scourging Ulpianus, Urbanus had him stretched on a rack until nearly all his bones were broken and his joints dislocated. Still not satisfied, the heartless judge ordered that the teen be sewn up in a calfskin bag with a dog and a snake and thrown into the sea.

Exercise: St. Ulpianus no doubt found courage during his ordeal by singing or praying the Psalms, perhaps even the one I chose above. The Psalms are known as a "School of Prayer," and are well worth taking the time to read and study. Spend a few minutes today reading a Psalm and reflecting on what it can teach you about prayer. St. Ulpianus had nearly all his bones broken, but you can prevent broken bones by strengthening them through weight-bearing exercises such as weight lifting, running, and walking. Calcium is very important for bone health. Good sources include low-fat milk, cheese, yogurt, and dark leafy greens like spinach, kale, or collard, mustard or turnip greens.

St. Isidore of Seville
Patron Saint of Computers and the Internet

The fear of the Lord is the beginning of knowledge; wisdom and instruction fools despise.   *Proverbs 1:7*

Learning unsupported by grace may get into our ears; it never reaches the heart. But when God's grace touches our innermost minds to bring understanding, his word which has been received by the ear sinks deep into the heart.   *St. Isidore*

St. Isidore is honored as a Doctor of the Church, but he had a bit of a rough start in his educational journey. As a child, he was raised and educated by his brother, St. Leander (March 13). Leander was a harsh taskmaster and Isidore was not the best student. He ran away in frustration but prayed for help, returning home with a new zeal for his studies. When Leander died, Isidore succeeded him as Archbishop of Seville. During his 37 years as Archbishop, he accomplished more than most men could do in centuries. He converted many heretics and Barbarian Visigoths, required seminaries to be built in every diocese of Spain, founded many schools, and encouraged learning and study especially in science. In fact, he is known as "Schoolmaster of the Middle Ages" due to his immense contributions to educational growth in Spain. St. Isidore was also known for his voluminous writing on a variety of topics, including a dictionary and a history of the world. His most influential work was a summa of universal knowledge called *Etymologies* in which he basically recorded everything that was known at that time. It included 448 chapters in 20 volumes! In true charity, St. Isidore's last act before his death was to give all his possessions to the poor.

Exercise: Before you surf the web, say the following prayer:

Lord, through the intercession of Saint Isidore, during our journeys through the internet, help us to direct our hands and eyes only to that which is pleasing to you and to treat with charity and patience all those souls whom we encounter. Amen.

St. Vincent Ferrer (1350-1419)

You are not your own. You were bought with a price. So glorify God in your body.
                                                                1 Corinthians 6:20

Whatever you do, think not of yourself, but of God.   *St. Vincent Ferrer*

We've already seen that St. Vincent Ferrer teamed with St. Colette (March 6) to help heal a schism with three claimants to the papacy. This saint was also quite the miracle worker and apostle for Christ, preaching and converting souls from Spain to Switzerland, from Italy to Scotland, and in many European countries in between. Indeed, he learned the Scriptures by heart and converted many infidels and heretics. He also converted many of the Jewish faith, and under his influence, the Jews of Valencia, Spain converted their synagogue into a church. St. Vincent usually prayed extensively to prepare for his sermons, but once, in preparation for a homily in which a very important nobleman would be in attendance, he studied extensively instead. The nobleman was not particularly impressed. Later, unbeknownst to St. Vincent, he came to hear another homily and was deeply moved by the saint's message. When told this story, St. Vincent replied that he had given the first homily, but Jesus himself had given the second!

Exercise: Physical exercise provides us a wonderful opportunity to transform an activity most often performed with eyes on the self into one performed with our eyes turned toward God. Jesus bought our salvation with his own bodily sacrifice. How little we are asked in return to be stewards of our bodies and to glorify him in them. Though we can never return that glorious favor in full, we can do our share to pay him back in small measure for that great price he paid.

So what will you do *today*, to glorify God in *your* body? "Think not of yourself, but of God!"

St. Juliana of Liege (1193-1252)
Saint of the Corpus Christi Feast

St. Juliana was born in Belgium and was orphaned at the age of five. She was entrusted to the care of Augustinian nuns and received an excellent education. Juliana joined the order at the age of 13. She worked in the convent-run hospital and became very devoted to adoring Jesus in the Blessed Sacrament. As a young woman, she received the first of many visions of a full moon with a dark diagonal stripe across its surface. She gradually understood that the moon represented the Church on earth and the diagonal line showed the absence of a feast to honor the Blessed Sacrament. Juliana kept these visions a secret for over 20 years before finally confiding them to her confessor who then approached the bishop. The bishop liked the idea, and the feast of Corpus Christi (Body of Christ) was celebrated in 1247 in the diocese of Liege, Belgium. St. Juliana and her new feast were not popular with everyone, and she endured much persecution and several false accusations. She was driven out of Liege and spent the remainder of her life in quiet and prayerful seclusion. It was not until after her death that Pope Urban IV instituted the Feast of Corpus Christi for the entire Church. He also commissioned St. Thomas Aquinas (Jan. 28) to write the text for the feast's Office and Mass. Today the feast of Corpus Christi is celebrated on the first Thursday after Trinity Sunday (one week after Pentecost). In the United States, the feast is transferred to the Sunday after Trinity Sunday.

Exercise: Make a visit to the Blessed Sacrament. Stay for at least 15 minutes. To strengthen your knees, work the muscles that act on the knee—the quadriceps, hamstrings, calves and shin muscles. One good exercise is a partial squat: Stand about 12" in front of a chair with your feet shoulder-width apart. Slowly lower yourself halfway to a sitting position, checking to make sure your knees stay behind your toes. Hold briefly and return to standing. Repeat 8-10 times. As you get stronger, add weights and/or more repetitions.

St. John Baptist de la Salle (1651-1719)

That your words may produce their full effect on your students, preach by example and practice what you wish them to accept.

St. John Baptist de la Salle

St. John Baptist de la Salle was born in Rheims, France to a wealthy and noble family. He became a priest, a respected church canon, and a doctor of theology. In his early thirties, he would give $400,000 of his fortune to the poor during a famine. He would go on to leave his position as canon and devote his life to the education of the poor. A brilliant man with a true gift for teaching, he formed a group of lay teachers, the Christian Brothers, which eventually went international and helped pave the way for universal education of the poor. His innovative reforms included the spread of literacy by teaching the children to read in their own language before introducing Latin, grouping children in grades according to age and ability, and forming the first schools designed to train teachers to teach.

Exercise: Back in my (Kevin's) days of Catholic grade school education, our physical education was anything but formal. After all, they'd just recently invented the ball. Seriously though, our "recess" time was spent on a blacktop playground playing kickball, "red rover," four-square, football, and the like. At times our teachers, not Christian Brothers, but Dominican Sisters, would indeed practice what they preached, a couple of them kicking a pretty mean kickball in their full black-and-white habits. We lacked equipment, but not fun, sportsmanship, or plenty of exercise. If you're not a teacher, perhaps you still have the opportunity to train children in the joys of playful exercise as a parent, grandparent, aunt, uncle, etc. So, April's here. Why not think of some ways to get them outside and have some fun through some old-fashioned sports and games?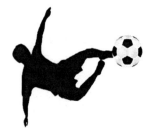

St. Julie Billiart (1751-1816)
Patron of the Sick and Impoverished

[The Lord] said to me, "Assemble the people for me; I will have them hear my words, that they may learn to fear me as long as they live in the land and may so teach their children."   *Deuteronomy 4:10*

I ought to die of shame to think I have not already died of gratitude to my good God.   St. Julie Billiart

As a little girl of seven, Julie had already memorized her catechism and was eagerly teaching and explaining it to other children in her hometown of Cuvilly, France. Her parents lost their fortune during her teenage years, and she labored in the fields to help support her family. Julie continued to teach catechism to young children in her spare time and encouraged devotion to their faith. In her early 20's, she was paralyzed by shock during the attempted murder of her father and was confined to bed for over 20 years. St. Julie refused to change her habits of daily prayer and of teaching the local children, gathering them around her bed each day to continue their education in the catechism. When the French Revolution broke out, she used her home as a hiding place for priests. When her plan was discovered, friends hid her from the authorities, carrying her from house to house. During this time she had a vision of nuns surrounding Calvary and knew she should start a religious order. She established the Sisters of Notre Dame, devoted to teaching the poor and training catechists. Julie was miraculously cured of her paralysis and spent the rest of her life in service to God and the poor.

Exercise: If you have children or godchildren, ensure that they are very familiar with the Catechism of the Catholic Church. The *New St. Joseph Baltimore Catechism* series is a good choice for younger children. Older children can read *Youcat*. There are also many online resources for worksheets, crossword puzzles and other activities to make learning more fun. To make your workouts more fun, find some new music to listen to during exercise. A simple MP3 player is very inexpensive, and you can upload songs from your favorite CDs.

St. Mary of Egypt (344-421)

The body is not meant for immorality, but for the Lord, and the Lord for the body....Do you not know that your body is a temple of the Holy Spirit within you, which you have from God? 1 Corinthians 6:13, 19

From the age of 12, for more than 17 years, St. Mary of Egypt treated her body and the bodies of her customers as anything but temples of the Lord. She lived openly and shamelessly as a prostitute in Alexandria throughout her teens and twenties. Later, she embarked on a ship headed for Jerusalem on a pilgrimage, though her intentions were anything but holy. To her surprise, when she was with a group celebrating the Feast of the Exaltation of the Cross, she found herself unable to enter the door of the church. The realization of the wickedness of her life suddenly overcame her. Seeing then a statue of the Virgin Mary, she vowed that if she were allowed to enter and venerate the relic of the sacred cross, she would renounce the world and do Mary's bidding. This she did, removing herself from temptations; she eventually led a solitary life as a desert hermit for more than 47 years. A monk named Zozimus then chanced upon her in the wilderness. He brought her communion and she asked him to return in one year to do the same. When he returned, he found her corpse with a note requesting her burial.

Exercise: Has our modern culture lost its sense of shame? Sadly, some modern critics, including "new atheists" and secularists of various sorts, proclaim that the Church believes that our bodies are shameful, that sexuality is dirty, when this could not be further from the truth. The Church recognizes that God made us as embodied souls, and that those bodies are good, *very good.* (Gen 1:31). Indeed, as St. Paul often notes, our bodies are the very temple of the Holy Spirit. We should feel shame when we denigrate our bodies, treating them as mere flesh alone. But the good news is that even those who mistreat and dishonor their bodies most gravely can always be redeemed through their repentance, reform, and God's mercy. They may even become saints.

Blessed Anthony Neyrot (1425-1460) Martyr

The saint is the person who is so fascinated by the beauty of God and by His perfect truth as to be progressively transformed by it. Because of this beauty and truth, he is ready to renounce everything, even himself. *Pope Benedict XVI*

We read about many martyrs who choose to die rather than renounce their faith. Blessed Anthony actually did renounce his faith, at least for a time. He was a Dominican priest who became bored and restless in his monastery in Italy and requested a transfer to Sicily. He didn't care for that location either and transferred again to Naples. On the voyage, his ship was captured by Muslim pirates and taken to North Africa. He resented his imprisonment and converted to the Muslim faith in order to buy his freedom. He even married a high-ranking Turkish woman! The death of a beloved Dominican friend and teacher, St. Antonius, caused him to begin to question his new life. A few days later St. Antonius appeared in a vision and urged Anthony to return to his faith and the Dominican order. Knowing that such actions would result in certain death, he sent his wife back to her family, found a Dominican priest and confessed his sins and was restored to the order. He publicly proclaimed his Catholic faith on the Muslim king's palace steps and was sentenced to death by stoning.

Exercise: It is easy to get bored and restless if your prayer life and exercise routine never change. Mix things up a bit and learn a new prayer devotion or search through a Catholic bookstore (brick and mortar or online) for a new book that interests you. Your parish might have a library with books or DVDs you can borrow. Add some variety to your workout routine by trying a new piece of gym equipment. Medicine balls, stretch cords, kettle bells or stability balls are available in most gyms. They are fairly inexpensive and can be purchased for home use as well. Ask a gym staff member for help if you're not sure how to use them or search for exercises online.

St. Pope Leo the Great (400-461)

Stand therefore, having girded your loins with truth, and having put on the breastplate of righteousness...   *Ephesians 6:14*

St. Leo was the first pope to be labeled "the great" for his accomplishments in the papacy. He battled heresies including Pelagianism and Manichaeism, the one holding that original sin did not taint our human nature, the other, that the material world was evil. St. Leo strengthened the primacy of the bishop of Rome as the successor of Peter and head of the universal Church on earth. He is a theological doctor of the church and was known for facing and persuading Attila the Hun to turn away without sacking Rome.

Exercise: St. Leo the Great was indeed both leonine and great—a lion-hearted warrior, willing to don the armor of Christ to face even the ruler of the Huns. In a sense, our skeletal muscles can act as our body's armor, protecting our bones and internal organs from harm. And beneath every breastplate are the pectoral muscles of the chest. Here is a specialized chest workout for the "pecs" employing the brief, intense, and efficient method of "pre-exhaustion." (See glossary.) If you have access to strength machines, first perform a set of 8 to 12 repetitions to failure or near failure on a chest "fly" machine that isolates those muscles. Then immediately, without rest, perform at least 3-5 repetitions, to failure, on a chest press or incline press machine. The relatively rested front shoulder and triceps muscles will take the "pre-exhausted" pectorals over the threshold to growth stimulation—and you'll feel the "pump" and "burn."

That's it—a 3-minute chest workout for men or women. You would simply attempt to do more repetitions or add a little more weight the next time you do that workout. Alternative methods are to use dumbbells for chest flyes followed by bench presses or incline presses, or a "chest crusher" type spring exerciser immediately followed by pushups on handles that allow a full stretch.

St. Teresa of the Andes (1900-1920)
Patron Saint of Young People

I have called you friends, for all that I have heard from my Father, I have made known to you.   *John 15:15*

So dearly does His Majesty love us that He will reward our love for our neighbor by increasing the love which we bear to Himself, and that in a thousand ways.   *St. Teresa of the Andes*

S t. Teresa was born in Santiago, Chile, to a wealthy family. She was given the name Juanita at Baptism and lived a life of privilege, riding horses and going on vacations. She was a spoiled, conceited child until her older brother taught her to pray the Rosary, which profoundly changed her life. Young Juanita promised to pray the Rosary every day, forgetting only once during her short life. She longed to receive her First Holy Communion and was able to do so at age 10, but only after much careful preparation. She wrote in her diary, "I prepared myself for one year. During that time the Virgin helped me to purify my heart from all imperfections." As a young teen, Juanita read *The Story of a Soul* by St. Thérèse of Lisieux (who at the time was not yet a saint; see entry for Oct. 1). The book helped her to realize that she wanted to devote her life to God as a nun. At age 19, she became a Discalced Carmelite novice, taking the name Teresa of Jesus. (Religious in discalced orders do not cover their feet, either going barefoot or wearing sandals.) Teresa focused on prayer and sacrifice. She wrote many letters to friends and family about her faith. Less than a year after entering the convent, Teresa contracted typhus and died on April 12, 1920. She is Chile's first saint.

Exercise: Write a letter to your own children, a niece or nephew, or another young person telling them about your faith and its influence in your life. St. Teresa never knew how much she enjoyed tennis until she tried it. Follow her example and try a new sport or a new mode of exercise this spring.

Blessed Ida of Lorraine (1040-1113)

...from you shall come forth for me one who is to be ruler in Israel...
Micah 5:2

The wife of Eustace II, Count of Boulogne, in what is now France, Blessed Ida of Lorraine would give birth to Eustace III, the next Count of Boulogne. She would also bear two sons who would be rulers in Israel—Godrey of Bouillon and Baldwin, the first and second rulers of the Kingdom of Jerusalem won back in the early crusades. Though a countess herself, and the daughter, granddaughter, and sister of dukes, this noblewoman showed her dedication to her young children in her insistence on breastfeeding them herself. Her dedication to Christ and the Church was shown in her generosity to the poor, her generous funding of the first crusade, the founding of five monasteries, and her own vow, after her husband's death, as a Secular Oblate of the Benedictine Order. She corresponded with St. Anslem (April 21) and some of his letters to her are still extant.

Exercise: That Blessed Ida was busy doing God's work is quite fitting, given that the very name Ida derives from the Old Germanic *id*, meaning labor or work. So, in her honor today, why not tend your bodily temple by performing some "house aerobics," some house or yard work timed and done vigorously as a workout? And why not tend for your children and their temples at the same time? Kathy and I (Kevin) have sometimes set a kitchen timer for everyone in the household to get in such a "workout," and it can be amazing what a whole family can get done when everyone is racing the clock to see how much cleaning can be accomplished before that buzzer goes off in a half-hour or so. Your house is already too clean and organized to need such a family workout?—well then, make your workout the preparation of a healthy dinner while the rest of the crew does the cleaning. For some added twists, observe a period of monastic-like silence and prayer while everyone works, or put on a Gregorian chant CD.

St. Peter Gonzalez (1190-1246)

Survey the path for your feet, and let all your ways be sure. Turn neither to right nor to left, keep your foot far from evil. *Proverbs 3:26-27*

I t is a common saying that pride goes before a fall; in the case of St. Peter Gonzalez, the maxim can be taken literally. St. Peter, like many before his day and since, saw the clerical life as a way to climb the social ladder, thinking that the priesthood would be an easy way to cement his self in the ranks of high society. A few years into his ordination, on a citywide Christmas Day procession, all of that (along with St. Peter himself) was upended, when his horse became startled and threw Peter onto a dung heap. Rather than being horrified, the peasants (some of whom had been paid to cheer him on) instead cackled with glee at his humiliation. This was a wake-up call for Peter, who began to consider his vocation no longer as a means for self advancement, but as a Christ-centered calling to save souls. From that point forward, he stopped being enamored with positions of high esteem, and actively sought ways to aid in the salvation of those traditionally neglected by society.

There is a strong parallel between the "pre-fall" St. Peter Gonzalez and those of us who initially chart physical goals out of a sense of vanity. The appeal of beauty and status, especially in a narcissistic culture, can be deceptively strong. How, and why, do we want to improve our appearances? Does the idea that we can rise in social status, or perhaps make others jealous of our bodies, hold too much of a grip on our desire to attain physical fitness? In a youth and beauty-obsessed society, many of us can relate to St. Peter before his (literal) downfall, dwelling on superficial reasons for pursing the plans God has laid out for us.

Exercise: As you engage in your daily physical activities, consider your motivations. Are you trying to lose weight or tone muscle because you crave the positive opinions of others, or because you realize that your body is a temple of the Holy Spirit, and it should be cared for out of reverence for God?

April 15

St. Damien of Molokai (1840-1889)

Truly I say to you, as you did it not to one of the least of these, you did it not to me.
Matthew 25:45

My greatest pleasure is to serve the Lord in his poor children rejected by other people.... Be severe toward yourself, indulgent toward others.
St. Damien of Molokai

In 1873, this young Belgian priest embarked on his first three month rotation to the island of Molokai, established as a colony for lepers seven years before. He would soon volunteer to stay there permanently, tending to the physical and spiritual needs of these very least of the brethren of Hawaii. He tended the lepers' diseased bodies, planted gardens, developed irrigation, and worked for an increase in governmental aid for them. He tended to their spirits as well, erecting a church, a school, and orphanage, and attracting an order of Franciscan sisters. Fr. Damien himself became the subject of abuse from ill-informed and ill-willed detractors. The celebrated author Robert Louis Stevenson would come to visit and staunchly defend this Christ-like saint's work. After several years, Fr. Damien himself would contract leprosy (Hansen's disease), and would die from it at age 49. In 1959, the newly admitted State of Hawaii would have his statue erected in the U.S. Capitol. Pope Benedict XVI would celebrate his canonization on October 11, 2009.

Exercise: Imagine how acute and penetrating was St. Damien's vision, enabling him to see that those deformed, decaying, and dying bodies he tended, remained holy temples, housing Christ within each afflicted breast. He was so indulgent toward them and so severe on himself, that he sacrificed the health of his own body for those whom he loved. To what extent then are we willing to suffer minor discomforts and inconveniences to tend for the robust bodies with which we have been blessed? Or perhaps you too are afflicted in physical health. Are there still lessons you can learn from this great saint?

St. Benedict Joseph Labre (1748-1783)
Patron Saint of the Mentally Ill and Homeless

My Good, my All, sole Object of my love, O come! I long for Thee, I sigh after Thee, I wait for Thee! Every little delay seems a thousand years! Come, Lord Jesus, and tarry not."   St. Benedict Joseph Labre

Misfits of the world can find a holy example in St. Benedict Joseph Labre. He desperately wanted to become a monk, but was constantly rejected by each monastery he sought to enter. He was well-educated, sweet, humble, cheerful, and very pious but also a bit odd and perhaps mentally disabled. Undaunted by his inability to formally enter the religious life, he became a wandering pilgrim, visiting shrines and holy places throughout Europe. Benedict wore simple clothes and begged for food and lodging, willingly sharing what little he was given with others. Many people thought he was insane, and he was mocked, ridiculed, and pelted with stones and garbage. He lived a life of silence, praying constantly and was often drawn to adore the Blessed Sacrament in the European churches. He became known as "The Beggar of Perpetual Adoration." Benedict often went into a state of ecstasy while worshipping, and a heavenly light seemed to shine around him. An Italian artist named Antonio Cavallucci painted a portrait of the saint deep in prayer, his face illuminated with a supernatural light. Benedict collapsed on the steps of a church during Holy Week and died a few hours later. Within just three months of his death, 136 miracles were worked through his intercession.

Exercise: Think of St. Benedict when you encounter someone who is odd, eccentric or mentally ill. God calls people from all walks of life to become saints. Although you probably can't devote years to pilgrimage, you can visit one of the shrines or holy places in the United States. Pilgrims in Europe walk to the holy sites, but that's not always practical. Instead, calculate the distance to a chosen place of pilgrimage and make a pledge to walk the same number of miles on a treadmill or in your neighborhood before you visit.

Blessed Kateri Tekakwitha (1656-1680)
Patroness of Ecology, The Lily of the Mohawk

Now I rejoice in my sufferings for your sake and in my flesh I complete what is lacking in Christ's afflictions for the sake of his body, that is, the Church.

Colossians 1:24

Jesus, I love you.

St. Kateri Tekakwitha's last words

Blessed Kateri was born in New York to a Mohawk chief and a Christian Algonquin mother who had most likely been captured in war. Throughout her short life, Blessed Kateri Tekakwitha passionately adored Christ and gladly bore abundant sufferings, and self-mortifications, while showering those around her with acts of service and kindness. Smallpox took her parents and left her with a pockmarked face and damaged vision at the age of only four. After a brief visit from three "blackrobes," (French Jesuit priests) when she was ten years old, young Kateri burned to seek out Christ. At age eighteen, despite the displeasure of her uncle, also a chief, and a hater of the blackrobes and Christianity, she sought instruction when a Fr. de Lamberville came to her village. She was baptized at age 20. Her name Kateri is the Mohawk adaptation of her namesake, St. Catherine of Siena (April 29). Kateri suffered great mockery among her tribe for her devotion, later moved to a Christian Mohawk settlement, and consecrated herself to a life of virginity for Christ. Weakened throughout her life from smallpox, she died at 24. Witnesses reported that her pockmarked face was healed at her death on April 17, 1680. On June 22, 1980, she became the first beatified Native American. Her feast day is celebrated on July 14 in the United States.

Exercise: It appears that Blessed Kateri practiced a rosary workout of sorts, circling a cornfield while reciting Hail Mary's even during harsh winter months. Well, if it's April 17 (or especially July 14) while you're reading this, why not pick up that rosary and go for a walk in the great outdoors today, saying a prayer to our patroness of the environment as well?

Blessed Mary of the Incarnation (1566-1618)
Patron of Parents Separated From Their Children

Be careful to heed all these words which I command you, that it may go well with you and your children after you forever, when you do what is good and right in the sight of the Lord your God.
Deuteronomy 12:28

I am a poor mendicant who begs of you the divine mercy, and that I may cast myself into the arms of religion. *Blessed Mary of the Incarnation*

When Blessed Mary's mother was pregnant, she vowed that she would offer her child to the Blessed Mother. A healthy young girl was born and christened Barbara. She was pious, modest, and sweet-natured. She had planned to enter a convent, but her parents insisted that she marry. Barbara bore six children and passed on her devout lifestyle; all three of her daughters became nuns and one of her sons became a priest. Her home became a center of religious life in Paris. People gathered there for daily Mass and lively discussions on Church doctrine and spiritual matters. One regular visitor was St. Francis de Sales (Jan. 24), who became Barbara's confessor and dear friend. During this time, she began to read the works of St. Teresa of Avila (Oct. 15). The saint later appeared to Barbara in a vision and instructed her to bring the Discalced Carmelite order to France. Barbara helped found several convents and joined the order herself as a lay sister after her husband died. She took the name Mary of the Incarnation. Ironically, her own daughter became the Mother Superior, but Blessed Mary obeyed her, glad for the opportunity to practice humility.

Exercise: Paris Catholics benefited from Blessed Mary's generosity in opening her home as a type of religious center. Sadly, many US Catholic parishes do not promote groups where adults can gather to discuss spiritual matters. Consider starting such a group in your parish. If you encounter road blocks, then invite others to your home. Perhaps the group members can take turns hosting. You can even encourage a healthy lifestyle by going for a group hike or walk and discussing a topic along the way, or afterward over a healthy snack.

St. Alphege (954-1012)

One thing you still lack. Sell all that you have and distribute to the poor, and you will have treasure in heaven; and come, follow me.

Luke 18:22

What reward can I hope for if I spend upon myself what belongs to the poor? Better to give up to the poor what is ours than to take from them the little which is their own.

St. Alphege

S t. Alphege had lived as a monk, an anchorite, an abbot, and a bishop before his appointment as Archbishop of Canterbury in 1005. He worked tirelessly in converting raiding Danes to Christ. In 1011 a particularly brutal band of Viking raiders sacked and pillaged Canterbury, taking many captors, including Archbishop Alphege who had stayed in Canterbury to support his flock. After seven months of captivity in foul conditions, his captors agreed to leave the land for a huge "Danegeld," a tribute of 84,000 pounds, collected through taxation. St. Alphege infuriated them, however, by refusing to allow the people to be burdened by another 3,000 pounds for his own ransom. His drunken, enraged captors beat him brutally with ox bones until his life was ended with the blow of an ax, delivered, some say, to end his agony, by a man the archbishop had baptized.

Exercise: St. Alphege gave all that he had to the poor in a most courageous and unusual manner. He gave his life rather than see them robbed of their sustenance. How easy in comparison is modern life for us. We are able to live in comfort, with so much surplus food that most of our bodily temples bulge in the middle. Will you consider fasting for one meal today and setting aside the money you save to share with a food bank for the poor?

St. Agnes of Montepulciano (1268-1317)

S t. Agnes' birth was announced by lights encircling the house where she lived, causing the townspeople to wonder just what sort of woman she would grow up to become. When she was very little, Agnes knew she wanted to devote her life to God. At age nine, her parents allowed her to enter a Franciscan convent in Montepulciano, Italy. The little girl was overjoyed to live with the other sisters, and she willingly worked hard and prayed often. At the age of fifteen, she was asked to move to a new convent in another town and was immediately put in charge. Another supernatural event marked this occasion—tiny white crosses rained down over the church and the people in it as Agnes was consecrated as the abbess. She returned to Montepulciano and built a Dominican convent, using three stones that the Blessed Mother had given her for that purpose. She lived on mainly bread and water and slept on the hard ground. The Blessed Mother allowed her to hold the Infant Jesus, and she received Holy Communion from an angel. According to many sources, she brought a drowned child back from the dead. Agnes was also known to levitate several feet in the air while praying. Her body is incorrupt even to this day.

Exercise: Jesus said that we must be like children to enter the kingdom of heaven. Children trust and depend on their parents, and we must do the same with God. Practice praying with childlike trust and faith. Although you probably can't levitate like St. Agnes, you can get up in the air and strengthen your legs through step-ups. Use a step-stool, bench, an aerobic step or just about anything that is stable and will support your weight. The best height allows your knee to bend at a 90-degree angle, although a slightly lower step is still beneficial. Using one leg at a time, place your foot in the center of the step. Push through the heel and step up, just lightly touching the step with the opposite foot. Return to the starting position and repeat 5-15 times, then switch to the other leg. As you get stronger, hold weights in your hands or on your shoulders.

April 21

St. Anslem (1033-1109)

Brethren, do not be children in your thinking; be babes in evil, but in your thinking be mature.
1 Corinthians 14:20

God cannot be conceived not to exist. – God is that, than which nothing greater can be conceived.—That which can be conceived not to exist is not God.
St. Anslem

St. Anslem was a later successor to St. Alphege (April 19) as Archbishop of Canterbury. He was loyal to the pope, refusing to yield to British kings' claims to the right to invest him as archbishop, he was twice exiled. Anslem is best known, however, as a profound philosopher and theologian. He championed the idea that faith comes first, but reason can elaborate upon faith's foundation. He is considered the Father of the Scholastics, inspiring the likes of St. Albert the Great (Nov. 15) and St. Thomas Aquinas (Jan. 28), and is a Doctor of the Church. He is best known in philosophical circles for his famous "ontological proof" of God's existence (an excerpt from which is cited above.)

Exercise: St. Anslem had quite a head on his shoulders, opening the way to centuries rich in mature and sublime scholastic thinking. But for now, let's think about our own shoulders. For a change of pace you can build a thorough upper body workout around shoulder work. The fundamental compound shoulder movement is some form of overhead press. After one set to failure or near failure, move right along to a dumbbell or machine lateral for the side deltoid muscles, next do a "bent lateral" or bent over reverse fly motion with dumbbells or cable for the posterior deltoids (rear shoulder muscles), finishing with an upright row, and then a barbell shrug for the trapezius. You can also "pre-exhaust" your deltoids sometime by doing a lateral movement immediately before a press, and pre-exhaust your trapezius by doing a shrug immediately before an upright row.

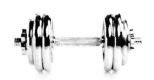

St. Gianna Beretta Molla (1922-1962)
Saint of Mothers, Physicians and Unborn Babies

Love your children. In them you can see Baby Jesus. Pray for them a lot and every day put them under Holy Mary's protection. St. Gianna

* Note: St. Gianna's feast day is actually celebrated on April 28th, the same day as St. Louis de Montfort.

Today's "Supermoms" have nothing on St. Gianna! Not only was she a practicing doctor in 1950s Italy, she was also a devoted wife and mother, a gifted athlete, and a selfless volunteer. She managed to "do it all" and to do it well, giving modern women an example of how to be holy and virtuous. As a young woman, Gianna spent much time in prayer and serving people in her community. She became a pediatrician and was especially devoted to the poor, waiving payment for her services if they could not be afforded. In 1955, she married Pietro Molla and soon gave birth to three beautiful children. She suffered two miscarriages then became pregnant with her fourth child in 1961. When a fibroma (benign tumor) developed on her uterus, doctors gave her the choice of abortion, a hysterectomy or surgery to remove the growth. She chose the surgery rather than sacrifice the life of her tiny baby. The surgery was successful, but a difficult pregnancy lay ahead. Before delivering her baby, St. Gianna firmly instructed the doctors to save the life of her child over her own life. A baby girl, Gianna Emanuela, was born on April 21, 1962, but St. Gianna died a week later due to complications from an infection that developed during delivery.

Exercise: Pray a Rosary today for protection for the unborn. Better yet, pray your Rosary in front of Planned Parenthood or an abortion clinic. You don't need a permit or permission, simply stay on the public sidewalk. If this isn't possible, donate time or money to a pro-life group. St. Gianna found time for exercise in her busy life because she knew it was important for her health. Pray for her assistance if you struggle with fitting workouts into a hectic schedule.

St. George (275-303)

Awake, awake, put on strength, O arm of the Lord, awake, as in days of old, the generations of long ago, Was it not thou that didst cut Rahab in pieces, that didst pierce the dragon? Isaiah 51:9

The historical record of St. George is slim, but in stories of his life, deeds, and apparitions, (including one to King Richard the Lionheart), he has left an enduring, worldwide legacy in legend and in art as a model of Christian fortitude. This bold dragon-slayer, this patron of England, of Malta, and many other lands, was born in Cappadocia, and was a favored soldier in the army of the Roman Emperor Diocletian, being raised to the status of a tribune. When the Emperor began to persecute Christians, George rose up to boldly defy and rebuke his actions. For this, he would endure torture and a martyr's death through beheading, but he would come to inspire countless Christians throughout the millennia (and even Saracens who revered this "White-Horsed Knight") for his godly courage.

Exercise: Inspired today by the physical and moral courage of St. George, let's consider a simple workout to strengthen our own arms, (as in days of old, if it's been awhile since you trained them!) Either as a stand-alone workout for a change of pace, or following one chest and one back exercise as part of a complete upper body strength workout, try this: First perform a two-arm biceps exercise like a barbell or machine curl. Do one set of 8-12 repetitions in normal fashion or 3-5 repetitions in super-slow fashion, to the point of failure. Next, do a two-arm triceps exercise like a French press, pushdown, or triceps machine to failure. Now, perform a biceps exercise like a concentration curl with a dumbbell or a biceps machine, using only one arm at a time. After completing one set with each arm, finally perform a one arm triceps exercise, one arm at a time. Training only one limb unilaterally allows for peak concentration and maximum neuromuscular connection between the brain and the brawn. Your arms should know and feel like they've done something after this workout, and you will have slain the dragons of sloth and inertia!

April 24

St. Mary of Clopas and St. Salome (1ˢᵗ Century)
Followers of Jesus

Standing by the cross of Jesus were his mother, and his mother's sister, Mary the wife of Clopas, and Mary Magdalene. John 19:25

When the Sabbath was over, Mary Magdalene, Mary the mother of James, and Salome brought spices so that they might go and anoint him. Very early when the sun had risen, on the first day of the week, they came to the tomb. Mark 16:1-2

Mary of Clopas and Salome were devout followers of Jesus. Although we have few details about their lives, Biblical scholars agree on several points. Mary of Clopas is likely the same Mary mentioned in the gospels as the mother of James (the Less) and Joseph. She is probably not an actual sister of the Blessed Mother, but more likely her sister-in-law, married to St. Joseph's brother. It is also possible that she was one of the travelers on the road to Emmaus (Luke 24:13-35), along with her husband Clopas (also called Cleopas). They met Jesus after he had risen from the dead but didn't recognize him until he broke bread and gave it to them to eat.

Salome is probably the mother of James (the Greater) and John. She is sometimes known as the original "helicopter mom" since she boldly asked Jesus to save a place in heaven at his right and left hand for her two sons (Matthew 20:20-28). Salome and Mary of Clopas traveled with Jesus and the Apostles. They probably cooked, sewed and cleaned, willingly offering their assistance to make life easier for their sons and the Messiah. On Easter Sunday, they awoke very early to go to the tomb in order to anoint the body of Jesus but were surprised to see the stone rolled back and an angel present who told them that Jesus had risen from the dead. According to Matthew's Gospel, Jesus himself appeared to them near the tomb.

Exercise: St. Mary of Clopas and St. Salome willingly devoted several years of their lives to humbly serving Jesus and his followers. Today, serve someone you love in true humility.

St. Mark the Evangelist (?-68)

Now a young man followed him wearing nothing but a linen cloth about his body. They seized him, but he left the cloth behind and ran off naked.
Mark 14:51-52

Get Mark and bring him with you, for he is helpful to me in the ministry.
2 Timothy 4:116

There is a tradition that says that St. Mark appears once in his own Gospel, as the young man running naked from the scene at the arrest of Jesus. Mark wasn't one of the twelve Apostles, but if this particular tradition is true, he was certainly one of the followers of Jesus who abandoned him in his darkest hour. We hear nothing else about Mark until Acts 12, when this man who once used his energies to run from Christ can be seen using those energies to assist St. Paul (June 29) and Barnabas in their missionary journeys. In fact, when St. Paul writes to the Colossians from prison, we see him sending Mark's greetings to the Church at Colosse along with his own.

St. Mark is a great example of someone who learned how to use his strength to bring himself toward Christ rather than away from him. The saint that fled naked from Jesus in the garden of Gethsemane went on to become the first bishop of Alexandria, and the first Gospel writer. Indeed, it is from St. Mark that we get the very term "Gospel," meaning "good news," from the first words of his biography of Jesus: "The beginning of the Gospel of Jesus Christ (the Son of God)" (Mark 1:1).

Exercise: Take time during today's workout to think about whether or not your fitness efforts are taking you away from Christ or moving you toward him. As you grow in strength, what are some specific ways that you can use your increasingly healthy body to help in those efforts that further the Kingdom of God? What acts of charity do you have the energy to support, and who could use your gifts to help them spread the Gospel?

St. Pedro Betancur (1619-1667)
"St. Francis of the Americas"

We serve God better by carrying a sick person from one room to another, than by submitting ourselves to excessive penances.
St. Pedro Betancur

Pedro was born in the Canary Islands and lived a simple life as a shepherd. He loved being outside in nature and spent his days in prayer and contemplation. A conversation with a relative about America inspired Pedro to become a missionary to the New World. Unfortunately, he never made it that far. By the time he reached Guatemala, Pedro had run out of money and had to beg for food at a Franciscan monastery. There he met Friar Espino, who would become a lifelong friend and counselor. The friar realized that the poor young beggar was a holy man and encouraged him to study for the priesthood. Again, Pedro failed to reach his goals. The academic demands exceeded his abilities, and Pedro withdrew from the Jesuit college. He finally found his calling as a lay brother, or tertiary, and became a Third Order Franciscan. He established and built a hospital, homeless shelter, several churches and a school for the poor of Guatemala. Pedro's holy example and genuine concern for the poor and destitute inspired other men and women to join his efforts. He organized them in a new order called the Bethlehemite Congregation. St. Pedro is the first saint who worked and died in Guatemala.

Exercise: St. Pedro teaches us to bloom where we are planted. His grand plans often went astray, but he adapted quickly. He didn't look at setbacks as failures but as opportunities. Remember that God sometimes puts roadblocks in our paths because we are not on the right road. Through frequent prayer, we can discern God's will. Be open to changes in your physical life and your spiritual life. If you eat the same meals every week, try something new. Mix up your exercise routine as well. Walk your usual route backwards or try a new cardio or weight machine at the gym. Change can give us a new perspective.

April 27

St. Zita (1218-1272) Patron of Homemakers, Domestic Workers and Lost Keys

Whatever your task, work heartily, as serving the Lord, not men, knowing that from the Lord you will receive the inheritance as your reward.
                                                            Colossians 3:23-24

[St. Zita] considered her work as an employment assigned her by God.
                                                  From Butler's "Lives Saints"

St. Zita's life bears many similarities to the tale of Cinderella. At age 12, she was sent to be a servant for a well-to-do Italian family. Although she worked hard and without complaint, her employer and fellow servants despised her. The cheerful young girl patiently bore the physical and verbal abuse, offering up her sufferings to Christ. She willingly took on extra work and completed chores that her lazy fellow servants left undone. Zita rose early every morning to attend daily Mass and shared her meager food rations with the poor who came to beg at the kitchen door. One day St. Zita lost track of time while praying after Mass and returned home too late to complete her daily bread baking. The other servants saw that she was late and rushed to tell the master. Imagine their surprise when they led him to the kitchen and found angels busily buttering perfectly-formed loaves of crusty bread. The family and servants realized that Zita was a holy woman and finally treated her with kindness and respect. She continued to cheerfully and humbly perform her duties until her death in 1272.

Exercise: Consider that your daily work can be a form of prayer. As Catholics, we are called to "pray constantly," (1 Thess. 5:17), yet even Jesus had to work. By offering our work to God, no matter how dull or menial, we are placing ourselves in His presence and giving our work a deeper meaning. Bake a loaf of bread today. I can't guarantee angelic assistance, but there's nothing quite like fresh bread right out of the oven. If you're uncertain about using yeast, there are many great recipes for quick breads such as zucchini bread, banana bread and other sweet or savory versions. Bread should be eaten in moderation, but it contains fiber and other healthy nutrients.

St. Louis de Montfort (1673-1716)

[If] we are establishing devotion to our Blessed Lady, it is only in order to establish devotion to our Lord more perfectly.
From Montfort's "True Devotion to the Blessed Virgin"

Canonized in 1947, St. Louis Marie is known the world over because of the above quoted work. Blessed Pope John Paul II said that reading the book marked a decisive turning point in his life and that it was "from Montfort that I have taken my motto: 'Totus tuus' ('I am all thine [Mary]')." If you have seen a statue of St. Louis Marie, then you know that calling him "fit," is an understatement. When he left for seminary he declined the offer of a horse and instead chose to walk the 180 miles from the family home to Paris, tending to the poor he met along the way. Once ordained, he spent the next 16 years walking from one assignment or parish to the next. At one point early in his priesthood, when he found his ministry seriously impeded, Louis Marie walked 1,000 miles to Rome, to ask Pope Clement XI if he was in fact on the path God wanted. The Pope's response was to send him back to France with the title Missionary Apostolic. We find the content of his preaching crystallized in *True Devotion*. He displayed a keen penetration into Sts. Peter and Paul's teaching: "We, though many, are one body in Christ, and individually *members of one another*" (Romans 12:5). "Like living stones be yourselves built into a spiritual house...to offer spiritual sacrifices acceptable to God through Jesus Christ" (1 Peter 2:4). The grace that the Holy Spirit poured out upon Mary, the grace that allowed her to give her continual "fiat," or "let it be done unto me," *is still available to the rest of the Body*; and in prayer we can ask God to participate in it (2 Kings 2:9)!

Exercise: If you live close enough to the market, walk to it and carry your bag of groceries home. Instead of taking the elevator or escalator, opt for stairs. Offer these choices to Jesus as a small gift, a tending of this magnificent temple. Ask the Holy Spirit to join your heart to Mary's and flood it with the faith, hope, and charity He lavished upon her.

St. Catherine of Siena (1347-1380)

We know that in everything God works for good with those who love him, who are called according to his purpose.   *Romans 8:28*

Love transforms you into what you love.   *St. Catherine of Siena*

In a century marked by wars, bubonic plague, and decadent corruption within the Church, this semi-literate twenty-fifth (yes, twenty-fifth) child of a humble, Italian wool-dyer would become a bringer of peace, a counselor to popes, and one of three female Doctors of the Church. At a time when religious sisters were cloistered, Catherine, who had consecrated her virginity to the Lord, followed the unique and active path God laid out for her. She joined the lay Dominicans at age 15 and spent three years cloistered within her own room in her house, studying, praying, and experiencing visions, and visitations from Christ. She emerged from her cell as a dynamo for Christ, writing letters to church leaders to encourage them to reform, travelling across Italy to broker peace among warring parties, convincing Pope Gregory XI to leave Avignon, France and return to Rome, counseling Pope Urban VI, and chastising cardinals who had elected an antipope. She died at only 33, and had experienced the stigmata of the crucified Christ.

Exercise: We think about and act upon that which we love, and it truly does transform us. What then shall we love? If our love is for food or for inactivity, it will transform us in ways that dishonor and bloat our bodily temple. If our love is for money, the transformation it brings will make our spirits shrink. St. Catherine of Siena loved Christ and that love made her Christ-like. Despite her most humble of beginnings, through her faith, her good works, and her total openness to God's graces, she acquired the love and the wisdom of Christ, and shared it to her fullest, until, at the same age as her Spiritual Spouse, she left the earth and ascended into heaven, serving as model and intercessor for countless saints to follow.

Pope St. Pius V (1504-1572)
Apostle of Our Lady of the Rosary

Born Anthony Ghislieri, the future pope was fittingly a shepherd in his youth. He longed to become a priest, but his family could not afford to send him to school. Fortunately, a group of traveling Dominican priests met the young boy. They were impressed by his holiness and offered to educate him. He took the name Michael and became well known for his active defense of Church teachings against various heresies. He was ordained a bishop and cardinal and became Pope Pius V in the year 1566. He was responsible for implementing the changes of one of the most important councils in Church history, the Council of Trent. He published a new missal, breviary, catechism and established Confraternity of Christian Doctrine (CCD) classes. His reign was not without controversy due to the Inquisition and his decision to excommunicate Queen Elizabeth I. He is probably most famous for the Battle of Lepanto. In 1571 he organized the Holy League, a Christian naval force, to defend Europe against an invasion by the Turkish navy. Outnumbered, the Christians had little hope of victory, but they did have a secret weapon—the Rosary. Pope Pius V prayed the Rosary daily for victory and encouraged the sailors and Christians throughout Europe to do the same. Miraculously, the Christians won a decisive victory, preventing Muslim control of Europe. He established what is known as the Feast of Our Lady of the Rosary. It is celebrated on October 7th.

Exercise: Pray a Rosary for victory over your own sins. Do V-for-Victory sit-ups. Lie on a mat on your back and bend one knee. Raise the opposite leg straight in the air at a 45-degree angle. Press your lower back into the floor and do not arch it during the exercise. Slowly do an ab crunch, lifting both arms up until they're parallel with your raised leg. Slowly lower your head to the floor and repeat 5-10 times. Switch legs and repeat the sequence.

St. Joseph the Worker, Patron Saint of Laborers

He came to his native place and taught the people in their synagogue. They were astonished and said, "Where did this man get such wisdom and mighty deeds? Is he not the carpenter's son?

Matthew 13:54-55

Saint Joseph taught Jesus human work, in which he was an expert. The Divine Child worked beside him, and by listening to him and observing him, he too learned to manage the carpenter's tools with the diligence and the dedication that the example of his foster father transmitted to him.

Pope Blessed John Paul II

I (Peggy) was thrilled to discover that John, my wonderful husband, has a birthday that falls not only on the first day of the Month of Mary but also on the feast of the greatest of earthly husbands and fathers. Today is the second time the Church has honored St. Joseph (March 19) in the last two months, because next to Mary, he is the greatest of saints. The feast of St. Joseph the Worker is a relatively recent addition to the Church calendar. It was instituted by Pope Pius XII in 1955 as a Catholic response to the "May Day" worker feasts in Communist countries. As a humble carpenter who worked hard to provide for the Holy Family, St. Joseph was the obvious choice as the patron of workers. He lived in poverty but devoted his life to providing a good home for Jesus and Mary. When you get tired, bored, or restless on the job, turn to St. Joseph's holy example for inspiration. Work can be a form of prayer, and imitation of St. Joseph's quiet and dignified labor can unite us with Christ and bring us closer to heaven.

Exercise: As you work today, think of St. Joseph and imagine that the young Christ child is by your side, watching you carefully and trying to imitate your work. That should certainly help you see your daily labor from a new perspective! In honor of St. Joseph, try an exercise called a hammer curl, which will work the biceps muscles in the upper arms while limiting strain to the wrist. Hold two dumbbells with your arms at your sides, as if they were hammers, with your palms inward, facing each other. Slowly raise and lower the dumbbells, bending your arms. Repeat eight to ten times.

St. Athanasius (296-373) Doctor of Orthodoxy

I and the Father are one.   *John 10:30*

A man's personality actuates and quickens his whole body. If anyone said it was unsuitable for the man's power to be in the toe, he would be thought silly, because, while granting that a man penetrates and actuates the whole of his body, he denied his presence in the part. Similarly, no one who admits the presence of the Word of God in the universe as a whole should think it unsuitable for a single human body to be by Him actuated and enlightened.   *St. Athanasius*

Athanasius persevered through a lifetime of lawsuits, harassments, and five exiles, defying four Roman emperors, all to champion the orthodox Catholic faith as defined in the Nicene Creed. Indeed, in 325, when but a young deacon, he wowed the members of that very Council of Nicea with his knowledge and eloquence in defense of the faith. Later, as a bishop and patriarch of Alexander, he travelled throughout the east, fighting for 46 years against Arian himself and the Arian heresy that denied Christ's full divinity. When St. Jerome (Sept. 30) would translate the Scriptures into the Latin Vulgate, he used only the books that St. Athanasius had listed as canonical. St. Athanasius is the earliest of all the 33 Doctors of the Church. His first of three citations in the *Catechism of the Catholic Church* is in article 460, "For the Son of God became man so that we might become God."

Exercise: Note well that the "Doctor of Orthodoxy" is a saint who so forcefully spoke out for the goodness of the body as evidenced by the choice of God Himself to take on our human nature through the Incarnation. Today, still so early in this month of Mary, the Mother of God, do two things: 1) Read and study paragraphs 456-483 of the *CCC* on Article 3: "He was conceived by the power of the Holy Spirit, and was born of the Virgin Mary." 2) Honor her who gave Christ flesh with a rosary workout.

The Finding of the Holy Cross

When they came to the place called the Skull, they crucified him and the criminals there, one on his right, the other on his left. Luke 23:33

Behold the wood of the cross on which the Savior hung.

Good Friday hymn

I (Peggy) read a fascinating book about the story of St. Helena and how she discovered the True Cross, which had been buried and concealed for 300 years. The book is called *The Living Wood* and is written by Louis de Wohl, and I highly recommend it. St. Helena was the mother of the Emperor Constantine, the first Roman emperor to become a Christian. She felt urgently compelled to search for the True Cross and traveled to Jerusalem. Helena finally found three crosses and some nails after destroying and digging under a temple to Venus that the Roman pagans had built to conceal the site. The bishop of Jerusalem had each of the three crosses carried to a critically ill woman. The cross that immediately and miraculously healed her was determined to be the True Cross.

My parish is blessed to have a relic of the True Cross. It is venerated on this feast (also celebrated on September 14th) and Good Friday. It is quite a humbling experience to venerate the actual wood on which our Savior hung.

Exercise: Do you have a crucifix in your home? If not, today would be a good day to purchase one. Visit your local Catholic bookstore or search online. Many Catholics hang a crucifix over each bed in their home. When Catholics venerate the cross, they often genuflect in respect. To strengthen your legs for genuflections, do walking lunges. Take a big step forward with one leg and bend both knees so that your front knee is over your ankle and your back knee is nearly on the ground. Then push off with your back leg, bringing your back leg forward to take a big step and repeat the movement with the opposite leg. Work up to 10 repetitions on each leg, and then start adding weights in each hand. To avoid stress on the knee, ensure that your knee does not go forward over your toes.

St. Monica (333-387)

Is any among you suffering? Let him pray. Is any cheerful? Let him sing praise. James 5:13

St. Monica suffered and prayed for many years while her husband Patritius and their son remained outside the Church. A year before his death, Monica's suffering turned to joy and her prayers to praise when the formerly pagan Patritius came to Christ and His Church. Her son, though, would be lured from the faith by the heresies of the Manichees and by pagan philosophy. He would travel to Italy to free himself from his mother's untiring efforts to draw him back to the Church. Here too though, St. Monica's prayers would eventually be answered, granting to the Church one of its most profound theologians and fathers. He would come tell his own story in his timeless *Confessions*, and to tell the story of mankind as a whole in his *City of God*. He would become a highly influential bishop in his own day, and his works would be cited dozens of times in the *Catechism of the Catholic Church*, produced 1600 years after his death. This answer to his saintly mother's prayers is himself profiled on August 28th. He is, of course, St. Augustine of Hippo.

Exercise: St. Augustine knew well how the yearnings of the flesh can lead us away from the goods of the spirit. He knew as well how the lure of reason and knowledge might lead away from the faith. Ultimately, though, through the persevering prayers of his caring mother, St. Augustine would achieve integrity and freedom of body and spirit, of reason and faith. We must never underestimate the power of a mother's prayers. As I (Kevin) travel the country, discussing my own reversion story, I am blessed to encounter many a modern St. Monica. I always encourage these women to persevere in prayer for their prodigal sons and daughters. Today, let's add our prayers to theirs. God will work wonders in accord with His own time table.

St. Judith of Prussia (1200-1260)
Patron Saint of Prussia and Widows

Religion that is pure and undefiled before God and the Father is this: to care for orphans and widows in their affliction and to keep oneself unstained by the world.   *James 1:27*

Three things can lead us close to God. They are painful physical suffering, being in exile in a foreign land, and being poor by choice because of love for God.   *St. Judith of Prussia*

St. Judith lived in what is now central Germany and modeled her life on the example of St. Elizabeth of Hungary. She married a nobleman at age 15 and convinced her worldly husband to live a simple life so that they could use their money and aid the poor. When he suddenly died during a pilgrimage to the Holy Land, Judith became a single mother, devoted to teaching her children how to live a holy life. After each one entered the religious life, Judith sold all her possessions to help the poor. She journeyed on foot to Prussia (eastern Germany) and became an anchoress. An anchoress is a holy woman who is willingly locked into a tower or fortress. She lives the life of a hermit and receives food, Holy Communion, visitors, and news from the world through a small window in the fortress. St. Judith died of a fever in 1260.

Exercise: Today, follow St. Judith's lead in changing her husband's dependence on worldly goods by making a conscious effort to cultivate heavenly treasures rather than earthly ones. Do not buy anything other than what is absolutely necessary all day. St. Judith was a sort of voluntary prisoner as an anchoress, so we'll do prisoner squats today. They are similar to regular bodyweight squats, except that your hands are placed behind your head so that your elbows extend to each side. This helps keep your shoulder blades aligned and your chest up during the movement. Place your arms as described above then slowly sit back as if you are sitting down in a chair, keeping your knees behind your toes, until your thighs are parallel to the ground. Slowly return to the starting position. Repeat 10-12 times.

St. Petronax (670-747)

After this I will return, and I will rebuild the dwelling of David, which has fallen; I will rebuild its ruins, and I will set it up, that the rest of men may seek the Lord...   *Acts 15:16-17*

St. Petronax was the first great rebuilder of the Abbey of Montecassino. This was the home of the Benedictines, the first of the Western monastic orders, established around 529 by St. Benedict of Nyssa (July 11). In 717, more than a century after the monastery's destruction by the Lombards in 584, Pope Gregory II advised Petronax to make a pilgrimage to St. Benedict's tomb. There Petronax found some hermits among the ruins, living lives of prayer and labor (*ora et labora* being the Benedictine motto, after all). They elected him their prior and he proceeded to gather new monks and new funds, including a generous gift from the Duke of Beneventum, himself a Lombard. Soon the Abbey would stand again. Despite subsequent destructions and sackings over the centuries from the likes of the Saracens, an earthquake, Napoleon's troops, and even Allied forces in World War II that had been led to think it was a Nazi stronghold, Montecassino would be rebuilt many times, and stands today as a magnificent monument to the persistence of the Benedictines and for the glory of God. St. Petronax would head the monastery until the end of his life on earth on May 6, 747.

Exercise: Even if we do strive to develop the virtues of fitness and to exercise regularly, sometimes the vicissitudes of life, perhaps excessive commitments or an unexpected illness, get in the way, our training lapses, and our bodily temples end up in need of repair. No need to worry, though, if you're familiar with the phenomena of "muscle memory." Once you've built up your muscles, if weeks or months of inactivity allows them to shrink or atrophy somewhat, they tend to rebuild quite quickly when you're back in your routine. So, the next time some Lombards, Saracens, an earthquake, Napoleonic or Allied troops interfere with your training, be like St. Petronax. Just clear away the rubble and get rebuilding that temple!

St. Rosa Venerini (1656-1758)
Foundress of the Venerini Sisters

St. Rosa was the well-educated and devout daughter of an Italian physician. Like many other female saints, she consecrated herself to God as a young child and worked hard to put prayer and meditation above worldly goods. She entered a Dominican convent as a young woman, but the death of her father caused her to leave the order to care for her heartbroken mother. After her mother died, she opened her home to the women in the area so that they could find companionship as they prayed the Rosary together. Rosa quickly realized how little education these poor women had in spiritual or practical matters. After consulting with her spiritual advisor, she opened the first public school for women in Italy in 1685. Classes included reading, writing, religion, and sewing. There were many critics of this new school, including the local clergy who thought that only they should teach catechism. Rosa persevered despite the sometimes violent opposition. Eventually the critics acknowledged the benefits of her approach, and she was asked to open more schools throughout Italy and to train other women as teachers. She opened a school in Rome but it failed, causing Rosa much distress. She tried again several years later, and this time Pope Clement XI and several cardinals attended her classes. After just a few hours, Pope Clement declared, "Signora Rosa, you are doing that which we cannot do. We thank you very much because with these schools you will sanctify Rome." Today, the group of women St. Rosa founded is known as the Venerini Sisters.

Exercise: Take time this week to write a nice note, send flowers, or show some sort of appreciation to a teacher who has impacted your life or the life of your children. Be sure to pray for that person as well. Continue your own education through the purchase of a book that teaches about fitness in a faith-filled way. Kevin's book *Fit for Eternal Life* and Peggy's book *The Rosary Workout* are great places to start!

St. Pope Boniface IV (550-615)

What agreement has the temple of God with idols? For we are the temple of the living God... 2 Corinthians 6:16

St. Boniface was the son of a physician, a student and deacon under St. Pope Gregory the Great (Sept. 3), and a Benedictine monk, before becoming the 67th pope in 608. He helped expand and strengthen the Church in England and was recipient of a rather remarkable letter of both deferential praise and rather harsh theological criticism from the bold and headstrong St. Columban. It speaks of Pope Boniface's saintly humility, that relations between the fiery Irish saint and the Holy See remained strong. Pope Boniface was also famous for converting the pagan Roman Pantheon into a Catholic Church. First built by Marcus Agrippa in the first century AD, and reconstructed by the Emperor Hadrian in 126 AD, Pope Boniface IV, with the permission of the Eastern Roman Byzantine Emperor Phocas, rededicated the majestic Pantheon as the Church of St. Mary and the Martyrs on May 13, 609. He would also convert his own house into a monastery in his last years.

Exercise: St. Petronax (May 6) rebuilt the great Catholic edifice of the Abbey of Montecassino. Pope Boniface rededicated one of Rome's greatest architectural wonders from devotion to Jupiter, Venus, Mars, and literally in the Greek, to *pan theos* (all gods), to the devotion to the one true God. Appropriate to our theme for the month of May, he consecrated it to Mary and all the holy martyrs. How fitting too that he essentially rededicated his own house as a temple to God as well. Here, then, is a theme to keep in mind as we tend our own temples. In practicing a truly Catholic approach to fitness, we dedicate our temples, not to glorification of the god of self, but to the one true God, born to the mother of us all. So, if perhaps we've persisted in our physical training, but have lost focus on its spiritual ends, let's pray to St. Boniface IV today and ask that we be given strength to rededicate our homes and our bodies as temples of the Holy Spirit.

St. Isaiah (c. 742-687 BC) Old Testament Prophet and Patron of Striving to Do God's Will

[Isaiah] was more of an Evangelist than a Prophet, because he described all of the Mysteries of the Church of Christ so vividly that you would assume he was not prophesying about the future, but rather was composing a history of past events.   *St. Jerome*

D o you know that there are saints in the Bible? My (Peggy's) good friend, Theresa Doyle-Nelson, has written two books on this topic, *Saints of the Bible* and *More Saints of the Bible.* I was surprised to discover that several holy men and women from the Old Testament have their own feast days and are listed in the *Roman Martyrology,* the Church's primary resource for saints. The prophet Isaiah is one of these select few. He lived during a time of great fear for the chosen people of Israel. Their once great kingdom was divided in half, and the Assyrian empire had taken over the northern region. Isaiah and his people in the southern region of Judah constantly feared the enemy, now so close to their own homes. Isaiah was called by God in a dramatic scene during which a seraph touched his lips with a burning coal, thus cleansing him from sin. He became an influential prophet who tried to convince the people of God's great love for them. The prophet also emphasized that the Israelites would incur God's wrath by worshipping pagan gods and continuing to live sinful lives. Isaiah is known as an evangelist because of his many Messianic prophecies (chapters 6-12), written in a beautiful and poetic style.

Exercise: Read the four Suffering Servant Songs in the book of Isaiah: Isaiah 42:1-4, Isaiah 49:1-7, Isaiah 50:4-11, and Isaiah 52:13-53:12. Meditate on the Passion and Crucifixion of Jesus. Use these verses as inspiration to suffer a bit during your workout today. (You don't want to feel real pain which can lead to injury.) Exercise for a longer period of time or increase the intensity of your workout a bit. Or if you weren't planning on exercising today, change those plans!

St. John of Avila (1500-1569)

This is how one should regard us, as servants of Christ and stewards of the mysteries of God.   1 Corinthians 4:1

Dear brothers and sisters, I pray God may open your eyes and let you see what hidden treasures he bestows on us in the trials from which the world thinks only to flee. Shame turns into honor when we seek God's glory. Present affliction become the source of heavenly glory. To those who suffer wounds in fighting his battles God opens his arms in loving, tender friendship.   St. John of Avila

St. John of Avila's ancestors in Spain had been Jewish converts to Christianity. He studied law, and later philosophy and theology, before his ordination to the priesthood. His parents having died during his training, he gave his inheritance to the poor, and set his sights on missionary work in the Spanish New World of Mexico. The Archbishop of Seville had other plans for John though, and at age 30, he began his missionary work closer to home in the Andalusia region of southernmost Spain. The Moors had claimed the region and the need arose for a new Christian Apostle. A great preacher, mystic, theological writer, and advisor of many saints, including the likes of St. Teresa of Avila (Oct. 15) and St. John of God (March 8), St. John of Avila would become that Andalusian fisher of men, reeling in a region that had gotten away. St. John would at one point be charged and brought before the Inquisition, and the last fifteen years of his life were marked by constant, serious bodily illness, but he would know spiritual health like few others before or since.

Exercise: A favorite saying among weightlifters goes, "No pain, no gain!" The philosopher Spinoza expressed a similar idea with the more elegant phrase, "All things difficult are as excellent as they are rare." Let's meditate today on the extent to which we are willing to do the difficult, to bear hardships, setbacks, and failures, never losing sight of that most excellent of all goals: serving Christ with all our hearts and all our minds and all our strength.

May 11

Blessed Vivaldo (died 1320) Hermit

There is nothing on this earth to be prized more than true friendship.
St. Thomas Aquinas

Blessed Vivaldo is a shining example of a true friend, one willing to sacrifice two decades of his life to care for another. He met Blessed Bartolo Buonpedoni, a local priest and Franciscan tertiary, in his hometown of San Germignano, Italy. Vivaldo became Bartolo's assistant and was very devoted to serving the priest and his parish. When Bartolo contracted leprosy, he was taken to a leper's hospital. Vivaldo stayed with his friend, caring for him until his death 20 years later. At that point, he became a hermit, living in the hollow trunk of a chestnut tree for the next 20 years. On the day of his death, the church bells in a nearby village began to ring incessantly of their own accord. As villagers ran to the church to discover the source of the constant ringing, a hunter emerged from the woods with an interesting story. His dogs had circled a tree and began to bark excitedly. Inside the tree was the dead body of Blessed Vivaldo, kneeling in prayer. As soon as the hunter finished his story, the bells stopped ringing. Realizing that the hermit must have been a very holy man, the villagers retrieved his body and buried it beneath the church altar. Many miracles were worked through his intercession, and the tree which had been his home was used to build a new chapel in honor of the Blessed Mother.

Exercise: A true friend is a treasure that must not be taken for granted. Pray for your friends, and let them know how much you value their friendship. In honor of Blessed Vivaldo, send a card to your closest friends today, either by snail mail or email. A nice touch would be to add that you arranged to have a Mass said for them. Contact your parish to find out dates available and the suggested donation. As for the exercise—you might not ever live in a tree, but you can use one to get more fit! Hang from a sturdy tree branch and do pull-ups or hanging leg raises to work your abs. If you don't have a suitable tree at home, try this exercise the next time you go to the park or take a hike.

St. Epiphanius of Salamis (310-403)

Therefore, my beloved brethren, be steadfast, immovable, always abounding in the work of the Lord, knowing that in the Lord your labor is not in vain.

1 Corinthians 15:58

God gives not the kingdom of heaven but on the condition that we labor; and all we can do bears no proportion to such a crown.

St. Epiphanius

St. Epiphanius is yet another of the early Eastern Church Fathers who championed Catholic orthodoxy against various heresies. A monk, an abbot, and a bishop of Salamis and Metropolitan of Cyprus for nearly 40 years, he wrote a book called *Anchoratus*, "The Well-Anchored," against the heresies of Arian and Origen, and also the *Panarion*, "Medicine Chest," providing antidotes to over 80 heresies! He is venerated today in Catholic and in Orthodox Churches.

Exercise: St. Epiphanius was very well-anchored in his Catholic beliefs. Through his ecclesiastical and theological labors, he helped many others in his own time and centuries hence remain steadfast in theirs as well. If we are to keep our own feet firmly planted, immovable and steadfast, yet ready to carry us forth in the abounding labors of God, then we'd be wise to build some powerful legs both to anchor and to propel us!

Running, biking, walking, elliptical machines and such give our legs, as well as our hearts and lungs, something good to think about, but if at all possible for you, consider at least a minimal strength training routine as well for those pillars of strength upon which we stand. At a bare minimum, one slow, meticulous, intense set to failure or near failure on a squat or a leg press machine will enhance the power and form of your quadriceps, hamstrings, and gluteus maximus muscles. If time and energy permit, include from time to time a set of some form of calf raise, a leg curl, leg extension, or hip adduction/abduction motion and you will be superlatively well-anchored indeed—and reap rewards far exceeding your labors!

Blessed Imelda Lambertini (1322-1333)
Patron Saint of First Communicants

Tell me, can anyone receive Jesus into his heart and not die?

Blessed Imelda

Blessed Imelda yearned to receive her First Holy Communion as a young child, but the traditional age was 12 years old. She begged to be given an exception, but the local priest stuck to tradition. She created a little prayer corner in her home with flowers and pictures of Jesus and Mary. At age nine, she asked to enter a Dominican convent in her hometown of Bologna, Italy, so that she could be taught by the nuns. She was so holy and sweet that the nuns quickly fell in love with the little girl. Imelda spent a good deal of time in the chapel, on her knees in front of the tabernacle. On May 13, 1333, Imelda and the nuns attended Mass for the vigil of the feast of the Ascension. The young girl, now 11, watched with a heavy heart as the sisters received Communion. She was still too young and would have to wait. After Mass, she knelt in front of the tabernacle in fervent prayer. A nun who was leaving the chapel turned toward the altar and gasped in surprise. A sacred host was suspended in front of little Imelda. The priest was quickly summoned, and he realized that he was being given a sign to give the girl her First Communion. He took the host and gave it to Imelda. As soon as she consumed it, she fell to the floor in ecstasy. When the nuns tried to lift her, they discovered that she was dead. She had died of happiness. Today is also the feast of Our Lady of Fatima.

Exercise: The next time you receive Communion, think of Blessed Imelda. Remember to pray fervently before approaching the altar. You might not be able to experience ecstasy like Blessed Imelda, but remember that moderate exercise triggers a chemical in your body called endorphins, which create a feeling of euphoria. This feeling can be achieved during a run, a very brisk walk, or a challenging aerobics class.

May 14

St. Mary Dominica Mazzarello (1837-1881)

She was full of good works and acts of charity. *Acts 9:36*

Good-bye. I am going now. I will see you in heaven.
St. Mary's last words

Mary Mazzarello was a go-getter from the get-go. As a child, she loved to study for weekly contests in religion class, taking special relish in regularly beating the boys! As a teen, her ability to labor in the fields and vineyards near the town of Mornese in northern Italy put all the others to shame, even the grown men! She labored in those fields until she contracted typhoid fever while tending to the ill during an outbreak. Weakened, she continued to work indoors, starting a dress-making business in which young girls would learn to sew and weave and to love God through the very act of sewing. In 1864, the great saint John Bosco (Jan. 31) would come to town investigating a possible school for boys. That did not pan out, but he did meet Mary. Under his saintly guidance, she would soon start a school of her own for girls and head a new congregation of Salesian Sisters called The Daughters of Mary Help of Christians. Today, more than 16,000 sisters wear the Salesian habit, tending schools in more than 50 countries.

Exercise: St. Mary's joyful zeal for work and challenges calls a couple of ideas to mind. She certainly knew that "real work works!" Let us, then, do an intense "house or yard aerobics" workout today. Let's set a timer for at least 30 minutes and do some kind of cleaning, vacuuming, mowing, car washing, etc., with true zest and gusto, working up a sweat! Here's one more training idea she calls to mind that might especially appeal to men. St. Mary had to switch from farming to sewing when weakened by typhoid. Whether totally fit or wheelchair bound, if your hands are in good shape, there is a whole art and science to training the fingers, hands, and wrists with special grippers and apparatus of various sorts. Try your hand at www.ironmind.com for a sample!

St. Dymphna (7th Century) Patron of
Those Suffering from Mental Illness and Depression

Bless the LORD, my soul; do not forget all the gifts of God, Who pardons all your sins, heals all your ills, delivers your life from the pit, surrounds you with love and compassion, fills your days with good things...   *Psalms 103:2-5*

Neither a difference of death nor any distance of place can separate those who are united in the bonds of the true faith and who are one in the love of Christ.   *Last words of St. Dymphna*

I (Peggy) first "met" St. Dymphna in a Catholic bookstore. I was simply browsing, but she kept popping up everywhere. First, I saw a medal with a relic, then a chaplet, and finally a small book about her life. I laughed and said, "OK! Who are you?" and flipped through the book. Imagine my surprise when I discovered that this Irish saint was the patron of depression and mental illness. I suffer from a hormone condition which causes me to have cyclical bouts of depression, and I had been praying for help in battling this disorder. Even more surprising was the fact that her feast day was exactly nine days away—just enough time to pray a novena for her intercession. I bought the book, chaplet, and medal and looked forward to learning more about this interesting saint. Dymphna was the daughter of an Irish chieftain. When his wife suddenly died, he went insane and made advances on his young daughter. She fled, taking refuge in Belgium with a priest who was a friend of her family. Her father pursued her and eventually found her, killing her in a violent rage.

Exercise: If you suffer from depression or another type of mental illness, St. Dymphna is a wonderful patron. Prayer can certainly help, but it is also important to seek medical attention for any type of mental disorder. If you are given medication, take it as directed. Discuss any side effects with your doctor and ask for different medication if needed. Exercise can help relieve symptoms of depression, but it does not replace medical help. Ask your doctor about the best type of exercise for your particular condition.

St. Brendan the Navigator (486-578)

St. Brendan is amongst the most colorful of those ancient Irish saints about whom the facts are so sparse, but the lore is so lusciously rich. Brendan founded many monasteries and served as abbot at Clonfert in western Ireland. Some say his famous voyage to the "Isles of the Blessed" describes his discovery of America, nearly a thousand years before Columbus, and this in a small wooden-framed and ox-hide covered boat! Behold now a favorite St. Brendan tale. He spies two whales fighting in the waters off the western coast of Ireland. The smaller is taking the brunt of it and calls out in a human voice for the intercession of St. Brigid (see Feb. 1st)! The larger whale immediately swims off, leaving Brendan wondering why the whale called out for that land-loving saint on the other end of the Emerald Isle, while he was standing right there! He decides that this experience merits a trek across Ireland to make St. Brigid's acquaintance. When he arrives at her hut, just in from tending her sheep, Brigid hangs her cloak upon a sunbeam. Amazed, Brendan tries to do the same and his cloak hits the floor. In fact, it took the great saint *three tries* before he too succeeded!

Exercise: St. Brendan so wonderfully demonstrates the virtue of magnanimity, a greatness of soul that dares great deeds – with the help of God. Indeed, though the extent of some of Brendan's voyages may be the stuff of legends, a group of recent adventurers have proven that they can be done, sailing from Ireland to Newfoundland in a simple leather boat made of and with materials available in the sixth century. (See Tim Severn's *The Brendan Voyage.*) But magnanimity is never complete without the companion virtue of humility. St. Brendan did, after all, seek the wisdom of St. Brigid. Our exercise for today? Can you endure a little longer, adding a few minutes to your cardio workout, in honor of St. Brendan? Better yet, can you perform some grand act of kindness today, and perform it in the spirit of humility? (It's easier than hanging your coat upon a sunbeam.)

St. Paschal Baylon (1540-1592)
Patron Saint of Shepherds and Cooks

Meditate well on this: Seek God above all things. It is right for you to seek God before and above everything else, because the majesty of God wishes you to receive what you ask for. This will also make you more ready to serve God and will enable you to love him more perfectly.
St. Paschal

St. Paschal lived in "The Golden Age of the Church" in Spain, when great saints including Ignatius of Loyola, Francis Xavier, Teresa of Avila, and John of the Cross significantly influenced both their native country and the Church as a whole. Paschal was a poor and pious shepherd who prayed as he tended his sheep. He taught himself to read and began to find books on the saints and meditations on the life and teachings of Christ. Paschal eventually became Franciscan tertiary and continued his devotion to poverty and penance. As porter, gardener, cook, and beggar for the order, he was very careful not to waste a single morsel of food that the brothers were given. Yet he was very generous to the poor who begged at his monastery. (So much so that his fellow brothers asked him to cut back a bit so that they could have some food too!) St. Paschal was very devoted to the Blessed Mother and prayed the Rosary daily. He also spent much of his time adoring the Blessed Sacrament and encouraged devotion to the Eucharist in his community. So great was his love of the Eucharist that in 1897, Pope Leo XIII declared him patron of all Eucharistic confraternities and congresses.

Exercise: This week, follow St. Paschal's example and be very careful about not wasting any food. Buy just enough food to meet your basic needs. Serve yourself a small portion at each meal. You may still feel hungry when you finish eating, but give yourself 15 minutes or so to digest. Distract yourself, and you may find that your hunger has vanished. Of course, you can always eat more if you are still hungry, but it is not a bad thing to feel a little hungry after a meal. The practice of eating until you are about 80% full is very common in Okinawa and is called *hara hachi bu*. Okinawans are well known for their healthy weight and longevity due to this practice.

St. Eric of Sweden (died 1160)

Behold, a king will reign in righteousness, and princes will rule in justice.
                                                                    Isaiah 32:1

Eric IX, King of Sweden, is also known as "Eric the Lawgiver," and "Eric the Holy." This holy king established a code of law in Sweden: "Eric's Law" or "The Code of Uppland," incorporating Gospel principles. Legends have it that King Eric also led the First Crusade of Sweden, leading to the evangelization and Christianization of the natives of Finland to the east. King Eric would pay the martyr's price (and reap the martyr's reward). Certain nobles (in name only) would despise the tithes to the Church included in the king's laws. On May 18, 1160, after leaving Mass on Ascension Sunday, said "nobles" would capture, torture, and behead the holy king. Legend holds that a fountain sprang from the place where his head hit the ground. Further kings would descend from the House of Eric, and St. Eric's image, even today, graces the third seal of the City of Stockholm.

Exercise: Brave King Eric gave his life to glorify God and to make his laws, and his people's laws, the laws of God. Let's reflect just a bit today on the fundamental laws of nature that God provides us. The natural world operates according to just and reasonable laws of cause and effect, founded upon natural principles. In *Fit for Eternal Life*, I (Kevin) listed seven fundamental principles of strength training as progression, intensity, duration, frequency, rest, form, and order. If we understand these basic principles and apply them, our training will be simple, "principled," and effective. God has ordained that positive physical results will surely follow in this world for those who learn and follow His natural principles of bodily function. Ever greater still are the rewards in this kingdom and the next, for the holy principles of the Gospel.

Pope St. Peter Celestine V (1210-1296)
Patron of Bookbinders

St. Peter Celestine V is the only pope in history to resign. He was the 11th of 12 children, and his father died when he was young. His mother, though poor, ensured that Peter was well-educated. He became a priest and lived in a cave as an ascetic in imitation of John the Baptist (Aug. 29), attracting many followers. He founded the Celestine order but wanted no glory for himself and moved to a new cave where he could be alone in prayer and penance. When the former pope died, the conclave spent over two years bickering over his successor. Outraged, St. Peter sent them a letter and told them that God was not pleased with such a long delay. The conclave replied by appointing Peter as the new pope! At the time, the saint was 80 years old, had lived his life primarily in seclusion, and was in poor health. He tried to refuse the appointment but eventually agreed to become pope, taking the name Celestine V. He was taken advantage of, made poor decisions and resigned after a mere five months, humbly apologizing for his lack of leadership. Peter wanted to return to his cave in peace, but his successor put him under guard in a nearby castle where he died 10 months later. Some accounts say this was done to prevent a division in the Church, others say he was imprisoned willingly, and still others say he was murdered.

Exercise: You might be in the wrong career/vocation like St. Peter Celestine. If so, pray for guidance. Certainly we want our careers to be exciting and rewarding, yet sometimes we must do work in the interim that is difficult, boring, or unfulfilling. Do these undesirable tasks well, for the glory of God. If you spend most of your day at a desk, try these easy stretches: Sit up straight with shoulders relaxed and tilt your head so that your ear is toward your shoulder. Hold 10-15 seconds and repeat on the other side. Slowly circle one arm at a time both forward and backward. Repeat 6-8 times on both arms. Relax your shoulders and squeeze your shoulder blades together and hold for 5-10 seconds, then relax. Repeat 3-5 times.

St. Bernardine of Siena (1380-1444)

Therefore God has highly exalted him and bestowed on him the name which is above every name, that at the name of Jesus every knee should bow, in heaven, and on earth and under the earth, and every tongue confess that Jesus Christ is Lord, to the glory of God the Father.   *Philippians 2:9-11*

Glorious name, gracious name, name of love and of power! Through you sins are forgiven, through you enemies are vanquished, through you the sick are freed from their illness, through you those suffering in trials are made strong and cheerful. You bring honor to those who believe, you teach those who preach, you give strength to the toiler, you sustain the weary.   *St. Bernardine*

In the midst of a sermon, powerful orator St. Vincent Ferrier (April 5) told the crowd that a young Franciscan in their midst would one day outshine him as a preacher. Preaching missionary Bernardino degli' Albizzechi was that man. Raised by an aunt, for years he cared for her during her illness, when blind and so bereft of strength, all she could do was repeat the Holy Name of Jesus, and here Bernardine found his own holy devotion. He ended his stirring sermons by displaying on a tablet, letters that Catholics will find most familiar—IHS—a contraction of Jesus' name based on the first three letters in Greek (IHΣ), upon the background of a blazing sun. St. Ignatius Loyola (July 31) would later use IHS as the emblem of the Jesuit Order.

Exercise: Borrowing inspiration from St. Bernadine and his ailing aunt, we suggest renaming HIT (High Intensity Training) strength workouts done in the manner of tending the temple as "HIS" (High Intensity Strength) workouts, employing as well those same three letters in Jesus' name, and also implying that our strength workouts are indeed HIS workouts, done in the honor of Jesus' Holy Name. Let's offer up our next HIS Workout then, to His Holy Name!

May 21

St. Cristobal Magallanes and Companions (died 1915-1937) Mexican Martyrs

I am innocent and I die innocent. I forgive with all my heart those responsible for my death, and I ask God that the shedding of my blood serve the peace of our divided Mexico. *Last words of St. Cristobal*

St. Cristobal was a shepherd as a young boy and enrolled in a seminary at age 19. He became the parish priest for his hometown of Totatiche and was very active in the community. He helped found schools, a newspaper, carpentry shops, and an electric power plant, along with missions and catechism centers for both children and adults. When an anti-Catholic regime took over the government, churches and seminaries were closed. Priests were arrested for celebrating Mass, and it was illegal to be baptized. Undaunted, St. Cristobal gathered all the seminarians he could find and established a clandestine seminary in his hometown. It was discovered and closed, but he found ways to educate the future priests in private homes. He started what was known as the Cristero movement. He and his fellow priests bravely ministered to those Catholics determined to practice their faith during the persecution. Cristobal was arrested in 1927 on his way to celebrate Mass in a farmhouse and was executed without benefit of a trial. Between 1915 and 1937, St. Cristobal, 21 other priests, and three laymen were martyred by shooting or hanging.

Exercise: I (Peggy) once read a thought-provoking message on a country church marquee: "If you were arrested as a Christian, would there be enough evidence to convict you?" Spend some time contemplating whether or not you live your faith each day. Do others know that you are a devout Catholic? Do you leave your faith at the office door or do you follow Christian principles at work? If others visit your home, will they see crucifixes, statues of the saints, or religious art? You don't have to be pushy, but be proud of your faith! In honor of St. Cristobal, play a game of soccer, Mexico's favorite sport. Can't play or find a group for a game? Work on some soccer skills. Kick a ball through some cones or practice kicking a ball into a goal or between two cones.

St. Rita of Cascia (1381-1457)

And plaiting a crown of thorns they put it on his head, and put a reed in his right hand. And kneeling before him they mocked him, saying, "Hail, King of the Jews." Matthew 27:39

My dear cousin, there is nothing impossible to God. St. Rita

This patroness of lost causes desired to become an Augustinian nun, but her parents had arranged for a marriage to a man who turned out to be cruel, violent, and unfaithful throughout most of the eighteen years of their marriage. Shortly after he had converted from evil ways, her husband was murdered and their two sons sought revenge. The sons were dissuaded and repented due to Rita's beseeching and prayers. Rita entered the Augustinian Convent at Cascia after all, living a devout, religious life for the last 42 years of her life. Rita acquired an open ulcer on her forehead that was said to represent a wound from Christ's crown of thorns, so intense was her meditation on his passion. The wound never healed, and for fifteen years she received mystical experiences and cared for ailing sisters, before she succumbed to tuberculosis.

Exercise: Are there any "lost causes" or "impossible cases" in your own life? Sometimes when we are down and depressed, causes seem impossible that are anything but the case. Perhaps you feel this way even about your pursuit of spiritual and physical fitness. We must allow that God-infused virtue of hope to flow within us, so that we will seek to do God's will on earth, inspired by our heavenly reward, assured that God will provide us with the help we need along the way. We need also to heed St. Rita's example of the wonderful power of prayer and of the virtues of patience and perseverance. During your next workout, why not meditate upon Christ's passion and ask God for His strength?

St. John Baptist de Rossi (1698-1763)
The Apostle of the Abandoned

Are not five sparrows sold for two small coins? Yet not one of them has escaped the notice of God... Do not be afraid. You are worth more than many sparrows.   *Luke 12:6-7*

St. John was a poor but pious Italian boy. He attracted the attention of a visiting nobleman who offered to arrange for his education, so John moved to the nearby city of Genoa to live with him and his family and attend school. He continued his studies at a college in Rome and was frequently praised for his brilliance and holiness. Unfortunately, he took on too much work, and the combination of his intense studies, epileptic seizures, and severe penance practices caused a breakdown. Despite his poor health, he received a dispensation and became a priest. John remained in Rome and founded a homeless shelter and hospice, under the patronage of St. Aloysius Gonzaga (June 21). At first, he didn't want to perform his priestly duties in the confessional out of fear that he might have a seizure, but his bishop convinced him otherwise. St. John quickly became known as a great confessor, and long lines formed for his absolution. He is known as the "Apostle of the Abandoned."

Exercise: Do you pray for your parish priest? Priests very much need our prayers! Many of them live isolated lives and experience loneliness. If others gossip about or criticize your pastor, don't join in. Priests are human and sinners like the rest of us. You'll make a priest's day if you send him a card, thanking him for his service to the Church and your parish. It would be a nice touch to include a gift certificate for a local restaurant, movie theater, or video rental store. Today's workout will help you find more balance in your life. Stand up tall, lift one foot off the ground, and balance for at least a minute on one leg. Close your eyes and try to maintain your balance. Open your eyes and bend forward to pick up an object from the floor while still balancing on one leg. Repeat this action with the opposite leg.

St. David of Scotland (1085-1153)

Behold, a king will reign in righteousness, and princes will rule in justice.
                                                                    Isaiah 32:1

Did you know that good King David, born in 1085, spoke in a Scottish brogue? King David of Israel, born in 1085 B.C., had a saintly namesake, you see, born around 1085 A.D., and he is our saint of the day! The Prince of the Cumbrians since 1113, David became King of the Scots in 1124. He helped civilize and unify Scotland in a barbarous time of bloody battles between various earls and other nobles in Scotland and in England. King David was also a prince of the Church. He would be eulogized at length by St. Aelred of Rievaulx (Jan. 12) for his good works in strengthening the Church of Scotland in its ties to Rome, by adding and revitalizing bishoprics, strengthening the parochial and monastic systems, and ruling that fierce land with "royal gentleness."

Exercise: All fathers are called by God to reign as kings within their own households, but as kings who lovingly help and serve their families in thrall to the Heavenly King. Mothers then are queens, and both parents are tasked with the raising of godly princes and princesses. Let us as fathers and mothers, then, reflect on the nature and atmosphere of our own little royal courts. Have we allowed the guards to admit barbarous intruders—electronic scenes and voices that would inflame the hearts of our own royal children with images of lust and violence, of disregard and disrespect for the very bodily temples that house their souls and God's own Holy Spirit? Even King David of Israel succumbed and sinned greatly when his eyes had seen what was not rightly his to see. What lesson then can we learn today from this great Scottish king and saint, so that our physical and spiritual descendents will not fall for the snares of the world, but like young St. Aelred raised in his court, grow in spiritual friendship with Christ? Let's take a minute or two to meditate on that several times today.

St. Mary Magdalene de Pazzi (1566-1607)
The Ecstatic Saint

Christened Catherine at Baptism, this saint was a very unusual child. At age nine, she was taught meditative prayer and spent at least half an hour in daily meditation. Catherine experienced her first ecstasy while looking at a beautiful sunset at age 14. She became a contemplative Carmelite nun, taking the name Mary Magdalene, but soon became deathly ill. She made her vows from a cot in the chapel and immediately fell into ecstasy. This began a series of 40 daily ecstasies during which the saint had many insights into divine truths. Following this time of extreme closeness to God, she experienced five years of desolation, spiritual dryness, extreme temptations, great physical sufferings and depression so severe that she almost committed suicide twice.

The trial ended with an ecstasy on the feast of Pentecost. St. Mary was often embarrassed by the attention her ecstasies brought. She tried to go to her room if she felt one coming on and genuinely felt that these ecstasies were needed to save her soul. Her relationship with Jesus was almost playful at times. In some of her writings, she tells how He teased her and bantered with her, no doubt revealing part of His human personality.

Exercise: If you are experiencing spiritual dryness, reading stories of saints like Mary Magdalene de Pazzi can provide comfort during times like these. Tell your confessor and seek advice on how to overcome this difficult period. You can literally pull yourself up when you're down by performing a great upper body exercise, the negative chin-up (especially helpful if you can't do a standard chin-up). Jump up or use a chair to bring your chin above a pull-up bar, using an underhand grip. Slowly lower your body back down, taking about 5 seconds, until your arms are fully extended. Repeat 5-10 times. This is a great exercise to do at a playground if you don't have access to a pull-up bar.

May 26

St. Philip Neri (1515-1595)

We are fools for Christ's sake, but you are wise in Christ.
1 Corinthians 2:10

Cheerfulness strengthens the heart and makes us persevere in a good life. Therefore the servant of God ought always to be in good spirits.
St. Philip Neri

Philip Neri was born in Florence, experienced a powerful conversion to Christ in his late teens, and headed out to Rome. He would study theology and philosophy there for three years, and though a brilliant student, he would drop his classes, sell his books to raise money for the poor, and set about the special plans God had in mind for him. Later known as "The Apostle of Rome," and "The Humorous Saint," Philip literally roamed Rome, chatting and spreading goodwill to passersby, and gradually bringing their conversation to the things of God. Known for his personal charm and humor, this saint might shave only half his face or dress in bizarre clothing, making light of those who called him a saint, all the while spreading good cheer and demonstrating his saintly humility. With a pat on the cheek, a gentle yank on one's hair, and a smiling personal greeting, the people of Rome sought out his mere presence to gladden their hearts and lighten their spirits. He formed a group of laymen for spiritual discussions and was later called to the priesthood, doing much good work as a confessor.

Exercise: St. Thomas Aquinas (Jan. 28) taught that joy is an effect of charity, a blessed effect that is caused by the love of God. St. Philip, like St. Thomas, experienced great joy flowing from charity. St. Thomas shared his serene joy in his sublime writings. St. Philip shared his humorous joy in his interpersonal relationships and in good works of mercy. One of his favorite sayings was: "Well brothers, when shall we begin to do some good?" Let that be our question of the day. Tending our temples should make us feel good, and ready to spread our joy to all those we shall encounter today. Well then readers, shall we begin to do some good?

St. Augustine of Canterbury (died 605)
Patron Saint of England

Pray in the spirit and sentiment of love, in which the royal prophet said to Him, "Thou, O Lord, are my portion." St. Augustine of Canterbury

We don't often think of saints running away in fear, but such is the case with St. Augustine of Canterbury. Pope St. Gregory the Great (Sept. 3) asked Augustine to lead a group of 40 monks on a missionary trip to England to spread the Good News to the pagan Anglo-Saxons. When the party arrived at France and was about to cross the English Channel, they were told incredible stories about the fierceness of the natives they planned to evangelize. Terrified, the group sent St. Augustine back to Rome to request permission to abandon the mission. St. Gregory assured them that the rumors were unfounded, and the group gathered their courage and sailed to England. Fortunately, they landed in Kent, a territory ruled by the pagan King Ethelbert and his Christian wife. The kindly king set up accommodations for the group in Canterbury and was baptized a year later. Augustine prudently heeded the advice of St. Gregory and retained local customs as much as possible as he worked to convert the Anglo-Saxons to Christianity. He encouraged them to transform their pagan rites and festivals into Christian celebrations and worked to purify their temples rather than destroy them. St. Augustine was the first Archbishop of Canterbury.

Exercise: In carrying out our vocations as Christians, it is natural to experience fear. Find courage in reading about the saints. They too were often fearful, but relied on God's help to complete their missions. Increase the strength of your muscles and mix up your workout by doing a super set. A super set works two opposing muscle groups back-to-back with no rest in between. For instance, do a set of bicep curls followed immediately by a set of triceps extensions or a set of bench press followed by a set of lat pull-downs. Start with just one super set in a workout before adding more, and do these more intense exercises no more than once a week.

St. Bernard of Menthon (923-1008) Patron of Skiing, Snowboarding, Hiking, Backpacking and Mountaineering!

Before the mountains were brought forth, or ever thou hadst formed the earth and the world, from everlasting to everlasting thou art God.   *Psalms 90:2*

Did you ever see those old cartoons where a traveler stuck on a snowy mountain is rescued by a huge, courageous St. Bernard dog, complete with mini-keg of medicinal brandy attached underneath his collar? Those cartoons bear witness to one of the many acts of corporal mercy brought forth by our saint for today. Born to a rich and noble family in the southeastern French Alps, on the day before his arranged marriage, Bernard fled to the Italian Alps, where he became a Benedictine priest, an archdeacon administering the diocese of Aosta for its bishop, a preacher of the Gospel, converter of souls, and miracle-worker to the mountain people of northern Italy, many of whom clung to old, pre-Christian pagan traditions. Among his most famous achievements is the establishment of monasteries at the highest Alpine passes. With snow ranging from six to at times even 40 feet deep in places, European pilgrims would cross these extremely dangerous passes on the way to Rome. St. Bernard and his monks offered hospitality to the pilgrims and also ventured out, accompanied by their herding dogs (now known to all as St. Bernard's) to find and save victims trapped in the snows of the mountains.

Exercise: Do you live by any mountains or hills and do you have a dog? If so, today is the day to pop Fido on that leash and head out the door for a vigorous, prayerful hike. Have no hills or no dogs? No worries. It's still a great day for hiking and praying. Any why not meditate on the virtues of kindness and hospitality while you are at it? Can you pass on a wave or a smile to those who cross your path? Can you plan some little good deed for the family once you are safe and sound back at home? Of course you can!

St. Madeleine Sophie Barat (1779-1865)
Foundress of the Society of the Sacred Heart

The more we have denied ourselves during the day, the nearer we are each evening to the heart of our Lord.   St. Madeleine Sophie Barat

When St. Madeleine Sophie Barat was asked as a child what brought her into the world, she replied with one word: "Fire." Her mother delivered the future saint prematurely when she was badly frightened by a fire. Sophie (her preferred name) did not have a very fun childhood. Not only did she live during the Reign of Terror and the French Revolution, but she was also essentially locked up in her house by her older brother, a seminarian. He was so determined to educate his younger sister that he compelled her to study without interruption or the benefit of friends and a bit of relaxation. Even so, Sophie developed a love for learning and quickly mastered such difficult courses as theology and the teachings of the Church Fathers, while also becoming fluent in five different languages. She was very devoted to the Sacred Heart of Jesus and consecrated herself to Him under this title as a young woman. Sophie felt called to the religious life but wanted to help other girls and young women to receive an excellent education. She founded the Society of the Sacred Heart and opened schools for poor girls and boarding schools for wealthy young women. St. Sophie served as Superior General for the Society for 63 years, devoting her life to sharing her love of learning and her devotion of the Sacred Heart to girls throughout Europe, Africa, and America.

Exercise: Catholics devoted to the Sacred Heart like St. Sophie try to attend Mass on the first Friday of each month. If you can't make it to Mass, pray the Litany of the Sacred Heart of Jesus, easily found online. Cultivate a love of learning like St. Sophie by reading, taking a class that interests you, or finding a hobby that you enjoy. As we age, it is important to keep our minds active. Studies show that frequent physical activity helps prevent mental decline as we get older, yet another reason to exercise today!

St. Joan of Arc (1412-1431)

Plans are established by counsel; by wise guidance wage war.
Proverbs 20:18

Jesu et Maria.   *Inscription on Joan of Arc's banner*

God can fashion the mightiest of leaders from the humblest of shepherds, fishermen, and even illiterate, teenaged maidens. At age 12, Joan experienced her first vision of Sts. Michael the archangel (Sept. 29), Catherine of Alexandria, and Margaret of Antioch. Astoundingly, they counseled this poor peasant girl to help drive out the English from France and to restore the dauphin (eldest son of the King) to his throne. After four years of undaunted pleading she was allowed to don armor, leading the troops to military victories, most notably a triumph at the battle of Orleans. This led to the crowning of Charles VII. She was later captured by the English, and after an unjust mock trial, she was declared a heretic and burned at the stake at age 19. Two years later, the Church declared the trial an invalid travesty. Amidst gorgeous pomp and ceremony fit for the heavenly royalty of a saint, she was canonized by Pope Benedict XV in 1920.

Exercise: When St. Paul (June 29) enjoined us all to participate in spiritual combat, he advised us to "gird our loins in truth." (Ephesians 6:14). We'd also do well to learn how to gird our actual loins (groin and thighs) with bands of strong and flexible muscles. If you have access to an "adduction/abduction" machine, sit in the machine and position the stirrups and pads on the insides of your knees as far out as you can comfortably stretch. Then, slowly squeeze in and adduct (the inward motion—like "adding" to your body) until your ankles meet. Hold for a second and slowly return to the stretched position. Repeat until failure of near failure. Then switch around the knee pads to the outside, position the machine so your ankles touch and abduct (spread your legs outward) as far as you can go. Repeat until failure or near failure and you will know your loins and hips stand girded!

May 31

The Feast of the Visitation

During those days Mary set out and traveled to the hill country in haste to a town of Judah, where she entered the house of Zechariah and greeted Elizabeth. When Elizabeth heard Mary's greeting, the infant leaped in her womb, and Elizabeth, filled with the Holy Spirit, cried out in a loud voice and said, "Most blessed are you among women, and blessed is the fruit of your womb." Luke 1:39-42

Today we celebrate the Visitation of the Blessed Mother. This feast has been in existence since the 13th century, when it was instituted by St. Bonaventure (July 15). The Visitation is also the Second Joyful Mystery of the Rosary and teaches us the virtue of charity, or love of neighbor. Mary always acts in perfect charity. After she accepted her role as Mother of the Redeemer, the angel Gabriel (Sept. 29) informed her that her aging and previously barren cousin Elizabeth was six months pregnant. Mary went "in haste" to visit her cousin and offer assistance. Imagine that! Mary was told that she was to be the mother of the Savior, and she thought nothing of herself. Instead, she quickly prepared for a rather difficult journey to the hill country because she knew that her cousin would need plenty of help. Mary didn't need to tell Elizabeth her secret. The Holy Spirit did that for her and even informed the developing infant in her womb, John the Baptist. He jumped for joy as he recognized the Divine Presence, thus sanctifying this greatest of prophets. Elizabeth declares that Mary is "blessed among women." (Luke 1:42) She is God's masterpiece of human creation, and her soul magnifies His presence through her perfect humility and charity.

Exercise: Today, take some time to read and meditate on the Magnificat, Mary's beautiful canticle (song) of praise and thanksgiving (Luke 1:46-55) in response to her cousin's greeting. This feast also celebrates the sanctity of human life in the womb. Donate some needed items to a women's shelter or pregnancy help center. If you can't do that, then do a Rosary Workout, praying the Joyful Mysteries for a change of heart for women who are considering abortion.

St. Justin Martyr (103-165)

Truly, truly, I say to you, unless you eat the flesh of the Son of man and drink his blood, you have no life in you... *John 6:53*

And this food is called among us Εὐχαριστία [the Eucharist].
St. Justin Martyr

A studious and learned man, Justin had been immersed in the pagan Stoic and Platonic philosophies that recognized the existence of God through reason, but provided no way of intimately knowing and experiencing Him in a personal relationship. This Justin would find in the year 130 through God's revelation in the Scriptures and the Incarnation of the Logos in Jesus Christ. This early Church Father would write prolifically; two of his *Apologies* and his *Dialogue with Trypho* are extant today and available online. Interestingly, his first apology addressed to the Roman emperor includes an explanation that Christians were neither atheists nor criminals. (How sad and ironic that some avowed atheists strive to make Christian practices criminal in the public arena today). Justin's comment above on the Eucharist is but one of many glimpses at the beliefs and practices of the early Christians of the second century. The Roman prefect Rusticus ordered Justin to make sacrifice to the Roman gods. Justin answered that "no one in his right mind gives up piety for impiety." He was scourged and beheaded. Justin is then among the most powerful of early Christian witnesses who sought God with all their hearts, and minds, and souls, and gave their lives for Him.

Exercise: Christ is "the bread of life." Literal bread itself is a staple biblical food, yet some today would have us shy away from it for its purported fattening qualities. A couple of decades back, one study found that dieters who were advised only to **add** six pieces of whole grain bread to their daily diets lost fat. Why? Whole grain breads are high in fiber. Eat enough of them and you'll feel less hungry for low-fiber, high-calorie foods. Worried about the "carbs?" They are your temple's primary fuel of choice for your workouts!

St. Marcellinus and St. Peter (died 304) Martyrs

O, how much those men are to be valued who, in the spirit with which the widow gave up her two mites, have given up themselves! How their names sparkle! How rich their very ashes are! How they will count up in heaven!
                                        Edwin Hubbell Chapin

St. Marcellinus was a priest and St. Peter was an exorcist at the time of Christian persecutions by the Emperor Diocletian. Their skills were put to good use during their imprisonment. Peter expelled a demon from the jailer's daughter and the jailer, his family and the neighbors who witnessed the exorcism enthusiastically converted to Christianity. Peter brought the entire group to Marcellinus, who baptized them. When their actions became known, the two saints were separated and condemned to death. Marcellinus was confined naked in a dark cell covered in broken glass and was denied food and water. He and Peter were taken deep into a forest so that their bodies would not be discovered and venerated by their fellow Christians. The two holy men cheerfully went to work clearing a place in the forest for their execution by beheading. They must have made quite an impression on their executioner, as he too repented and became a Christian. He showed Church leaders where the two saints were buried so that their bodies could be moved to the catacombs. (Other accounts state that two women found the bodies based on a vision.) Peter and Marcellinus were popular saints in the early Church, and their names are included in the Roman Canon of the Mass.

Exercise: In honor of today's saints, try a great core exercise called "Wood choppers." Hold a medicine ball or one light dumbbell with both hands. Extend your arms up and diagonally to the right with your body turned slightly to the right. Slowly lower the weight diagonally across your body until it touches the ground beside your left foot, bending the knees slightly. Reverse the movement to return the weight to the starting position. Repeat 8-10 times and then again on the opposite side (high left to low right). During each repetition, pray, "St. Peter and St. Marcellinus, pray for us!"

St. Kevin of Glendalough (498-618)

Here we come to my namesake (Kevin's, of course!) I knew my mother gave me the middle name Gerard in honor of St. Gerard of Majella, patron of childbirth, because she'd had five miscarriages before I was born. What I found out just in the last year is that the name Kevin actually means "of fair or gentle birth!" I don't know if she knew that or not! In any case, I've found my namesake saint quite an inspiration. Legend has it that this beloved, hermit-like, monastic saint lived to be 120. One day a blackbird laid eggs in his outstretched hand while he was praying in an open-armed, cross-like position. This gentle lover of God's fair creatures (and saint of gentle births as well) stood there with outstretched hand until the baby birds hatched!

Exercise: Just imagine the strength and endurance it would have taken St. Kevin to hold his arm aloft for days. Here is a super-brief and simple 4-exercise arm workout using the "pre-exhaust" method that starts with an isolation exercise and is followed *immediately, without rest* by a related compound exercise:

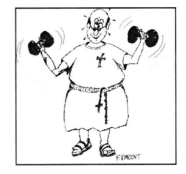

1. Some form of curl immediately followed by
2. Some form of chin or underhand pull down.

Next, catch your breath for a minute and then do this:

3. Some form of triceps exercise immediately followed by
4. Some form of dip or pushup.

Do each set until failure or near failure and in five or ten minutes you will know that not only have you given your biceps and triceps all they can handle, you have also strengthened your entire upper body. So, you may feel free to use this as change of pace workout for the entire upper body.

St. Francis Caracciolo (1563-1608)
"The Preacher of the Love of God"

Zeal for your house consumes me.   *Psalm 69:9*

Let us go, let us go to heaven!   *Last words of St. Francis Caracciolo*

S t. Francis was a very active child who enjoyed sports, especially hunting. He was also very dedicated to the Blessed Sacrament and to the Rosary. As a young man, he contracted a leprosy-like disease and made a promise to dedicate his life to God if he was cured. Almost miraculously, Francis was healed and made good on his promise. He became a priest and spent much of his time ministering to prisoners, especially those who were condemned to die. Francis founded a new order called the Congregation of the Minor Clerks Regular with a primary mission to care for prisoners and the sick. He wrote a book titled *Seven Stations of the Passion of Our Lord Jesus Christ*, and was known as "The Preacher of the Love of God" due to his advocacy of adoring the Blessed Sacrament, especially at night. He died at age 44 from a severe fever. According to several accounts, during his autopsy, his heart appeared to be burned and was imprinted with the words *"Zelus domus tuae comedit me." ("The zeal of Thy house has consumed me.")*

Exercise: St. Francis would be pleased if you made a visit to the Blessed Sacrament today. Spend some quiet time conversing with the Lord and lay your burdens at His feet. Time spent in front of the Blessed Sacrament will bring many blessings to your life. St. Francis is known as the patron saint of Italian cooks. Americanized Italian food can be very high in fat and calories, but genuine Italian cooking is quite healthy. You may have heard of the Mediterranean Diet, which includes fresh vegetables, fish, olive oil, beans, and grains. Check out some Italian cookbooks or search online for healthy Italian recipes to try and incorporate foods from the Mediterranean Diet.

St. Boniface (672-754) Apostle of the Germans

You shall have no other gods before me.   *Exodus 20:3*

As St. Patrick (March 17) was born in Britain, but would serve as Apostle to the Irish, so too would St. Boniface, born in Devonshire, serve as Apostle to the Germans. As legend would come to pair St. Patrick with the three-leafed clover as a teaching aid for the Holy Trinity, so too would facts and legends come to pair St. Boniface with some special trees. Later legends cite him as inventor of the Christmas tree. Older stories tell of how he chopped down a great oak tree dedicated to the old Norse god Thor. German natives, who worshipped the tree as an idol, were amazed when the thunder-god did not retaliate. In fact, St. Boniface would use the oak to erect a chapel at that spot. He would convert many Germans to Christ, organize the German Church, be appointed a bishop, found monasteries, and finally, when attacked with his 52 attendants by a band of armed pagans, suffer martyrdom under their swords.

Exercise: St. Boniface is obviously a model of the virtue of *fortitude*. His willingness, with the grace of God, to do hard and dangerous things for the pursuit of the worthiest of goals (the salvation of souls), should inspire us to face the much less difficult burdens of strength and cardiovascular training to achieve the goal of tending our temples. Let him also serve though as a model for the *temperance* that keeps us seeking the highest of goods, moderating our desires for lesser goods. He is a patron of brewers, for goodness sake. Beer, like wine, is one of God's blessings to us when imbibed in moderation (though it should not be consumed by those with addictive tendencies). So too is tending our physical temples a good, but one to be kept in its proper proportion, making sure that fitness training does not itself become a false idol. We might strive for the might of the mythical Thor, but must keep our hearts and minds focused on the one true God who died on the wood of a tree for us.

St. Norbert (1080-1134) Patron Saint of Peace

Do not be conformed to this world but be transformed by the renewal of your mind, that you may prove what is the will of God.

Romans 12:2

O Priest! Take care lest what was said to Christ on the cross be said to you: "He saved others, himself he cannot save!"   St. Norbert

St. Norbert did not take his duties as a priest very seriously when he was a young man. He entered the priesthood as a career move to increase his financial and social standing in the hedonistic German court. He lived a very worldly life until a Damascus-like experience dramatically changed his point of view. Norbert was out riding at night when lightning struck the path ahead. His horse bucked, knocking him unconscious. He immediately realized that his lavish lifestyle was offensive to God and quickly changed his ways. He became a traveling preacher, walking barefoot even in winter, and attracted many followers. Dissatisfied with the lack of discipline among his fellow priests, he founded a new order known as the Norbertines. He was appointed bishop of Magdebourg, and arrived at his new residence with ragged clothes and bare feet. The porter refused to let him in and tried to send him off to join the other beggars! When the porter was informed that he had just sent away the new bishop, he begged for forgiveness, but St. Norbert told him that he had in fact judged him correctly.

Exercise: St. Norbert is the patron saint of peace, so this would be a great opportunity to pray through his intercession for peace in your home, at your workplace, in our nation and throughout the world. A peaceful night's sleep is essential for good health. Growth hormone secretion, metabolism, and even weight gain can be negatively affected by a lack of sleep. Regular exercise, proper hydration, and a good diet help promote restful sleep. Try to go to bed and get up at the same time each day. Before bedtime, relax, read a book, or better yet, spend time in prayer. This will help you to unwind and fall asleep quicker.

St. Robert of Newminster (1100-1159)

Blessed is the man who walks not in the counsel of the wicked, nor stands in the way of sinners, not sits in the seat of scoffers: but his delight is in the law of the LORD, and on his law he meditates day and night.   *Psalms 1:1-2*

Born in northern Yorkshire, Robert studied at the University of Paris and reportedly wrote a commentary on the Psalms which is no longer extant. He became a parish priest and later a Cistercian monk, dedicated to the strict observance of St. Benedict's rule. He would become the first abbot of the Fountains Abbey in northern Yorkshire, living an austere life of self-deprivation within its glorious structures. The still-standing remnants are among the most magnificent monastic ruins in Europe. St. Robert would also send out three colonies of monks who established three additional monasteries. He was known for kindness and mercy. One story reports that he was accused by his own monks of improper relations with a village woman. When he took his case to the great Cistercian leader, St. Bernard of Clairvaux (Aug. 20), Robert's innocence and sanctity were apparent to him. St. Godric the hermit reported that on the day of St. Robert's death, he saw his soul ascend to heaven like a ball of fire, attended by angels.

Exercise: St. Robert of Newminster meditated day and night on the laws of God, and also on the Psalms. He walked in the counsel not of the wicked, but in the counsel of the wise, like St. Bernard. St. Robert fasted so intensely one Lent that his stomach eventually could hardly handle food. When he agreed to try some bread sweetened with honey, he changed his mind, fearing to set a bad example, so he sent it to the poor at the monastery gate. St. Robert certainly "walked his talk." Our typical lifestyles today are miles apart from the sacrificial austerities of the Cistercians, but might you be able to observe at least a partial fast today, depriving yourself of but a serving or two at lunch and dinner, in honor and remembrance, and praying for the intercession of St. Robert of Newminster?

St. William of York (died 1154) Archbishop of York

Wait for the Lord, take courage; be stouthearted, wait for the Lord!

Psalm 27:14

Patience is the companion of wisdom.

St. Augustine

St. William was in the center of several controversies. He was born into a powerful English family who may have helped him attain some of his positions in the Church. When he was appointed as Archbishop of York, he wasn't a popular choice, and the Archbishop of Canterbury refused to consecrate him. A few years later, he was consecrated by a neighboring bishop, but then the pope refused to approve it. It took 14 long years until William finally became Archbishop of York. Ironically, he was dead just two months later, probably from poisoning. Throughout all these ordeals, St. William was humble, patient, and pious. After his death, many miracles were worked through his intercession.

Exercise: It's important to be patient about reaching your goals in life, whether they are physical, spiritual, or work-related. Sometimes God delays in answering your prayers, but He always has a plan. Perhaps He wants you to learn lessons or skills that will help you later in life. Plenty of time spent in prayer and meditation can help you discern God's will and get you through these rough spots.

Be patient about your exercise program too. It can take weeks or even months to finally see results, but a consistent workout program will lead to better health.

St. Columba of Iona (521-597)

As for the saints in the land, they are the noble, in whom is all my delight. *Psalms 16:3*

Early Christian Ireland of the sixth century AD was bristling with saints aflame with missionary zeal. The massive Clonard Monastery alone was said to house 3,000 monastic scholars at a time. St. Finian would teach the so-called "Twelve Apostles of Ireland" there, and St. Columba (aka Columcille) was among the most prominent of them.

A physically powerful, intellectually brilliant, zealously passionate, and boldly outspoken man, his bones would one day rest with those of Sts. Patrick (March 17) and St. Brigid (Feb. 1). In an infamous, perhaps less than saintly dispute, after Columba had meticulously copied Finian's manuscript of the Psalms, intending to keep it, Finian declared that the copy also was his. Irish King Diarmaid judged in Finian's favor: "To every cow her calf, to every book its son-book."

Columba was not pleased and eventually a bloody battle ensued. Columba exiled himself to the small Island of Iona off the western Scottish coast, and with his group of twelve monks, evangelized the Picts of Scotland, and founded three more monasteries. One story holds that Columba vowed never to set foot on Irish soil again – so years later when his obligations brought him back to the Emerald Isle, he did so with clods of Scottish dirt affixed underneath his boots!

Exercise: The "Psalter" (Psalms) has played major roles in the lives of both St. Columba today and of St. Robert of two days ago. Perhaps then it's time for a Psalter Workout. Choose a favorite Psalm or perhaps use Psalm 16, cited above. Read it several times prayerfully and then meditate upon it while you walk, bike, run, or do house or yard work for 20 or 30 minutes today. Then perhaps you will say: "My heart is glad, and my soul rejoices; my body also dwells secure..." (Psalms 16:9).

St. Margaret of Scotland (1045-1093)
Patron Saint of Large Families

When [Margaret] spoke, her conversation was with the salt of wisdom. When she was silent, her silence was filled with good thoughts.
                    Turgot, St. Margaret's confessor

St. Margaret was an Anglo-Saxon princess who grew up in Hungary while her father was in exile. When the family returned to England, she was educated by the Benedictines and was renowned for both her beauty and her extraordinary virtue. In 1066, the arrival of William the Conqueror and the death of Margaret's father forced her family to flee England once again. Their ship was wrecked on the coast of Scotland, and King Malcolm III welcomed them to his castle. He was captivated by Margaret, and they married in 1070. Margaret gave birth to eight children, two of them future saints. As Scotland's queen, she promoted education and the arts, founded churches, and gave generously to the poor. She lived a simple and prayerful life and gave away most of her possessions to help the less fortunate. She practiced true charity, always putting the needs of others above her own. Her husband and son were killed in battle, and Margaret died just four days later.

Exercise: Like St. Margaret in the quote above, choose your words carefully. Pray to the Holy Spirit for the gift of wisdom and work hard today to speak wisely and to remember to think before speaking. Resolve not to say anything negative the entire day. The more you practice this virtue, the easier it will become. St. Margaret would often prostrate herself in prayer. You can do the same and work your core muscles by doing a plank exercise. Start in the "up" position of a standard push-up. Your back should be straight with no arch, and your head aligned with your neck so that you look down at the floor. Press your belly button toward your spine and hold the position for 20-30 seconds. Work up to a full minute. You can modify the exercise by resting on your forearms with your elbows bent. You can also place your knees of the floor. Prayer can help keep your mind off the discomfort of the exercise.

St. Barnabus (died 61 A.D.)
Apostle to Antioch and Cyprus

Thus Joseph who was surnamed by the apostles Barnabus (which means, Son of encouragement), a Levite, a native of Cyprus, sold a field which belonged to him, and brought the money and laid it at the apostles' feet.   *Acts 4:36-37*

Barnabus was a Hellenized Jew of the tribe of the Levites who served the Jewish Temple. He is first mentioned in Scripture in the verses above from Acts. He would go on to introduce St. Paul (June 29) to the Apostles and to accompany him on missionary trips of evangelization. He went to Tarsus and sought St. Paul's assistance in his evangelization and establishment of the Church at Antioch. Paul assisted him for a year and the two returned to Jerusalem. Barnabus was part of the Council of Jerusalem that decided to bring Gentiles into the Church. He then evangelized in Cyprus with John Mark until his martyrdom by stoning.

Exercise: St. Barnabus clearly earned that remarkable name bestowed on him by the Apostles: son of encouragement. Wouldn't it be wonderful to be regarded by others as a son or a daughter of encouragement? As a graduate of the Adler School of Professional Psychology, I (Kevin) always think of Alfred Adler's therapy when I hear the word encouragement, since he believed that it is the role of the therapist or of anyone who would help another achieve healthy mental functioning to "encourage" him or her in their strivings toward healing. Let's ask ourselves how we might serve as sons or daughters of encouragement to family and friends who would seek to serve the Lord and to properly tend His bodily temple. Indeed, St. Barnabus himself literally came from a long line of temple tenders! What can you do today to encourage a family member or friend to eat some healthy food, do some invigorating exercise, or join you in joyful prayers?

St. John of Sahagun (1419-1479)
Priest and Miracle Worker

A preacher must be prepared in his soul to speak the truth, both in denouncing and correcting shortcomings and in praising virtue, to such a point that he is willing in that cause even to face death.

St. John of Sahagun

St. John was born to wealthy parents who ensured that their son had a good education and a Christian upbringing. He became a priest, and could have lived comfortably in a wealthy parish, but he chose to serve the poor in a small community. When he suddenly became ill, John decided to join a community of friars. He continued to preach, and changed the hearts of minds of many through his inspiring homilies. Yet his straightforward manner in the correction of sinners angered those who did not want to change their ways. A local duke whom St. John admonished hired two assassins to kill him. When the would-be killers approached the saint, he was so calm and gentle that they immediately begged for forgiveness and refused to carry out the duke's order. The duke eventually repented and asked forgiveness as well. St. John had visions of Christ and worked many miracles. One miracle saved a child who had fallen into a well. St. John raised his hands and the water in the well rose, with the child floating to the top.

Exercise: St. John was not afraid to correct sinners and neither should we. One of the seven spiritual works of mercy is to "admonish the sinner." This must, of course, be done with charity and love. Admonishing a sinner is not the same as judging a person, and your gentle correction may very well put a sinner back on the path to heaven. Pray to the Holy Spirit to help you in this important work of mercy. You can take a similar loving and gentle approach to help a family member or friend lead a healthier life. Asking someone to quit smoking, start exercising, see a doctor, or adopt a healthier diet is not easy but can dramatically improve that person's quality of life. Don't nag, but kindly and gently explain how healthy habits can actually bring more enjoyment to life and provide more energy to meet worldly and spiritual needs.

St. Anthony of Padua (1195-1231)

The life of the body is the soul; the life of the soul is God.

St. Anthony of Padua

Fernando Martins de Bulhoes of Lisbon, Portugal is better known as St. Anthony of Padua. Perhaps best known in our day as the saint you pray to in order to find something you've lost, he was known in his own day as a wonder worker, a gifted preacher, and "the Hammer of Heretics." St. Anthony was born to a very wealthy family, but chose the religious life. He imbibed the learning of the Scriptures and the Latin classics deeply in his training as an Augustinian, but at age 26 became a Franciscan after he was inspired by the headless bodies of five brave Franciscan martyrs who had preached Christ in Morocco, North Africa. St. Anthony gladly did menial chores at a hermitage. When a learned group of Dominicans came for a visit, and expected a Franciscan to preach a homily, (to the surprise of the abbot), St. Anthony was chosen. He spoke with such a glorious voice, moving manner, and inspiring content, that he was from then on recognized as one of the age's most glorious preachers. When exhumed many years after his death, it is reported that while his body had turned to dust, his glorious preacher's tongue remained preserved! St. Anthony was canonized within a year of his death (the fastest ever!) and was proclaimed the Church's "Evangelical Doctor" in 1946.

Exercise: Why not honor St. Anthony, the "the Hammer of Heretics," by doing some "hammer curls?" Try doing dumbbell curls for a change of base with a neutral grip; in other words, with your hands positioned palms in toward your body, as if you were using a hammer. The biceps do not contract as fully in this position, but it gives an excellent workout to muscles in your wrists and forearms. Stay tuned for June 17, St. Gregory Barbarigo, and we'll examine a couple of other related hammer-like exercises for the hands, wrists, and forearms.

St. Lidwina (1380-1433) Patron Saint of Skaters

The story of St. Lidwina, whose name means "suffering," is difficult to read. Born in Holland to a poor family, she was very devoted to the Blessed Mother. At age 15, she was ice skating with friends when she slipped and fell, breaking a rib on a sharp piece of ice. The wound never healed, and gangrene set in. She developed ulcers on her body and in her lungs and was covered with sores. Poor Lidwina often vomited blood, which would also flow from her nose and ears. She slowly became paralyzed, and was eventually only able to move her head and her left arm. Confined to bed for 30 years, she had to be moved carefully by her family. Her body was wrapped in linen to literally keep it together due to the deterioration of her flesh. She lost parts of her skin, bones, and intestines. The local townspeople added to her physical suffering by gossiping that she was possessed by demons and that a priest had impregnated her. On top of all that suffering, she hardly slept or ate! One could hardly blame her if she had succumbed to utter despair. Although Lidwina did express some bitterness, she converted her negative thoughts and feelings to joy and consolation through constant prayer and meditation. She became a victim soul, offering up her suffering for others. Several miracles occurred by her bedside, and she had the gift of heavenly visions. According to some accounts, the Eucharist was her only food for over 19 years. She died at the age of 58 after receiving a vision of Jesus. Some scientists believe that St. Lidwina suffered from multiple sclerosis. Her intercession is often invoked by those suffering from MS and by their caretakers.

Exercise: Most of us will never suffer to the extent that St. Lidwina did, but we can follow her example by selflessly offering up our afflictions for others. It would be especially charitable to offer up your trials for your enemies or for the conversion of sinners who have no one to pray for them. In honor of St. Lidwina, patron saint of skaters, why not plan a trip to the local roller rink for some fun family fitness?

St. Vitus (died 303)

The door turns on its hinges, the sluggard, on his bed! *Proverbs 26:14*

God will not allow your foot to slip; your guardian does not sleep.
Psalms 121:3

The story of St. Vitus matches that of many fourth century Christian martyrs; he was raised in a pagan family, had a conversion experience and was eventually imprisoned for his newfound Christianity. Like many other followers of Jesus during the reign of the merciless Emperor Diocletian, there came a point when he was required to offer sacrifice to pagan gods; since he renounced them in favor of the true God, he was sentenced to a martyr's death, as part of a concentrated effort against Christians during Diocletian's term as emperor.

Catholicism has a long history of assigning patronages to saints based on the circumstances of their death, and St. Vitus is no exception. Since the mighty works Vitus had performed during his lifetime were falsely attributed to sorcery rather than to the power of God, he was subjected to a superstitious ritual against the magic arts, which involved being boiled in oil. The boiling ritual called for a rooster to be thrown into the pot along with him; and since roosters are associated with wake-up calls, St. Vitus has for centuries been invoked against oversleeping. Talk about a busy intercessor!

Exercise: Take time to reflect on how many of your spiritual and physical fitness goals are hindered or put off altogether due to your desire to sleep in. How much earlier would you have to wake up (or how many times fewer would you have to hit the snooze bar) to make even the smallest step toward starting your day with a manageable routine of prayer and exercise, in order to set the tone for the rest of the day?

St. John Francis Regis (1597-1640)
Patron Saint of Marriage and Illegitimate Children

For you have been a stronghold to the poor, a stronghold to the needy in his distress.
Isaiah 25:4

Brother, I see our Lord and our Lady opening the gates of Paradise for me. Into your hands, O Lord, I commend my spirit.
St. John Francis Regis on his deathbed

St. John was certainly an excellent catechist. While studying to become a French priest, he taught the children under his guidance so well that they brought their parents back to the Church! After being ordained, he traveled through France as a missionary, attracting quite a following with his simple, straightforward style of preaching. He ate very little, just an apple or a piece of bread, but he was a hearty soul, climbing the snowy mountains of France to hear confessions and preach to the people who lived far off the beaten path. John Francis helped prostitutes reform their lives and kept young girls from falling into this sinful lifestyle by teaching them skills such as needlework and embroidery so that they could stay busy and earn a living in a reputable manner. He established confraternities (voluntary associations) to honor the Blessed Sacrament, worked many miracles, and saw Jesus and Mary on his deathbed.

Exercise: Catechism is very important for both children and their parents. Many adults stop their faith formation after Confirmation and know very little about Catholic truths and teachings. It's never too late to resume learning about your faith. Ask your parish priest for guidance or stop by your local or online Catholic bookstore. If you have children, ask them what they are studying in faith formation and become actively involved in their catechism.

Today, your exercise is to take a day off! Rest is important so that your muscles have time to recover and grow stronger and to prevent boredom and burnout. Spend the time you would have spent exercising with researching catechism resources as outlined above.

June 17

St. Gregory Barbarigo (1625-1697)

Do not think I have come to abolish the law and the prophets; I have come not to abolish them but to fulfill them.   *Matthew 5:17*

Gregory Barbarigo was born to a wealthy Venetian senator, and would himself become a diplomat. He traveled with his father for the signing of the Treaty of Westphalia, ending the Thirty Years War that had ravaged Germany and much of the European continent. Providence would have it that Gregory would meet a papal nuncio there by the name of Archbishop Fabio Chigi, and through his influence, Gregory would become engrossed in the writings of great spiritual teachers, most prominently St. Francis de Sales (Jan. 24). Later, the archbishop would be known as Pope Alexander VII and Gregory would be known as Father Gregory, and then as the first bishop of Bergamo, and finally as a Cardinal at Padua. The learned Gregory had obtained doctorates in both canon and civil law, and would use his ecclesiastical authority to improve and enlarge seminaries in Bergamo and Padua and to establish both a library and a printing press in Padua.

Exercise: We saw that one great Paduan (St. Anthony, June 13) was "the Hammer of Heretics," and that's why we learned about "hammer curls." Since St. Gregory had two advanced degrees in law, let's use a judge's gavel to carry on our theme of hammer-like exercises for the wrists, hands, and fingers. If you have access to plate-loading dumbbells, take one very light plate (like a 2-1/2 or a 5 pounder.) and secure it near one end of the bar. Then stand with the dumbbell held down at arm's length and with a slight bend in the elbow, raise the dumbbell with wrist action only, as if it were a hammer. Complete a set and then switch arms. Next repeat the motions, but this time, bend your wrist toward your back to raise the loaded end up behind you. These gavel-like leverage exercises should do your wrists and forearms good—but you be the judge.

June 18

St. Osanna Andreasi (1449-1505)
Patron Saint of School Girls

He himself bore our sins in his body on the tree that we might die to sin and live to righteousness. By his wounds you have been healed.

1 Peter 2:24

And, my soul persevering in the demand, there appeared our Lady, the holy Mother of God, and standing before her Son she began to pray, and to help my soul that she might be consoled by the salvation of the pope, and by the renovation of Holy Church.

St. Osanna

Destined to be a saint since childhood, Osanna had her first vision at age five. She saw the Blessed Trinity, the nine choirs of angels, and Jesus as a five year-old boy carrying his cross. The life of St. Osanna bears many similarities to that of St. Catherine of Siena (April 29). Both miraculously learned to read and write, and rejected arranged marriages to become Dominican tertiaries. Both mystic saints were espoused to Christ with an invisible ring, barely ate any food as a form of penance, and received the stigmata (wounds of Jesus). St. Catherine's stigmata wounds were invisible until her death, but Osanna's could be seen by others on Wednesdays, Fridays, and during Holy Week. She willingly suffered greatly from these wounds, offering them up for the salvation of souls. St. Osanna was also a beloved spiritual advisor who spent most of her family's vast fortune in helping the poor and destitute.

Exercise: Does your parish have a library? If so, be sure to visit and check out some books to help you grow in your faith. If not, ask if one can be started. You might even set up a committee in your parish to oversee a new library. Many Catholics aren't sure which books can help them grow in their faith, and a carefully cultivated parish library could bring many blessings to your parish.

Have you been to your local library lately? If not, you are missing out on many free resources for health and fitness. Ask you librarian for help. Some libraries even have exercise DVDs that you can check out.

St. Juliana Falconieri (1270-1341)

I was sick and you visited me.   *Matthew 25:36*

Juliana was born to a prominent Florentine family, wealthy in both the things earthly and in the things of God. Her father died when she was young, and she was influenced towards sanctity by her uncle, St. Alexis Falconieri, one of the seven founders of the Servite Order, to whom the Blessed Virgin appeared and directed them in devotion to the sorrows she experienced at her Son's Passion. Juliana was so devout and so humble that she never looked at a mirror or held her gaze upon a man. She refused an arranged marriage at age 14 and dedicated her life to Christ. She would later found the Third Order of Servites, or the Mantellates, (from the Latin for cloak, *mantellum*), so named because of the short-sleeved habit the sisters wore to better enable them to actively serve the sick and perform other acts of mercy. They serve to this day in several countries in Europe and North America. Near the end of her life, this humble servant of the sick lay dying. Vomiting prevented her from taking the Eucharist, so she asked that the host be laid upon her chest. After she had passed from the earth, an image of the cross of the host was found upon her breast. This patroness of the sick is often depicted in her habit with the host.

Exercise: Let St. Juliana remind us that we are called not only to tend our own temples, but also to tend the holy bodily temples of our neighbors, regardless of their health or lack of it. Is there someone in your family, circle of friends, neighborhood, or parish who is ailing right now? Is there some kind of act of mercy you can perform? Remember that we are exercising our bodies to transform them into "dynamos of charity." Let's remain ever aware then of opportunities to "exercise" that charity.

Blessed Michelina (1300-1356)
Patron Saint of the Mentally Ill

I have prayed for you that your faith may not fail; and when you have turned again, strengthen your brethren. *Luke 22:32*

Do one's daily work in the spirit of Christ. *Pope Benedict XVI*

At the age of 12, Michelina married an Italian duke and gave birth to a son. She was very happy until her husband died when she was still just in her twenties. Now a single mom with a son to raise alone, Michelina tried to find comfort in parties, fine food, and a luxurious lifestyle. She soon realized that she was neglecting the person she loved best— her little boy. She befriended Syriaca, a Franciscan laywoman who taught her how to improve her prayer life and grow closer to God and in her faith. Michelina stopped going to parties and began to help and serve the poor, sick, and lonely people in her city. When her son died, she sold all her nice clothes and fine jewelry and became a Franciscan tertiary like Syriaca. Her family thought she was crazy and had her locked up in an insane asylum. They eventually realized that the simple life of a Franciscan was what made her truly happy and set her free. Michelina devoted the rest of her life to service of God and neighbor. It is said that she cured lepers by kissing their sores. After she died, the townspeople kept a lamp lit in her home which was later converted into a church.

Exercise: Sometimes we turn to food for comfort, when we should turn to God in prayer instead. If you are a person who seeks comfort in eating, keep a journal to find out what triggers these intense desires. Try to replace the food habit with a different habit like reading the Bible, taking a walk, or working on a hobby that you enjoy. Pray for help in overcoming the compulsion to eat for comfort. Of course, if you truly have an eating disorder or have been told that you might, seek professional help immediately.

St. Aloysius Gonzaga (1568-1591)

Let no one despise your youth, but set the believers an example in speech and conduct, in love, in faith, in purity.   *1 Timothy 4:12*

Man is born for action; he ought to do something. Work, at each step, awakens a sleeping force and roots out error. Who does nothing, knows nothing. Rise! to work! If thy knowledge is real, employ it; wrestle with nature; test the strength of thy theories; see if they will support the trial; act!   *St. Aloysius Gonzaga*

Born into a noble family that lived in a castle and travelled in circles of royal courts, Aloysius' father, a worldly man and compulsive gambler, saw a future of high office, perhaps in the military, for his young son Aloysius. God and Aloysius had other plans, however. Displaying great piety from his youth, (his first words were Jesus and Mary), at 18 he would renounce his inheritance to take the vows of poverty, chastity, and obedience within the Jesuit Order. Though brilliant in philosophy and theology, he desired to care for the sick and contracted the plague. He died at the age of 23.

Exercise: St. Aloysius of Gonzaga seems an extremely unlikely, yet extremely important, patron saint for our youth today. In an age that glorifies lust, violence, greed, sloth, and disrespect, we badly need the model of a young man who chose not to gaze unduly even upon the face of a woman (a counterpart to the feminine example of St. Juliana of June 19), one who was revolted by the violence of court life and local wars, who willingly gave up a huge fortune to obey superiors who would guide him toward Christ, and who would praise and practice intellectual, spiritual, and physical labors. His superiors, in fact, had to order him to eat more and to pray less! Let's ask ourselves what we can do, informed by St. Aloysius of Gonzaga to inspire the young people in our lives to a truly manly (or womanly) life of godly action that dares to fly in the face of the all-too-easy, and all too petty models of modern mass media.

St. Thomas More (1478-1535) A Man for All Seasons

For whoever would save his life will lose it; and whoever will lose his life for my sake, he will save it. For what does it profit a man if he gains the whole world and loses or forfeits himself?   Luke 9:24-25

We cannot go to heaven in feather beds.   St. Thomas More

S t. Thomas More has been immortalized in the play, "A Man for All Seasons" by Robert Bolt. As an author, scholar, lawyer, statesman, reformer, martyr, and devoted husband and father, he certainly deserves such an august title. His most famous written works are *Utopia* and *Treatise on the Blessed Sacrament*, but St. Thomas is best known for his refusal to recognize King Henry VIII as the supreme head of the Church of England. When Pope Clement II would not annul the king's marriage to Catherine of Aragon, Henry decided to break from Rome and establish his own church so that he could marry Anne Boleyn. St. Thomas resigned as the king's chancellor and was imprisoned in London Tower. He was tried and beheaded for treason, and his head was placed on a pike on London Bridge. St. Thomas is the patron saint of lawyers, politicians, and step-parents.

Exercise: The call to practice authentic Christianity can demand many sacrifices. Are you prepared to do what it takes to take up your cross and follow Jesus? Read and study the Bible and pray for strength to carry out your unique vocation on earth. Unite your suffering and sacrifice with Christ, and you will be richly blessed, either in this world or the next.

Keeping up a regular workout program also involves sacrifices. You may have to give up a movie or a night out for dinner in order to pay for your gym membership. You might have to walk when it's raining outside or lift weights in a garage with no air conditioning or heat. Offer up these little inconveniences and you will grow spiritually as well as physically.

St. Joseph Cafasso (1811-1860)

I was in prison and you came to me. *Matthew 25:36*

The body is insatiable; the more we give it the more it demands.
St. Joseph Cafasso

Joseph Cafasso was born with congenital problems that left him short in stature and with a twisted spine, but this determined saint would achieve great things that required a great deal of "backbone!" He taught at the Institute of St. Francis in Turin, Italy, and is known for his ministry to prisoners as "The Priest of the Gallows." In one bold act of mercy, the small, frail saint waltzed into a group of men condemned to die and grabbed the beard of the biggest and meanest of them, a man who had refused to go to confession. St. Joseph said he would not let go until he agreed to give his confession. The grizzled prisoner was won over and later wept with joy at the forgiveness of all his grave sins. St. Joseph would describe the men who repented sincerely and received absolution immediately before their executions as "hanged saints."

Exercise: St. Joseph made his small and crooked body serve his straight and powerful soul! I (Kevin) recall from my youth a multi-world record holder in the deadlift whose spine was twisted in two places. Another world champion squatter was a man who was born without kneecaps. Some physical impairments will seriously limit what we can do physically, and some can be overcome. If you are able to, in your next workout, do an exercise for your spinal muscles, like a "good morning," hyperextension, deadlift, or low back machine. Yet even if you are unable, remember that regardless of our physical woes, when our souls reign as masters over our bodies, we can do the works of God through our actions, words, or even simply our attitudes and demeanors, even if bound to a wheelchair or a hospital bed. St. Joseph of Cafasso would expect it of us!

Nativity of St. John, the Baptist Prophet

A voice cries out: In the desert prepare the way of the LORD! Make straight in the wasteland a highway for our God! Isaiah 40:3

This is the one about whom scripture says: "Behold, I am sending my messenger ahead of you, he will prepare your way before you." I tell you, among those born of women, no one is greater than John; yet the least in the kingdom of God is greater than he." Luke 7:27-28

Usually saints' feast days are celebrated on the date of their deaths, and only John the Baptist and the Blessed Mother are honored by the Church on their birthdays. Mary was born without Original Sin, and John was sanctified (cleansed of Original Sin) in the womb of his mother, St. Elizabeth, when Mary greeted her at the Visitation. John the Baptist is the "greatest of prophets," yet lived a humble life in the desert, eating locusts and wild honey. He was an inspirational preacher who baptized many people and convinced them to repent of their sins. When the Savior Himself asked him for baptism, John protested, stating that he was not even fit to tie Jesus' sandals. Yet Jesus insisted on being baptized to show us that Baptism is the way to salvation. John aroused the ire of Herodias, wife of King Herod, who convinced her comely daughter to perform a seductive dance for the king. When the king offered the girl anything in his kingdom, Herodias told her daughter to ask for the head of John the Baptist on a platter. Today's feast is tied to Advent, nearly five months away, because John's birth anticipates the birth of the Redeemer.

Exercise: We recently renewed our Baptismal Promises during the Easter season. Take some time today to reflect on those truths which we profess each time we pray the Nicene Creed. Do you understand what each line of the Creed really means? If not, refer to the *Catechism of the Catholic Church*. A good portion of this helpful reference aid is devoted to explaining each line of our profession of faith. It's easy to find online if you don't own a copy. In honor of St. John the Baptist, try some type of water exercise this week. Rent a canoe or kayak, go swimming or join a water aerobics class.

St. Prosper of Aquitaine (390-465)

Prosper of Aquitaine (today southwestern France) was very learned in world history and in sacred theology, and, though apparently a layman, devoted his energies to the refutation of heresies and the defense of Catholic orthodoxy. St. Prosper corresponded with St. Augustine (Aug. 28) and wrote treatises and even a 1,000 line poem on matters of grace and free will. He wrote a great historical chronicle covering the years from 379-455, which included descriptions of events like Attila the Hun's invasions of Gaul and Italy, and which remains to this day an important source of information on the fifth century. Prosper would become the secretary to St. Pope Leo the Great (April 11), the pontiff who would convince Attila to turn away from Rome.

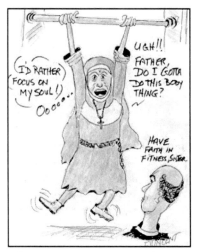

Exercise: An old term for physical fitness training, regrettably little-known today, was "physical culture," with those who trained their bodies being known as "physical culturists." In 1948, Pope Pius XII, a fitness-minded pontiff, declared to a group of athletes that "the Church, without any doubt whatever, approves of physical culture, if it be in proper proportion." We are to cultivate our bodies with just the right kinds and amounts of exercise, nutrition, and rest, just like a farmer cultivates his fields with the proper nutrients and water. We have to use our minds and wills whether cultivating our cornfields or our bodies, and we must cultivate within ourselves the proper habits in the proper proportion. Still, we must never forget that in both cases, it is the grace of God that has provided them in the first place, and that provides the growth. So, before, after, and perhaps during your next workout, include a prayer in thanks to God for giving you the growth!

June 26

St. Josemaría Escriva (1902-1975) Founder of Opus Dei

But as he who called you is holy, be holy yourselves in all your conduct.
1 Peter 1:15

We can all become saints just by staying where we are and doing just ordinary work, if we offer what we are doing, no matter how insignificant, to our Heavenly Father.
St. Josemaría Escriva

St. Josemaría is a very popular modern-day saint. Over 300,000 people filled St. Peter's Square on the date of his canonization in 2002. Pope John Paul II noted his connection to our own lives. "St. Josemaría was chosen by the Lord to proclaim the universal call to holiness and to indicate that everyday life; its customary activities, are a path towards holiness. It could be said that he was the saint of the ordinary." As a young boy in Spain, St. Josemaría knew that he would become a priest. He was ordained in 1925 and went on to earn a doctorate degree in law. He founded Opus Dei in 1928 to help ordinary people find more faith and holiness in their daily lives. During the Spanish Civil War, he had to work in secret to continue his mission. St. Josemaría was highly educated, very pious, and influential in matters at the Vatican. He died in 1975. Today, Opus Dei has nearly 100,000 members in over 60 countries.

Exercise: It's always helpful and inspiring to learn about saints who lived during our modern times. Like us, St. Josemaría Escriva flew in airplanes, ate at modern restaurants, watched TV, and was exposed to the same cultural influences that we are today. He managed to live a saintly and exemplary life during a time when secularism began to take over the world. Follow his example and try to live a holy and saintly life each and every day.

It's also important to try to live a healthy life. The saying goes, "garbage in, garbage out." If you eat a steady diet of junk food then you simply won't have the energy to meet the challenges of the day with enthusiasm. Try to change just one thing each week. If you usually eat a fast food breakfast, try to eat a bowl of whole grain cereal or a fruit and yogurt smoothie instead. Each week, replace an unhealthy habit with a healthy one, and you'll soon be reaping the rewards.

St. King Ladislaus of Hungary (1040-1095)

Kings of the earth and all peoples, princes and all rulers of the earth! Young men and maidens together, old men and children... Let them praise the name of the LORD...   *Psalms 148:11-13*

Ladislaus was a valued advisor to his brother King Geza I of Hungary, and after his brother's death in 1077, Ladislaus ascended to the throne. He would emerge victorious in a civil war against his cousin, King Salomon in Western Hungary, and would later extend his realm to Croatia after the death of their last royal heir. This would prompt armed reaction by the forces of Byzantine Emperor Alexios I, but King Ladislaus' forces would emerge victorious. Ladislaus strengthened the Church and set up a new bishopric at Zagreb. He strengthened the eastern border of Hungary by planting the Szekely people in Transylvania, who would guard against foreign attacks. Ladislaus was loved by his people and memorialized in their legendary sagas and poems as the model of a good and chivalrous Christian King. He was canonized on June 27, 1192.

Exercise: In honor of St. Ladislaus, how about today we learn how to strengthen our own eastern and western borders? I'm simply talking about the oblique muscles on each side of our waists. These muscles are involved in lateral bending from side to side and also in rotating the torso. The simplest lateral bending motion is the side bend. Grab a light dumbbell in your right hand, holding it down at arm's length. Now, simply bend to your right as far as you can comfortably bend. Slowly return to the standing position and repeat for your set. This works the oblique muscles on the left side of your waist. Then switch the dumbbell to your left hand and bend to the left for the set. This works the obliques on the right. We'll cover the twisting motion exercise a few days down the calendar.

St. Irenaeus (130-202) Early Church Father and Martyr

For as in Adam all die, so also in Christ shall all be made alive.

1 Corinthians 15:22

The glory of God is a human being fully alive; and to be alive consists in beholding God.

St. Irenaeus

We can thank St. Irenaeus every time we read the New Testament. He was the first to declare that the Gospels of Matthew, Mark, Luke, and John were canonical (divinely inspired writing). He also went through each of the books proposed for the New Testament and gave valid reasons for why they should be included or why they were not divinely inspired. St. Irenaeus certainly had the background and education to undertake this important task. He was taught by St. Polycarp (Feb. 23), a disciple of Jesus' beloved Apostle, St. John. Irenaeus was appointed bishop of Lyons, spending most of his time fighting the heresy of Gnosticism. He studied this heresy intently and wrote five books to refute it. Irenaeus used a gentle, thoughtful approach to lead the people away from this false teaching, but was not afraid to use strong language to get his point across. As a direct result of his efforts and prayers, the people began to turn away from Gnosticism and embrace the truths of their Christian faith. St. Irenaeus is believed to have died as a martyr in the year 202, but few facts are known about his death.

Exercise: Although Gnosticism is not as prevalent today as in St. Irenaeus' time, there are still plenty of heresies in our Church. Some people who claim to be Catholic support abortion, euthanasia, and contraception. Often these people are misguided and don't understand the truths of their faith. Follow St. Irenaeus' example and use a gentle approach so as not to alienate such people, but don't be afraid to use strong words when needed.

You might need a few strong words to motivate you to exercise today. Write a few motivational quotes and post them in places where you will see them so you don't abandon your workout.

Sts. Peter and Paul (died ca. 65)

I will give you the keys of the kingdom of heaven, and whatever you bind on earth shall be bound in heaven, and whatever you loose on earth shall be loosed in heaven.   *Matthew 16:19*

And take the helmet of salvation and the sword of the Spirit, which is the word of God.   *Ephesians 6:17*

God led both of these foundational saints, the head of Christ's Apostles and the "Apostle to the Gentiles," to spend their last days in Rome, establishing Christ's great Church that will prevail to the end of time. St. Peter is often depicted with keys, representing those papal keys to the kingdom bestowed on him by Christ himself. St. Paul is often depicted with a sword, as in the powerful statue outside the glorious Roman basilica known as "St. Paul's Outside the Walls." Peter was also the solid rock upon which the Church was formed, and Paul was much like a rolling stone, travelling from place to place, boldly winning countless souls to Christ. Though the world might question the choice of an unlearned, impulsive fisherman, and a self-righteous prosecutor of Christians to found and spread His Church on earth, the very history of the world's most enduring institution, the one, holy, apostolic, Catholic Church, shows that Christ's wisdom was the wisdom of God.

Exercise: Have you ever heard the old aphorism, "robbing Peter to pay Paul?" It may apply to some misguided efforts toward tending the temple. Some people who do show the fortitude to do aerobic training long and frequently enough to burn a lot of calories develop the habit of using it as an excuse to forgo temperance and take in too much food. "Sure I ate that box of chocolate chip cookies, but I just biked 20 miles!" Even the training of a marathoner or a tri-athlete cannot undo the negative health effects of a poor diet. Let's honor both the fortitude to exercise and the temperance to eat right, paying both Peter and Paul!

First Martyrs of the Church of Rome

When they lead you away and hand you over, do not worry beforehand about what you are to say. But say whatever will be given to you at that hour. For it will not be you who are speaking but the Holy Spirit.
Mark 13:11

Our hearts were made for You, O Lord, and they are restless until they rest in you.
St. Augustine of Hippo

Throughout this book, we have named many saints who were early Christian martyrs. There are quite a few facts known about some, very few on others, and some accounts are mostly legends. Today we honor those nameless saints who gave up their lives rather than renounce their faith. From the very beginning, the members of the new Church that Christ established were persecuted. In the year 64, the Emperor Nero famously composed music while the city of Rome burned. When the people learned that he was responsible for the fire, Nero was afraid that they might rise up and kill him, so he blamed the fire on the Christians. He had countless Christians tortured and put to death in very cruel ways. We honor those countless brave and unnamed men, women, and children today. Nero's efforts were in fact counterproductive. The more the people witnessed the bravery and unshakable faith of the Christians, the more people converted.

Exercise: Spend a few moments in prayer to these brave saints who paved the way for the spread of Christianity. Ask them for help in strengthening your own faith and resolve to defend it.

Today's exercise is a set of hill repeats. This will strengthen both your legs and your mental resolve. Find a hill that's about ¼ mile long. The steeper it is, the harder you'll work. If you are not very fit or if it has been a while since you have exercised, start with a relatively easy hill. Warm up for 5-10 minutes, then walk, jog, or bike to the top of the hill as briskly as possible; then catch your breath as you slowly return to the base of the hill. Repeat 2-4 times. Finish with a 5-10 minute cool-down. As you become stronger, increase the repeats until you can do 5. Then look for a steeper hill and start again with 2-3 repeats.

Blessed Junipero Serra (1713-1784) American Missionary

But how can they call on him in whom they have not believed? And how can they believe in him of whom they have not heard? And how can they hear without someone to preach? And how can people preach unless they are sent? As it is written, "How beautiful are the feet of those who bring (the) good news!" Romans 10:14-15

Blessed Junipero was born in Spain and became a Franciscan priest. He enjoyed reading stories of Franciscan saints and was especially captivated by St. Francis Solano, a South American missionary. Junipero decided that he too wanted to become a missionary and spread the Good News. He finally got his wish 20 years later, when he was sent to New Spain, or what is now part of Mexico and California. The first mission he established was Mission San Diego in southern California. The native people gathered at the Mission, and Blessed Junipero taught them all about Christ and his message of love and forgiveness. He also taught them useful life skills like farming and cattle-raising. Amazingly, Junipero founded nine missions throughout California (12 more were established after his death), and baptized over 6,000 people. He died peacefully at Mission San Carlos in beautiful Carmel, and is buried there.

Exercise: Since I (Peggy) lived in California for several years, I had the chance to tour quite a few missions. It is fascinating to see how the people lived and worked back then, and how the mission and its church were truly the center of life for the people. There are missions scattered throughout the US. If there's one nearby, arrange to take a tour. If not, perhaps you can plan a family vacation based on visiting one. Almost every mission in California is close to a major tourist attraction. Blessed Junipero had to be very fit to walk so many miles (around 25,000!) establishing missions throughout California. Walking is a great exercise because it can be done almost anywhere and requires no special equipment other than a good pair of shoes. If you are new to exercise, walking is the perfect place to start. What are you waiting for?

St. Acestes (died 65 AD)

When he entered Rome, Paul was allowed to live by himself, with the soldier who was guarding him.   *Acts 28:16*

Can you imagine what it would be like to live with the great missionary, St. Paul? Today's saint was a pagan soldier assigned to escort Paul to his death. He may or may not have been the same soldier mentioned in Acts above, but in any case, he was profoundly affected by the teaching of the apostle and became a Christian. The scant information available on Acestes states that he declared his faith after Paul's execution and was beheaded himself immediately afterward, along with two other soldiers.

Exercise: The words of St. Paul had such a great effect on St. Acestes, so take some time today to read one of Paul's epistles in the New Testament. Since we are also focusing our efforts on care of our bodily temples, then perhaps you'd like to read 1 Corinthians, the book that contains the famous quote that our bodies are temples of the Holy Spirit. In Corinthians, Paul was speaking to Greeks, known for their appreciation of the body and its strength, so he makes use of several athletic metaphors. In 1 Cor 6:20, Paul urges us to "glorify God in your body." Today, choose a cardio exercise and focus on how your body can give glory to God through your workout. I (Peggy) find the best way to do this is to pray the Rosary while I run, bike, swim or hike. Here's a fun variation, a "pyramid" Rosary Workout. (You might ask St. Acestes to join you.)

Warm up during the opening prayers: Apostles' Creed, Our Father and three Hail Mary's.

During the first decade, keep a fairly easy pace. Speed up during the second decade to a moderate pace. As you pray the third decade, increase the pace even more, close to a pace you'd use in a race. For the fourth decade, slow down slightly to a moderate pace, about the same pace you held during the second decade.

Return to a fairly easy pace for the fifth decade, the same as the first. Finally, cool down for at least 5-10 minutes and stretch.

St. Thomas (died c. 72) The Doubter

Then [Jesus] said to Thomas, "Put your finger here and see my hands, and bring your hand and put it into my side, and do not be unbelieving, but believe." Thomas answered and said to him, "My Lord and my God!"
                                                                    John 20:27-28

Thomas' unbelief has benefited our faith more than the belief of the other disciples; it is because he attained faith through physical touch that we are confirmed in the faith beyond all doubt.
                                                        Pope St. Gregory the Great

Everyone has heard the term "Doubting Thomas," but it downplays the fact that this Apostle was one of the 12 men chosen personally by Jesus to establish His Church on earth. In fact, Thomas demonstrates great courage in John 11:16. Jesus' life was in danger, but Thomas says to the other Apostles, "Let us also go, that we may die with him." Despite his brief and famous lapse of faith, Thomas was a great leader in the early Church. He traveled to Parthia, Persia, and India to spread the Gospel. He converted many people to Christianity and died a martyr's death, killed with a spear while kneeling in front of a cross.

Exercise: It is normal to doubt our faith at times. Yet the more we learn about and study our faith, the stronger it will grow. Remember to have the faith of a child (see Matthew 18:3-4) and try to simply believe. Pray for guidance and consult reliable sources on Catholic doctrine. There is a lot of false information and half-truths being disseminated, even by well-meaning Catholics. If you're unsure, consult a trusted and orthodox priest or reference the Catechism.

You won't doubt the strength of your biceps after completing this challenging exercise. It's called "21s" because you will do 21 repetitions. Hold a barbell or a pair of dumbbells in each hand, with arms extended. Slowly curl up just halfway, so that your arms are parallel with the ground. Return to the starting position and repeat 7 times. Then start with arms parallel to the ground and curl up toward your chest and return to the starting position. Repeat 7 times. Finally, complete 7 full biceps curls. Modify by doing fewer reps of each set.

Blessed Pier Giorgio Frassati (1901-1925) Rosary Athlete

Thus I do not run aimlessly; I do not fight as if I were shadowboxing. No, I drive my body and train it, for fear that, after having preached to others, I myself should be disqualified.   *1 Corinthians 9:26-27*

You ask me whether I am in good spirits. How could I not be, so long as my trust in God gives me strength. We must always be cheerful. Sadness should be banished from all Christian souls. For suffering is a far different thing from sadness, which is the worst disease of all. It is almost always caused by lack of Faith.   *Blessed Pier Giorgio Frassati*

Blessed Pier Giorgio is one of my (Peggy's) favorite Catholic heroes. I say a prayer to him every time I ride my road bike, as he too was an athlete devoted to the Blessed Mother's favorite prayer, the Rosary. Pier Giorgio provides a shining example of how a young man in our modern world can live a holy life. He was a handsome young Italian who was an accomplished athlete. He was a popular and very normal kid, even earning the nickname "Terror" due to his penchant for practical jokes. Pier Giorgio promoted devotion to the Eucharist, the Rosary, and to chastity before marriage. He became a Dominican tertiary and was known to walk through his little town, praying the Rosary and asking others to join him. His family was very wealthy, but he spent much of his money caring for the poor and sick. He contracted a disease as a result of his ministry and died at the young age of 24. On the day of his funeral, thousands lined the streets to pay tribute to this holy young man. Blessed Pier Giorgio is often called "The Man of the Eight Beatitudes" because he lived his life according to those words of Jesus in the Sermon on the Mount.

Exercise: In honor of Blessed Pier Giorgio, pray the Rosary on a walk today. Better yet, imitate him and ask a friend to join you. You can take turns leading the mysteries. When you're finished with the workout, treat yourselves to a cold beverage and spend a few minutes talking about how to be a saint in today's world. Read the Beatitudes (Matthew 5:1-11) for inspiration.

St. Anthony Mary Zaccaria (1502-1539)
Founder of Clerks Regular of St. Paul

That which God commands seems difficult and a burden. The way is rough; you draw back; you have no desire to follow it. Yet do so and you will attain glory.   St. Anthony Mary Zaccaria

Although St. Anthony's father died when he was very young, his mother encouraged her son to study hard and become a doctor so that he could serve the poor people of their town. He did so, graduating from medical school at the age of 22. Although he was a good and devoted doctor, Anthony was not happy in that occupation and began to study for the priesthood. He was ordained a priest and gave all his money and possessions to his mother. According to some accounts, during the first Mass he celebrated as a priest, he appeared to be illuminated by a heavenly light and surrounded by angels. He was especially interested in the writings of St. Paul and studied them intently. He started a new order of priests, calling them the Clerks Regular of St. Paul, and a religious order for women called the Angelic Sisters of St. Paul. They taught the people the message of St. Paul in simple terms and encouraged devotion to the Eucharist. Anthony began a custom of ringing the church bells at 3:00 on Fridays in honor of Jesus' death on the cross. St. Anthony became ill while on a mission, and died at the age of 37.

Exercise: In honor of St. Anthony, read a chapter from one of St. Paul's epistles. If possible, use a study Bible so that you can better understand the poetic words of this great missionary. You'll be able to study harder and start your day with energy if you eat a healthy breakfast. Many people make the mistake of skipping breakfast, but your body needs fuel to break the nighttime fast and jumpstart your metabolism. Good choices include whole grain cereal or toast, oatmeal made with old-fashioned oats, fresh fruit and yogurt, eggs, or a smoothie. If you don't like a traditional breakfast, try a European-style breakfast such as lunch meat, cheese, fruit, and bread or crackers.

St. Maria Goretti (1890-1902)

But the wisdom from above is first pure, then peaceable, gentle, open to reason, full of mercy and good fruits, without uncertainty or insincerity.   *James 3:17*

Young Maria Goretti's story is a singularly moving story of horrendously violent outrage and absolutely saintly gentleness, forgiveness, and redemption. While her mother and older siblings were working in the fields, this young Italian girl of 11, at home caring for her infant sister, was stabbed 14 times by the 20-year-old would-be rapist whom she had refused upon threat of death, desiring to avoid sin. She would die the next day, but not before forgiving him. She had known him, as his family had lived in the same building as her, and stated she wanted him with her in heaven. This young man was unrepentant for the first three years he spent in prison, until he was visited by a bishop and soon after had a dream in which Maria handed him lilies which burned his hands. He would seek and obtain forgiveness from Maria's mother, become a lay Capuchin friar, working and eventually dying in a monastery in 1970, 20 years after he had attended St. Maria Goretti's canonization. Maria's own three brothers were among those blessed by her miraculous intercessions.

Exercise: What a shocking story for our modern culture. Hardly over a hundred years ago, this young girl was willing to face a painful death rather than to have her bodily temple defiled. How sad that so many messages in the popular media today would have young girls throw away for nothing the dignity of body and soul, for which St. Maria would pay the price of her life. Our exercise for today is one of thought and prayer. What can *you* do to counteract our modern day culture full of its worldly wisdom of lust, violence, and death, with the kind of wisdom from above which gave St. Maria Goretti such peace, and gentleness, and mercy, so that even after death she keeps feeding us with her spiritual fruits? Let's pray to St. Maria herself for her loving intercession.

Blessed Roger Dickenson, Blessed Ralph Milner, and Blessed Lawrence Humphrey (16th Century) Martyrs

In this you greatly rejoice, though now for a little while, if need be, you have been grieved by various trials, that the genuineness of your faith, being much more precious than gold that perishes, though it is tested by fire, may be found to praise, honor, and glory at the revelation of Jesus Christ.   *1 Peter 1:6-7*

We always find that those who walked closest to Christ were those who had to bear the greatest trials.   *St. Teresa of Avila*

These three Englishmen lived during the terrible persecutions of the Catholic Church by Queen Elizabeth I. Blessed Roger Dickinson was a native of England who studied to be a priest in France. He was secretly sent on a mission to England and became a parish priest. He said Mass, heard Confession, and ministered to his flock in secret. Blessed Ralph Milner was a poor Protestant farmer who was so inspired by his Catholic neighbors that he converted. He was arrested on the day he made his First Communion, but befriended the jailer and was allowed to leave frequently on "parole." While out of jail, he helped Blessed Roger and other priests in their secret ministry. When Blessed Roger was finally caught, he and Blessed Ralph were brought to trial together. Blessed Lawrence Humphrey was also a convert who was arrested and tried for his faith. All three of these brave men were hung, drawn and quartered.

Exercise: Make it a goal today to do 10 good deeds or sacrifices. Collect 10 pennies, rocks, beads, or some other small objects and put them in your pocket (or someplace where you'll notice them throughout the day). Each time you do a good deed or make a sacrifice, take a trinket out of your pocket and put it in a separate pile so that you can see your good deeds growing. At the same time, say a short prayer to today's martyrs asking for an increase in the type of heroic virtue that they practiced. Find 10 minutes today for some simple body weight exercises. Push-ups, sit-ups, dips, squats, and lunges can be done anywhere—at home, the office or at the playground. Don't forget to stretch when you're finished.

St. Elizabeth of Portugal (1271-1336)

Let us then pursue what makes for peace and for mutual upbuilding.
Romans 8:19

The European monarchs of the Middle Ages were a most colorful mix of saints and sinners. This great Portuguese queen was the namesake of her saintly great-aunt, Queen Elizabeth of Hungary. Her husband, King Denis, however, was a lusty, suspicious, and power-hungry man before many years of virtuous influence won him over. Once a royal page intrigued against her by telling the king Elizabeth had been unfaithful with another page. Enraged, the king instructed a furnace-maker to throw within his furnace the next page to deliver him a message. He then sent forth the falsely accused youth. Denis, in his suspense of the outcome, soon after sent a second page, the originator of the slander, to report on the first's demise. The first page, however, from daily habit had stopped to attend Mass along his way, and his false accuser encountered the furnace-maker, and his furnace, first. Elizabeth herself made room for daily Mass and recitation of the divine office despite her many responsibilities of state and her ongoing acts of charity and mercy. Known as a peacemaker, she brokered peace between her husband and her son Alphonso, who had raised arms against him. She would also broker peace between her own children. Later in life, she became a Third Order Franciscan, and lived a life of spiritual exercise and active almsgiving.

Exercise: What can we do today to broker both peace between others and peace within our own souls? St. Thomas Aquinas (Jan. 28) notes that the harmony that is peace flows from a life ordered by the gift of wisdom from God. This wisdom enables us to focus on the most important things and to develop the daily habits that keep us in inner and outer harmony. Are there any new daily habits that you could establish to achieve closer union with God and your neighbor? Is daily Mass feasible, or perhaps an early morning 20-minute walk with the rosary after 10 minutes of spiritual reading? What will it be? See where God moves you on this and give it a try for at least the next week.

The Martyrs of Orange (18ᵗʰ Century)

Do nothing out of selfishness or out of vainglory; rather, humbly regard others as more important than yourselves, each looking out not for his own interests, but (also) everyone for those of others.
Philemon 2:3-4

Although martyrdom represents the high point of the witness to moral truth, and one to which relatively few people are called, there is nonetheless a consistent witness which all Christians must daily be ready to make, even at the cost of suffering and grave sacrifice.
Pope Blessed John Paul II

Today we honor 32 French nuns from four different orders who were imprisoned in the city of Orange during the French Revolution. They were asked to renounce their faith, but refused. During their time in jail, the women formed a strong bond, praying together and comforting one another. On July 6ᵗʰ, one of the nuns was taken away. She never returned; a victim of the infamous guillotine. Each day one or sometimes two nuns would be taken away to be executed. The sisters never knew who would be selected on any given day, but they helped one another to be strong and brave. They sang the Te Deum daily, an ancient hymn of praise. When the war was over, the judges who put these innocent nuns to death were found guilty and punished severely.

Exercise: Like the martyrs of Orange, we never know when we will die. We must live each day as if it is our last, because we "know neither the day nor the hour" (Matthew 25:13). In honor of today's martyrs, sing (or listen to) the Te Deum. You can find several versions on YouTube.

Eating more fruits and vegetables may not prevent you from dying, but they can protect you against many serious diseases. Try to include at least five servings of fruits and vegetables each day. Drink juice for breakfast, have a piece of fruit for a morning snack, a salad at lunch, a pick-me-up smoothie in the afternoon, and some veggies for dinner.

The Seven Holy Brothers (died 150)

The mother was especially admirable and worthy of honorable memory. Though she saw her seven sons perish within a single day, she bore it with good courage because of her hope in the Lord.

2 Maccabees 7:20

The devout Jewish mother of the seven sons described in the second book of Maccabees witnessed the horrendous torture and execution of all of her sons. Yet she died with the joyful knowledge that her sons had not bowed to the orders of Greek King Antiochus to violate the laws of God by eating forbidden food. She knew in her heart what she told her last son, that the Creator "will in his mercy give life and breath back to you again." A few hundred years later, in second century Rome, a devout Christian mother, by the name of St. Felicitas, would witness the horrendous torture and execution of her seven sons. Yet she died with the joyful knowledge that her sons had not bowed to the Roman Emperor Antoninus to violate the laws of God by sacrifice to pagan gods. The emperor had ordered that each son be sent to a different judge to receive different executions, from bludgeoning with clubs, whipping, being thrown off a cliff, and beheadings. Felicitas herself was beheaded four months later.

Exercise: Just imagine the divine fortitude required not only of these sons, but of their godly mothers, to endure such loss for the glory of God. It calls to mind the seven sorrows of our Blessed Mother, as well. Here are three sevens that require infinitely less fortitude and will also help build your bodily temple. Try a technique called "21's" on an exercise like the curl sometime. Select a weight slightly lighter than one you would typically use for 8-12 repetitions. First, do seven reasonably slow curls, going up only halfway and then back down. Next, curl the weight to your shoulders and do seven more, going only halfway down. Finally, strive to complete seven more, using a full range of motion. This will breathe new life into your biceps (or at least you will know they are there!) You can also experiment with this technique as a change of pace for other strength exercises.

St. Benedict (480-547) Founder of the Benedictine Order

Seek the LORD while he may be found, call him while he is near.
Isaiah 55:6

Idleness is the enemy of the soul; and therefore the brethren ought to be employed in manual labor at certain times, at others, in devout reading.
St. Benedict

St. Benedict, as a young man, was very adventurous and loved to learn, but he did not like the worldly ways of the people around him. As an adult, he wanted to be alone so that he could pray and reflect on the Word of God. He found a cave to live in and enjoyed his life of prayer and solitude. Benedict endured severe temptations from the devil and often longed to return to his comfortable life. He fought off the temptations, even so far as to roll around in a bush full of thorns! People heard of his holiness and came to his cave seeking his wisdom. He founded several monasteries, the most famous of which is Monte Cassino. He wrote a rule for his monks that has become very well-known and is followed worldwide. Not everyone was a fan of St. Benedict's rule, however. Several of his own monks found it too strict and tried to poison him! He and his fellow Benedictines performed many works of charity. He believed that our primary purpose on earth is to seek God, hence his motto, "Quaerere Deum." St. Benedict worked miracles, could foretell the future, read minds, and drive out demons.

Exercise: How do you handle temptation? Do you pray for help and resist, or do you give in frequently? The devil is alive and well and tempts all of us daily. Pray to your Guardian Angel, St. Michael the Archangel, and St. Benedict to help you overcome these attacks by the devil.

There is a saying that an idle mind is the devil's workshop. Keep your mind busy by reading good books, cultivating hobbies, and devoting time to volunteer work and regular exercise.

Saint Veronica (died 1ˢᵗ Century)

And there followed him a great multitude of people, and of women who bewailed and lamented him. But Jesus turning to them said, "Daughters of Jerusalem, do not weep for me, but weep for yourselves and for your children."   *Luke 23:27-28*

Among my (Kevin's) most harrowing and yet enjoyable questions when interviewed about the book *Memorize the Faith!* was when Greg Willits of "The Catholics Next Door," threw at me, out of the blue, "By the way, Dr. Vost, what is the eighth Station of the Cross?" With God's grace, I recalled exactly "where" that station was in my system of mental locations, and immediately fired back, "Jesus meets the women of Jerusalem." Greg said he was impressed, but then admitted (kiddingly, I'm sure) that he didn't know himself and might have believed me if I said it was, "Jesus meets the women in the supermarket!" Of course, the 14 traditional Stations of the Cross are also a very serious and very profound devotion. St. Veronica appears in number six, where she famously wipes the face of the suffering Jesus on his way to Calvary. Veronica is not named in the Scriptures, but is the subject of many pious legends and traditions. The name Veronica actually means "true image," designating the true image of Christ's face that appeared on the towel that she used to comfort him.

Exercise: What practical lesson for tending our neighbor's temple might we learn from Veronica's simple act of charity to ease the pains of Christ? Here is a very direct lesson. The next time you work out with a friend or family member, bring along a small hand towel for him or her. Come to think of it, just last summer, when I ran 10 miles with a couple of running partners and we finished at an indoor/outdoor restaurant for an ice cold drink, I was able to say to one of them, "You know you have a true friend when she willingly wipes the dead bugs off your face!" Another idea is to bring along and share an extra bottle of water. In any case, let St. Veronica embody the true image of gentle kindness in your life.

July 13

St. Henry II (972-1024) Holy Roman Emperor

By justice, a king gives stability to the land.   *Proverbs 29:4*

Present glory is fleeting and meaningless while it is possessed unless in it we can glimpse something of heaven's eternity.   *St. Henry II*

Henry was born into a royal family but really just wanted to become a priest. When his father, the Duke of Bavaria, died, he had no choice but to take his place. Shortly thereafter, he had a very strange dream. His childhood teacher, St. Wolfgang, appeared to him and pointed to some words written on the wall that read, "After six." Henry spent much time puzzling over the meaning of these cryptic words. He assumed they referred to his death. His first guess was that he would die in six days, but he was still alive and perfectly healthy a week later. Was it six months? No, still going strong. Six years after the strange dream, he became the emperor of Germany, and he finally grasped the dream's meaning.

As emperor, Henry ruled wisely and with great virtue. He was forced to fight many wars but was a good and respected leader. Henry often had visions of angels and martyrs leading his soldiers into battle. Eventually he and his wife, Cunegundes (also a saint) were crowned as the Holy Roman Emperor and Empress. He was one of the greatest emperors and brought peace and prosperity to Europe and to the Church.

Exercise: You might not see angels like St. Henry did, but you are surrounded by them. Your guardian angel is always with you, and it's a good idea to pray to your angel daily for guidance and protection:

O Angel of God, my guardian dear, to whom God's love commits me here. Ever this day, be at my side to light and guard, to rule and guide. Amen.

Your guardian angel can also be your workout partner. Talk to your angel while you exercise and ask him to help you grow in holiness and strength.

Blessed Humbert (1200-1277)

The dogs came and licked his sores. *Luke 16:21*

In one of the most intriguing and impassioned letters of the thirteenth century, the general of a religious order pleaded with a most esteemed and learned colleague to resist the desires of the pope, decline a bishopric, and remain a great professor within the order. He told this great man that he would rather hear that he had died than that he had accepted the bishop's chair! His friend would reluctantly heed the pope's call, restore a financial and spiritually ruined diocese in less than three years, and then return to his order for the last 18 years of his life. The bishop was St. Albert the Great (Nov. 15), an almost exact contemporary with his Dominican Master General, Blessed Humbert of Romans, who would lead the Dominicans for nine years, preserve their rights to teach at the University of Paris, strengthen their ties with the Franciscans, and oversee the production of a Dominican lectionary. Oh, and about St. Luke and the dogs. A medieval pun called the Dominicans "the dogs of God," playing on the Latin words *Domini* (of God) and *canis* (dogs). St. Albert would say that the wounds were men's sins and the healing licks and barks of the dogs were the preaching of the Dominicans!

Exercise: A Dominican motto is to share with others the fruits of contemplation. Please allow me (Kevin) to share a fruitful little strength training technique I've been contemplating (and sometimes doing) for about 30 years now, since I first chanced upon it in the writings of Nautilus inventor and HIT founder, Arthur Jones. Select an exercise machine with one fixed movement arm (both legs or arms work together to lift the same stack of weights). Let's use a biceps curl as our example. Use about 70% of your normal poundage. Curl the weight like normal, but then gently shift the weight to only your right arm and slowly lower it in about four seconds. Curl it up again with both arms and now lower it only with your left. Up again with both, down now with right, etc. until you can't lower the weight slowly. You'll find *"negative accentuated"* training a great strength builder. I'm positive!

St. Bonaventure (1221-1274) Doctor of the Church

I will pray with the spirit, but I will also pray with the mind. I will sing praise with the spirit, but I will also sing praise with the mind.
1 Corinthians 14:15

When we pray, the voice of the heart must be heard more than that proceeding from the mouth.
St. Bonaventure

S t. Bonaventure's unusual name comes from St. Francis of Assisi (Oct. 4th). When Bonaventure was very sick as a baby, his mother begged St. Francis to pray for his recovery. The saint foresaw the great holiness of the tiny baby and declared, "O Buona Ventura!" which means "Oh good fortune!"

Bonaventure joined the Franciscans at age 22 and continued his education in Paris where he befriended St. Thomas Aquinas (Jan. 28th). St. Bonaventure took a leadership position in the Franciscan order and was instrumental in bringing the order back to the original teachings and philosophy of its saintly founder. His writings, still widely read today, are so filled with the Holy Spirit that he is often known as the "Seraphic Doctor." He is a mystic, a theologian, and a Doctor of the Church.

Exercise: Like St. Francis, St. Bonaventure loved nature. There is nothing quite as inspiring as spending time in prayer and meditation when surrounded by the beauty of nature. Today, combine your spiritual and physical exercises by praying or meditating while you walk, hike, run, bike, etc. in the beauty of nature. Perhaps you will find extra inspiration for both your meditation and your workout!

July 16

Our Lady of Mount Carmel

"Do whatever he tells you."   *John 2:5*

Today is a another feast day in honor of the Blessed Mother. According to Carmelite tradition, on July 16, 1251, Our Lady appeared to St. Simon Stock and promised special graces for those who would wear a brown scapular. Interpretations of this apparition and of the Holy Virgin's message have been refined throughout the centuries. Wearing the brown scapular is a sign of one's special devotion to Mary through affiliation with the Carmelite Order. It implies as well one's intention to grow in virtue like Mary, particularly through virtues of chastity and humility, and spiritual practices including readings and days of fasting from meat, with special attention to Saturdays consecrated to Our Lady of Mount Carmel.

By living a life of prayer and virtue with devotion to Mother Mary, we intend to do what "He" (Jesus) tells us to, through His own father's words: "Honor your father and your mother," (Exodus 20:12), and through His own words to His beloved friend John about His mother Mary, who is also mother to us all, "Behold, your mother!"

Exercise: Since our feast for the day honors Our Lady and includes some abstention from meat, this may be a good day for a simple "guy" recipe, perhaps saving the lady of your house from having to make lunch! OK, take a piece of wheat bread, put some natural peanut butter on it, spread as many shredded carrots as you can fit on top, smoosh another piece of bread on top, and eat it, preferably with a glass of milk. Between the bread, the peanut butter, the carrots, and the milk, you've got a nice little combination of complex carbohydrates, quality protein, healthy monosaturated fats, fiber, vitamins A, B complex, D, calcium, and more, and even a guy who burns microwave popcorn can make it safely.

St. Pope Leo IV (died 855)

Keep watch over yourselves and over the whole flock of which the Holy Spirit has appointed you overseers, in which you tend the church of God that he acquired with his own blood.　　*Acts 20:28*

[Pope Leo IV] was a Roman; in him the courage of the primitive ages of the republic was revived, in a time of cowardice and corruption, like some beautiful monument of ancient Rome that is sometimes found amidst the ruins of the new Rome.　　*Voltaire*

St. Leo IV, a Benedictine priest who was educated in Rome, was well known for his holiness. Rome was in a state of panic when Pope Sergius II died at the same time that rumors were circulating about an armed invasion by the fierce Saracens. The Church desperately needed a pope to lead them through this crisis, and to Leo's surprise, he was selected. Although reluctant to assume the office, he turned out to be a very good leader. He not only strengthened the defense of the city of Rome to prevent future attacks, but also rebuilt the Basilica of St. Peter. This newly fortified part of Rome, which includes the Vatican, is known as the Leonine City in his honor. Pope Leo established rules to help priests live holier lives and spread the use of Gregorian chant in the Mass. He was humble, cheerful, kind, fair, and worked many miracles. He died in 855 of natural causes.

Exercise: Have you ever listened Gregorian chant? It is a beautiful way of praying the liturgy. You can search online to find many examples. Download a few and add them to your musical library. You might even try to learn a few Latin phrases.

Protein helps build muscle and is a very important part of a daily diet, but it is easy to eat too much or too little. If you eat too much protein, it will break down and be stored as fat. If you eat too little, you risk muscle atrophy (wasting away) as well as a shortage of essential amino acids. Most dieticians recommend that protein should be about 20-30% of your total calories, roughly 50 grams per day for an adult. Keep a food diary today and find out how much protein you are really eating. Avoid eating a lot of red meat. Good sources of low-fat protein are beans, chicken, fish, egg whites, and Greek yogurt.

July 18

St. Camillus de Lellis (1550-1614)

Do not lift a weight beyond your strength. *Sirach 13:2*

Why are you afraid? Do you not realize that this is not your work but mine? *The voice of Christ on a cross to St. Camillus*

Who would have thought that this strapping, young, twenty-something, 6'6," quarrelsome solider and professional gambler would, by his mid-30s, found a religious community to provide tireless care for the sickest of the sick in hospitals and within their homes? Blessed with a powerful physique, St. Camillus would bear his own cross of illness with recurring ulcers on the feet and ankles. Still, this did not slow him down. After several failed attempts to reform his life, accepting the work of a laborer building a Franciscan monastery would finally lead to his lasting conversion. Encouraged by his confessor, St. Philip Neri (May 26), he would become a priest. His order, the Servants of the Sick, would become well-known in Italy by the red crosses upon their cassocks. St. Camillus would be declared a patron of the sick and of nurses.

Exercise: The book of Sirach abounds in practical wisdom. We literally should not lift a weight that exceeds our capacity to handle it with safe, effective form. And yet, through the wonderful mechanisms of muscular growth God has planted in our bodies, the weight that stops us cold today may be the weight we consider child's play a few months down the road. But we must let our bodies and God take their own time. Even the young and powerful like St. Camillus are susceptible to 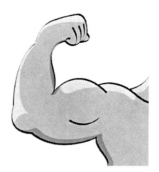 illness and injury. Teenage boys in particular should resist the urge to lift weights so heavy that proper form is compromised. It puts them risk of physical injury, and also at risk of pride and vanity. Better to take their time and grow in humility all the while.

St. Macrina (330-379) Saintly Sibling

By wisdom is a house built, by understanding is it made firm; And by knowledge are its rooms filled with every precious and pleasing possession.   *Proverbs 24:3-4*

[Macrina] reached the highest summit of human virtue by true wisdom.   *St. Gregory of Nyssa, brother of St. Macrina*

St. Macrina is the oldest daughter of two saints (Basil and Emmelia) and the sister of three more saints (Gregory of Nyssa, Basil the Great, and Peter of Sebaste). She was named after her grandmother, yet another saint as well as a martyr. What a holy and blessed home they must have lived in! Macrina helped to raise her nine brothers and sisters and influenced them greatly by her virtue and holiness. She was always sweet and cheerful, beloved by her siblings. Macrina was engaged to a young man who died before they could be married, and she decided to remain single and devote her life to God. Her brother, St. Basil the Great (Jan. 2), built a convent-like home for his mother, Macrina, and other young women to live in. After she died in 379, another brother, St. Gregory of Nyssa (Jan. 10), wrote about her life and holy example.

Exercise: If you have brothers and/or sisters, let them know how much you care for them. Give them a call this week and talk about a fond memory you shared. Pray for your siblings and their families. If you are estranged from a family member, pray for the grace of forgiveness. Swallow your pride and be the first to reach out to try to mend the relationship.

Carbohydrates are an important source of energy and should never be completely eliminated from the diet. You can certainly eat too many carbs, which will make you feel full at first but hungry again very quickly, as they are easily processed by the body. Too few carbs can be detrimental as well, leading to dehydration and loss of energy. Most nutrition experts recommend that a healthy diet should include 40-60% of calories from carbs. The key is to avoid highly processed and sugary carbs and to consume slow-digesting whole grains. Keep a food diary today to see if you are getting the right amount.

St. Joseph Barsabbas (1ˢᵗ Century)

And they put forward two, Joseph called Barsabbas, who was
surnamed Justus, and Matthias. Acts 1:23

St. Joseph Barsabbas could be unofficially considered a patron saint of runners-ups or also-rans. He appears in the New Testament when a group of about 120 of Christ's followers met to select the man to take the place of Judas Iscariot among the 12 Apostles. When lots were cast, Matthias won out over Joseph Barsabbas, but Joseph was no sore loser. Note his surname, Justus, "the just." Notice, too, that after all, we honor him today as a saint. St. John Chrysostom wrote that Barsabbas was full of joy for Matthias. Ancient church historian Eusebius wrote that he became one of the 72 disciples spreading the Gospel of Christ far and wide.

Exercise: The virtue of justice entails giving others their rightful due. While the general principles for tending our bodily temples with sensible exercise and nutrition applies to individuals of all ages, we should bear in mind that certain age groups should be paid their rightful due for their needs and concerns, as well as for the strengths and limitations that tend to be unique to them. Today, let's consider those in the "middle age," perhaps 40 to 60 or so. Some of these more fortunate folks can claim that they still weigh what they did in their 20s. Still, even for them, the odds are that their weight has remained stable because their accumulation of fat has been matched by their loss of muscle! If we don't use it, we lose it! Fortunately, God has given us muscles that can respond and grow, even in our 80s, and perhaps beyond.

OK, what are you going to do to do your own body justice and tend to your temple today? Whether a grueling HIT workout, a moderate Rosary Workout, a leisurely stroll, or a little focused "house aerobics," let's help build the virtue of justice within our own souls today.

July 21

St. Lawrence of Brindisi (1559-1619)
Apostolic Doctor of the Church

For God so loved the world that he gave his only Son, so that everyone who believes in him might not perish but might have eternal life.   *John 3:16*

God is love, and all his operations proceed from love. Once he wills to manifest that goodness by sharing his love outside himself, then the Incarnation becomes the supreme manifestation of his goodness and love and glory.   *St. Lawrence of Brindisi*

St. Lawrence was born as Caesar Rossi in Italy, but took the name Lawrence when he became a Capuchin Franciscan. He was sent to Padua to be educated and proved to be a brilliant scholar. He mastered six languages and studied the Bible extensively. Lawrence became a priest and was a sought after preacher because he spoke so many different languages. The emperor of Austria asked him to convince the German rulers to fight against the Turks. They agreed, but insisted that the saint accompany them in battle. Fearlessly, Lawrence led the soldiers into battle armed only with a crucifix. Inspired, the troops followed him and soundly defeated the Turkish attackers. St. Lawrence wrote many volumes of inspired letters and sermons. After his death, his fellow Capuchins published them. As a result, St. Lawrence was declared an Apostolic Doctor of the Church in 1959.

Exercise: As St. Lawrence showed, the power of the cross can work miracles. Try to spend some time each week, especially on Fridays, contemplating Jesus' Passion and death. Reflecting on His example of humility and suffering can help you deal with your daily trials. Many people think that fat is to be avoided in the diet, but this is not the case. Fat is an important source of fuel for endurance sports and activities, helps you to feel full after eating, and aids in the absorption of certain vitamins. The key is to avoid unhealthy, saturated fat and eat more unsaturated fat. Good sources are olive or canola oil, nuts, avocados, and natural peanut butter. Aim to eat no more than 30% of your total daily calories from fat. A food diary will help keep you on track.

St. Mary Magdalene (1ˢᵗ Century)

"Her sins, which are many, are forgiven, for she loved much."

Luke 7:47

Details regarding the identity and the life of Mary Magdalene have given rise to differing opinions among Greek and Latin Church Fathers and Protestant scholars as well. Recent writers of fiction (sometimes portrayed as fact) have gone beyond the pale with their unfounded speculations of her relationship with Christ. Of one thing all parties seem certain, and that is that she loved Jesus Christ and that He loved her as well. There are also other things we know from the explicit authority of the Scriptures and Church teaching; she appears in all four Gospels, seven demons had been cast out of her, she stood at the foot of the cross, assisted in Jesus' entombment, and was the first person to encounter the resurrected Christ. There are also reasons, when the narratives of the Gospels of Sts. Luke and John are compared, to identify her as the woman who washed Jesus' feet and anointed Him with ointment, with Mary of Bethany and with the sister of Martha and Lazarus. Her name, Magdalene, may derive from the gentile town of Magdala, but may also derive from a Jewish Talmudic term for adulteress.

In any event, her depths of repentance, contrition of heart, and devotion to Jesus Christ cannot be denied. She is a lesson to us all, that regardless of our past, God stands ready to forgive and welcome us with His loving arms.

Exercise: Mary's anointing the feet of Christ was an incredibly caring gesture of honoring and tending to his holy bodily temple. Indeed, she had wiped his feet with her long, flowing hair and her free flowing tears of repentance. Here is something to think about and act upon today: How can you show care and respect for the very bodies of your loved ones and friends today? Can you spare a non-hasty kiss or a backrub for your spouse, a hug for your child, a hearty handshake or pat on the back for a friend? If we would become as "dynamos of charity,' then today is the day we should start tending to some temples besides our own!

St. Bridget of Sweden (1303-1373)
Apostle of the Passion of Jesus

The Son of Man must suffer greatly and be rejected by the elders, the chief priests, and the scribes, and be killed and on the third day be raised.   *Luke 9:22*

There is no sinner in the world, however much at enmity with God, who cannot recover God's grace by recourse to Mary, and by asking her assistance.   *St. Bridget of Sweden*

I (Peggy) discovered St. Bridget of Sweden when a friend gave me a copy of the wonderful *Pieta Prayer Book*. I truly enriched my prayer life by praying her Fifteen Prayers daily for one year, and I am now very devoted to frequent meditation on Jesus' Passion.

St. Bridget had visions of Jesus at a very young age which would continue throughout her life. She married a Swedish prince who was also very devout. (Their daughter, Catherine is a saint.) When she received a message from Jesus, she spent much time and effort to ensure that the message was given to as many people as possible, gently explaining and encouraging the people to conform to God's will. When her husband died, St. Bridget left the royal life behind and founded the Order of the Savior, also known as the Bridgettines. Bridget encouraged everyone to meditate on the Passion and death of Christ. She went on a pilgrimage to the Holy Land, and Jesus appeared to her and told her of the events in His Passion and Crucifixion as she visited the holy sites. Her writings were published after her death and are still widely read today.

Exercise: You can easily find the Fifteen Prayers of St. Bridget online. After reading them, meditate on the Passion of Christ during your walk, run, or cardio workout today. If you meditate on each prayer for just two minutes, you'll easily complete a 30-minute workout. If you have trouble memorizing the general topics of the Fifteen Prayers, perhaps you might be interested in the wonderful book, *Memorize the Faith*, by one of my brilliant co-authors, Dr. Kevin Vost.

St. Christina the Astonishing (1150-1254)

Therefore, behold, I will again do marvelous things with this people, wonderful and marvelous.   Isaiah 29:14

There is more than one St. Christina. A third century saint of Tyre, Lebanon, St. Christina underwent brutally torturous martyrdom at the hand of her own father for her ardent devotion to Christ. St. Christina Mirabilis (the Astonishing) is unique among saints in that her saintly behavior is not exactly a model for imitation, yet the lessons of her strange, though saintly life, are nonetheless profound. Her story is told by Thomas of Cantimpre, a learned Dominican and student of St. Albert the Great (Nov. 15). Born in Belgium and orphaned at 15, at 21, St. Christina suffered such a massive seizure that she was believed to be dead. She astonished the crowd at the funeral, however, when she arose from her coffin. She astonished them all the more when she levitated to the rafters, told the crowd that she could not bear the smell of their sins, and commenced to tell them of her journey to purgatory, hell, and then heaven. She was known for violent fits of ecstasy. She would, for example, throw herself into the River Meuse and allow the currents to take her down to the mill which would whirl her around frightfully, but without bodily injury. A patroness of mental disorders and mental health workers, she calls our attention to the dignity of all of God's children, whether sound or not in mind and body.

Exercise: Since Christina flew up to the rafters, we might as well talk about "flies." Dumbbell flies are performed while lying on a flat, inclined, or declined weightlifting bench. Using lighter weights than what you would use for a pressing motion; press the dumbbells up at arm's length until your elbows are nearly locked. Then bring the dumbbells down to your sides in a wide, semi-circular arch until you achieve a mild stretch in your chest muscles and shoulders. Repeat for a controlled set until you are a repetition or so from failure. To achieve astonishing results while avoiding injury, these should always be performed in a slow and controlled manner.

St. Christopher (3ʳᵈ Century) Patron Saint of Travelers

He summoned the Twelve and began to send them out two by two and gave them authority over unclean spirits. He instructed them to take nothing for the journey but a walking stick—no food, no sack, no money in their belts.   Mark 6:7-8

Grant me, O Lord, a steady hand and watchful eye that no one shall be hurt as I pass by. You gavest life, I pray no act of mine may take away or mar that gift of thine. Shelter those, dear Lord, who bear my company, from the evils of fire and all calamity. Teach me, to use my car for others' need, nor miss through love of undue speed the beauty of the world; that thus I may with joy and courtesy go on my way. St. Christopher, holy patron of travelers, protect me and lead me safely to my destiny. Amen.   St. Christopher's Prayer for Travelers

My (Peggy's) family is very devoted to St. Christopher. Not only are we a military family who travels frequently, but we also spent four years on the road in an RV. We keep a St. Christopher medal in all our vehicles, and we pray the St. Christopher Prayer (above) before every trip. We have traveled hundreds of thousands of miles without incident. Little is actually known about St. Christopher, who was martyred sometime during the third century. Most of his story is legend. It is said that he was a very strong and well-built man who happened to meet a hermit living beside a dangerous stream. The hermit knew the water well and would guide travelers to the best place to cross. St. Christopher took the hermit's place and made crossing the stream even easier by carrying travelers across himself. One day a small child asked for a crossing, and St. Christopher figured it would be an easy trip. Not so! The child grew heavier with each step. When they finally reached the other side, the child revealed to Christopher that he was Christ and baptized the saint on the spot.

Exercise: Do you pray before you travel? If not, you are missing the protection and blessing of a very powerful intercessor. Pray for St. Christopher's protection for your family. The next time you travel, be sure to plan for workouts. Pack a pair of walking or running shoes. Stay in hotels with fitness centers or near a park where you can exercise.

Sts. Joachim and Anne (1ˢᵗ Century)

Honor your father and your mother.   *Exodus 20:10*

I must admit that I've never really reflected upon Blessed Mary as a child or Jesus as a grandson. That Mary had parents we can be certain of; that their names were Joachim and Anne we glean from traditions and apocryphal literature dating to the middle of the second century. The writings report, in a story that echoes the Scriptural account of the birth of Samuel, that Joachim, a godly man, was rebuked for being childless when he attempted to offer sacrifice at the temple. An angel appeared to both of them and foretold that Anne (Hannah, meaning "grace" in the Hebrew) would be cured of her sterility and would bear them a child that would be blessed by the entire world. They would name her Miriam (Mary) and blessed she would be, above all women and mortal men. St. Anne would, over the centuries, become venerated in the East and in the West, indeed, so far west that she is the patroness of Brittany, and also Quebec in Canada.

Exercise: Being full of grace and without sin, we can imagine that Mary must have honored her parents in the greatest abundance. We can imagine the joy this godly couple took in their sinless child, and perhaps the way she parented Jesus was patterned on lessons she learned from her saintly parents. What lessons are we teaching our children in terms of tending their temples? In psychology the "Premack Principle" is sometimes called "Grandma's Law" – first you work, then you play! Do we allow our children to sit in front of electronic devices for hours on end, rarely ever getting up to exercise body parts besides their thumbs? Do we allow them to gorge on convenience foods, rarely getting around to the fruits and vegetables? It is up to us to set up sedentary pleasures and sweet or salty delights as limited special treats, as icing on the cake, not as complete replacements for the cakes of invigorating exercise, outside play, and consumption of wholesome, hearty foods, the kinds that Jesus, Mary, and Joseph (and Joachim and Anne) would have consumed.

St. Pantaleon (275-305) Martyr

S t. Pantaleon was a Christian doctor from Asia who was so well-known that the pagan Emperor Maximilian requested him as his personal physician. Pantaleon was lured by the lavish lifestyle of the emperor and began to express interest in the pagan gods, eventually renouncing his faith. When a kind and holy priest began to gently question his turning away from Christ, Pantaleon repented and began to work among the sick, healing many with prayer rather than science and never asking for payment for his services. When the emperor began to persecute Christians, Pantaleon was arrested. He and a pagan doctor were both told to cure a paralyzed man. The pagan doctor's incantations were ineffective, but Pantheon worked a miracle and the man was healed. Many pagans converted to Christianity because of his very public miracle. The enraged emperor decreed that the saint should be put to death, but this was easier said than done. First, Pantheon was tortured on a rack and burned with torches. During his torments, Christ appeared to him and gave him strength. Then he was lowered into a pot of molten lead, but the fire went out and the lead became cold. Next, he was tied to a huge stone and thrown into the sea, but the stone miraculously floated. When he was bound to a wheel, the ropes snapped and the wheel broke. Wild animals were brought in to kill him, but they calmly lay down at his feet. Finally, he was then nailed to a tree and beheaded.

Exercise: In this world of New Age spirituality, it's easy to be led astray. Be firm in your faith and avoid influences that could sway it. Pray for guidance if you are tempted to explore other religions. It's also best to avoid New Age exercise like yoga. Although the Church has not officially "banned" yoga, it has emphasized discernment. I (Peggy) used to take yoga classes, but discontinued them as I read more about how they can become a negative influence. If you enjoy yoga, read more about it to ensure that you are not being led down the wrong path. It can be helpful to consult a priest or spiritual advisor.

St. Samson (died-565)

*Out of the eater came something to eat. Out of the strong came
something sweet.*   *Judges 14:14*

This St. Samson is not the Herculean Hebrew of the
book of Judges, but a holy, sixth century Welshman.
St. Samson became a priest and a monk, and like
many of his Celtic counterparts, imbued a great missionary
zeal for winning souls to Christ and founding monasteries
to God's glory. When travelling Irish monks visited his
monastery on their return trip from Rome, he was moved
by the holiness of the abbot and travelled to Ireland, where
he was caught up in the holy ardor of so many missionary-
minded Irish saints. He was made a bishop in 521, and he
travelled to Cornwall, the Channel Islands, and Brittany,
establishing monasteries at Cornwall and at Dol in Brittany.
He was known as a miracle-worker and was also known for
his powerful strength of self-discipline, refraining from
alcohol and meat at all times, and frequently fasting.

Exercise: The Biblical Samson is an incredible model of
fortitude, of the ability to do hard things through the strength
derived from God (like defeating 1,000 Philistines with the
jawbone of an ass as his weapon – nicely portrayed by Victor
Mature in the old *Samson and Delilah* movie, by the way.) I (Kevin)
recall that in the muscle magazines of my youth, they ran ads for
these "Samson" cables, or chest expanders as they used to be
called. Cables or "stretch cords" are simple tools that can still be
incorporated in one's home training for muscles like the biceps,
triceps, and shoulders. St. Samson is an equally powerful model
of temperance in his dietary self-control. I've have recently
decided to follow the Church's ancient precept of fasting from
meat on all Fridays for its spiritual and physical benefits. St.
Samson will be my intercessor as I strive to maintain this
discipline for tending the temple, making it something like a
monastery in honor of the Holy Spirit it houses. (Oh, and see
Judges 14 for the answer to Samson's riddle in our quotation du
jour.)

St. Martha (died c. 82) Friend of Jesus

The Lord said to her in reply, "Martha, Martha, you are anxious and worried about many things. There is need of only one thing. Mary has chosen the better part and it will not be taken from her."

Luke 10:41-42

Martha had the supreme honor of being a close friend of Jesus, but she still managed to complain. One day while Jesus and his followers were staying at her house, she was busy in the kitchen preparing food for everyone. Someone had to feed all these hungry men. Her sister Mary, however, chose to stay with the men and listen to what Jesus had to say. Martha didn't bother to nudge her sister or whisper that she needed help. Instead she went right to Jesus and asked Him to make her sister help her! Jesus gently rebuked her and told her that her sister had made a better choice. I (Peggy) always wonder if she just took off her apron at this point and sat down to listen too. We do know that later she expressed faith that Jesus was the Son of God before Jesus raised her brother Lazarus from the dead. According to some accounts, after Jesus' Ascension into heaven, Martha, Mary, Lazarus and other followers of Jesus were captured by the Jews, put in a boat with no sails or oars, and set out to sea. They arrived safely in Marseilles, France. Martha lived with a group of holy women, worked many miracles, and died peacefully. St. Martha is often depicted with a dragon at her feet due to an interesting legend. Apparently a beast of some sort was terrorizing the town where she lived. Martha fearlessly approached it, threw holy water on it, held up a crucifix, and bound it with her girdle so that it could be slain.

Exercise: It's important to get the house clean, the dishes done, the laundry folded, the grass mowed, and the car washed, but prayer is even more important. Pray FIRST, and then take the time to finish your chores. Better yet, pray WHILE you're doing them! Do your chores vigorously, and you'll even get some exercise.

St. Mary of Jesus Venegas de la Torre (1868-1959)

Be fruitful and multiply, and fill the earth...   *Genesis 1:28*

Here is a classic test case for our modern secular Planned Parenthood mentality. What possible good could come from the twelfth-born child of a poor Mexican family? Well, how about a saint who established a holy religious order to care for the sick? St. Mary of Jesus is but one of countless saintly examples of the fruits that can flow from the families who follow God's first commandment to humanity, "be fruitful and multiply!" (Even despite my [Kevin's] first-born pride, I thank God regularly that Ladolfo and Theodora of Aquino were open to the birth of their seventh-born, Thomas.) Maria Navidad Venegas joined the Association of the Daughters of Mary in 1898. She went to Guadalajara to join a community of sisters caring for the sick in a hospital, and in 1921, she was elected its superior general. She renamed it Sisters of the Sacred Heart of Jesus and professed her vows as *Maria de Jesus Sacramentado*, Mary of Jesus in the Sacrament. She was canonized by Pope John Paul II on May 21, 2000.

Exercise: St. Mary was deeply devoted to the Sacred Heart of Jesus and to caring for the sick. Of course, in our day, in our affluent culture, heart disease is among the most common kinds of sickness. Though our genetics certainly play a role, through proper diet and exercise, we can recognize that our own literal hearts and the hearts of our loved ones are sacred parts of our bodily temples. So absorbed in writing that I'd become overly sedentary and had let my dietary habits slip, I found myself with a cholesterol reading of over 200 a couple of years ago. After several months of daily intake of oats (through hot and cold oatmeal, Cheerios, and even added oats to protein drinks in a blender), I dropped it 40 points and required no medication. From thenceforth, I've vowed to tend with care the Sacred Heart of Jesus and the sacred heart of my temple!

St. Ignatius of Loyola – Founder of the Jesuit Order

Trust in the LORD with all your heart, on your own intelligence rely not; In all your ways be mindful of him, and he will make straight your paths.   *Proverbs 3:5-6*

Act as if everything depended on you; trust as if everything depended on God.   *St. Ignatius of Loyola*

St. Ignatius had quite an exciting childhood. He served as a page in the Spanish court of King Ferdinand and Queen Isabella. He wanted to grow up, marry a beautiful princess, and become a soldier. He joined the military and fought bravely but was injured in battle when a cannonball broke his leg. During his recovery, Ignatius became bored and wanted to read. The only books available were the Bible and lives of the saints, so Ignatius reluctantly decided to read them. They changed his life, making him realize that he no longer wanted glory, riches, or beautiful women but to imitate the virtues of the saints. He left the military and made a pilgrimage to the Holy Land. Ignatius continued his education and became a priest, later founding the order of the Society of Jesus, or the Jesuits. His famous "Spiritual Exercises" are still widely read and studied today.

Exercise: Learn more about St. Ignatius' spiritual exercises at IgnatianSpirituality.com. The publisher of this book, Cheryl Dickow, was profoundly influenced by a class she took on this subject. The emphasis is on deeper prayer, service to others, and good decisions based on keen discernment.

Reading about Jesus and the saints made St. Ignatius happy. One easy way to improve your physical health is to smile. Look at the bright side of life and thank God for your blessings. People who are happy are healthier and have less stress in their lives. Laughter really is one of the best medicines.

St. Alphonsus Liguori (1696-1787)

If any man would come after me, let him deny himself and take up his cross daily and follow me.   *Luke 9:23*

When we try to avoid a cross that the Lord has sent to us, we often meet with another, and a much heavier one.   *St. Alphonsus Liguori*

Modern-day Liguorians certainly share in the holy and forgiving spirit of their founder. I (Kevin) had hoped there would be no ill feelings when the illustrator of my *Memorize the Faith!* depicted this great saint as a tipsy elephant standing on two legs, holding a bottle of liquor in a brown paper bag! You see, the intent was to honor him as a representation of a great saint born in the seventeenth century, and "elephant-liquor" was simply a very concrete and memorable visual image that sounded like Alphonse Liguori! And I knew I'd been forgiven (or that they'd never seen it) when I had the honor of writing an article, *Tending the Temple: On Faith and Fitness,* for the May 2011 issue of *Liguorian Magazine*! Its great namesake held degrees in both canon and civil law, organized a religious order, The Congregation of the Holy Redeemer (Redemptorists), wrote 60 books, and became bishop at 66. He pledged not to waste a minute of time that could be used to do God's work. He persevered despite many physical ailments, including rheumatism.

Exercise: Let's focus on two of this great Doctor's themes – suffering and use of time. There is an old saying that those who can't make the time to care for their health will eventually have to find the time to be sick. Though there may be mild suffering involved in doing a hard strength or cardio workout, or in passing up a second helping of a desert, they reduce our chances of being laid low by an illness or plain-old lack of energy. They provide no guarantees, though. But let's bear in mind that in bearing our suffering patiently and offering it up to Christ; we can glorify God even when it's time for resting and mending the temple.

St. Eusebius of Vercelli (c. 283-371) Bishop

My sheep hear my voice; I know them, and they follow me. I give them eternal life, and they shall never perish. No one can take them out of my hand. My Father, who has given them to me, is greater than all, and no one can take them out of the Father's hand. The Father and I are one.   *John 10:27-30*

With his sound formation in the Nicene faith, Eusebius did his utmost to defend the full divinity of Jesus Christ, defined by the Nicene Creed as "of one being with the Father."   *Pope Benedict XVI*

S t. Eusebius was the son of a martyr who lived a holy life and became a priest. The people of his town approved of his pious lifestyle and asked him to become their bishop. He combined monastic and clerical life, renewing the priesthood in the Western Church. Eusebius was very eloquent and solved many problems. Pope Liberius asked him to talk to the emperor who was practicing the Arian heresy, telling the people that Jesus was not God. Eusebius tried to convince the emperor of the error of his ways, but he refused to listen and sent the saint to Palestine. The Arians later kidnapped Eusebius, dragged him through the streets and locked him in a cell with very little food and water. He was eventually released when the Arian emperor died. Eusebius spent his remaining days preaching about the truths of Christianity. He hand-wrote a copy of the Gospels, which is still preserved in a cathedral in Vercelli.

Exercise: Today is my son (Peggy's) birthday. Like St. Eusebius, he is very eloquent and explains complicated ideas in a very simple manner, perhaps an influence from the saint who shares this day with him.

Do you pray with your family? There's a saying that: "The family that prays together stays together." A good time to do this is right before bed. Make it a habit, and your children will likely do the same with their own children. You'll be spreading the blessings of this habit through future generations. It's also important to be sure your children exercise regularly and eat a healthy diet. Be a good example for them and they will someday do the same for their own children.

St. Lydia (1ˢᵗ Century)

One who heard us was a woman named Lydia from the city of Thyatira, a seller of purple goods, who was a worshipper of God. The Lord opened her heart to give heed to what was said by Paul.

Acts 16:14

This lay businesswoman, born in Thyatira, Lydia (modern-day Turkey), was a trader in expensive purple-dyed goods (hence also known as *St. Lydia Purpuria*) and was also St. Paul's first known convert! God made her heart receptive to Paul's teaching and she responded by embracing God, seeking baptism for her entire household, and also by extending her hospitality to St. Paul, allowing him to stay at her house in Philippi, Macedonia. Soon after, Sts. Paul and Silas were placed in jail. After their escape, they visited St. Lydia before they departed from the town. Certainly St. Lydia's story spoke to St. Brigid's (Feb. 1) own heart – so enterprising, devout, courageous, generous, and a trusted friend of other saints!

Exercise: Christ tells us in the St. John's Gospel (3:5) that we must be born "of water and the Spirit" to enter the kingdom of God. Note well how St. Lydia sought this baptism for her entire family, and St. Paul obliged them in the local river. Water is the essential material, earthly element in the holy sacrament of baptism. Water is, of course, essential to our bodily health as well. Let's remember, then, to take in plenty of water before, after, and during longer workouts. Studies have shown as well that drinking two cups of water before a meal is likely to help people feel full, even while taking in less food and fewer calories. Indeed, drinking very cold water also burns calories in itself, because the body uses food energy to maintain the good old 98.6° inside! While we must constantly replenish our water supplies, bear well in mind that the water of our baptism carries an indelible spiritual mark that cannot be washed away. What acts of kindness and hospitality might we do for others today that will show we've not forgotten that saving, indelible mark?

St. Jean-Marie-Baptiste Vianney (1786-1859)
The Curé of Ars

This humble patron saint of priests was sent away by his superiors to Ars, an insignificant little farming village in France, because of his poor academic performance in seminary. There he found the people living immoral lives with no regard for God. With firm resolve, he lived a life of consistent devotion and holy purity, which gave great example to the people of Ars. Moved by his life of holy integrity, they flocked to hear him preach. By God's grace, this humble priest converted the entire town, packing the once-empty church with newly devout souls, while the once-full taverns closed down for lack of patronage! Word spread quickly and penitents came to him by the hundreds each day from the surrounding villages. He heard their confessions for 13-17 hours a day, telling them hidden facts about their lives and sometimes predicting the future. He sobbed in misery at the thought of unrepentant souls losing the gift of salvation forever, and imposed great deprivations upon his own body in order to win the grace of forgiveness for them. For more than 30 years, he was visited by Satan, who attacked him nightly with great physical torments, and unsuccessfully tried to win him over through pride in his accomplishments. After 41 years of service, his body was finally laid to rest in the little town. 500,000 pilgrims visit Ars each year, asking his intercession and marveling at the sight of his body, which lies incorrupt to this day.

Exercise: Let's pray today for those who are disabled, especially those who desire to be in the presence of Our Lord in the Blessed Sacrament, but are not able. Every disability is a sign of the temporary nature of our bodies. We are all imperfect, awaiting the glory of the Resurrection. The very aspects of ourselves that appear to others as limitations are signs from God, drawing us into deeper awareness of our need for Him, in Whom we find completion.

Dedication of St. Mary ad Nives (358-present)

He gives snow like wool; he scatters hoarfrost like ashes. *Psalms 147:16*

Today is the feast of a dedication of a very special temple, the Basilica of Mary Major in Rome. My (Kevin's) family and I were blessed to see this magnificent tribute to Mary, gold ceiling and all, in 2005, the week of Pope John Paul II's funeral. The fascinating story of this church goes back just about 1,647 years before that visit, though. Legend has it that a Roman patrician named John, and his wife, had no heirs. They vowed to Blessed Mary to give her their possessions and they prayed for guidance on how to bestow them. The story goes that Mary came to John in a vision and a miraculous summer snowfall fell on the Esquiline hill on the night of August 4th and 5th, in the year 358, during the pontificate of Pope Liberius. We do know as fact that it was dedicated by Pope Sixtus III around the year 435; shortly after, at the Council of Ephesus, the Virgin Mary was declared "Theotokos," the Mother of God. (Photos of this incredible basilica are certainly worth a view on the internet.)

Exercise: Snow provides all kinds of opportunities for exercise. Cross-country skiers have been found to have, among all athletes, some of the greatest aerobic capacity, and some exercise machines have been designed to replicate their motions, involving the arms and legs and a great majority of the body's muscles. Snow also provides dangers. We had the heaviest snowfall I can recall just two weeks ago here in Springfield, IL. Perhaps you have heard of the proverbial case of the sedentary, middle-aged man who goes out to shovel his driveway and dies of a heart attack. Well, we had at least one such case this time. The combination of heavy exertion and cold can prove deadly to the unconditioned or those with heart disease. If you have strengthened your skeletal muscles and perhaps become adapted to the cold by some outdoor walking or running in the winter, your risk should decrease, but you should still always exercise caution and never use snow shoveling as your high intensity workout to failure!

Feast of the Transfiguration

[Jesus] took Peter, John, and James and went up the mountain to pray. While he was praying his face changed in appearance and his clothing became dazzling white. And behold, two men were conversing with him, Moses and Elijah, who appeared in glory and spoke of his exodus that he was going to accomplish in Jerusalem.
Luke 9:28-31

For a moment Jesus discloses his divine glory... He also reveals that he will have to go by the way of the cross at Jerusalem in order to "enter into his glory." Moses and Elijah had seen God's glory on the Mountain; the Law and the Prophets had announced the Messiah's sufferings. Christ's Passion is the will of the Father: the Son acts as God's servant; the cloud indicates the presence of the Holy Spirit.
Catechism of the Catholic Church, Section 555

Today we honor the day when Jesus showed His three chosen Apostles a glimpse of His glorified body. He knew that these men would be leaders in His new Church, so He wanted to strengthen their faith before His Passion and death. In this scene, Moses represents the Law and Elijah represents the prophets. They disappear, leaving only Jesus to show that He is the fulfillment of the law and that the prophets have pointed to Him. To make this clear, a voice from heaven says, "This is my beloved Son. Listen to HIM." Jesus is now the authority, not the prophets or the Mosaic law. The details of the Transfiguration are recorded in Matthew 17:1-8, Mark 9:2-9, and Luke 9:28-36. Most biblical scholars believe this event took place on Mount Tabor. The Feast of the Transfiguration was put on the Roman calendar by Pope Callistus III in 1457.

Exercise: In honor of this feast, pray the Luminous Mysteries of the Rosary today. Fervently pray for discernment to listen to the voice of Jesus and tune out all the distractions that prevent you from doing this. There are 4,300 steps on Mount Tabor, which were built in the 4th century for Christian pilgrims. It takes roughly 2,000 steps to walk a mile (1,400 if you're running). Make it a goal to walk, run or climb (on stairs or a Stairmaster) 4,300 steps as you meditate on the mystery of the Transfiguration. This may require several exercise sessions. For inspiration, read the three Gospel accounts of the Transfiguration, as listed above.

St. Cajetan (1480-1547)

If I am delayed, you may know how one ought to behave in the household of the living God...   1 Timothy 3:15

Gaento die Conti di Tiene was born to a wealthy, noble family at Vicenza in the Republic of Venice. He obtained a double doctorate in canon and civil law, and headed off to Rome to work as a diplomat for Pope Julius II. In 1516, he became a priest, and in 1523, he withdrew from the papal court to establish an association of priests called The Oratory of Divine Love. This was a most tumultuous time in Church history. With clerical morals at low ebb, many Christians had chosen to rend asunder that one, holy, catholic, and apostolic Church of the Creed. Indeed, Rome was sacked in 1527, and St. Cajetan was scourged. Our saint, however, strove to strengthen the Church's pillars and to shore up its 1,500-year-old bulwark. For example, to counteract the divisiveness of the groups that had split from the Church, he initiated the Forty Hours Adoration of the Blessed Sacrament. He expressed a special devotion to the Virgin Mary, and he chose to work with the poorest of the poor and tend to the sick. He sought to reignite the regular clergy with the spirit of monastic self-discipline and works of active, caring ministry.

Exercise: A pillar supports something, and a bulwark protects it from harm. That is the role played by the Church in supporting and defending the truth of God. What might we say is the pillar and bulwark of our bodily temples? Speaking on a purely physical level, this would be our skeletal muscles. We cannot stand without the pillars that are our legs. It is muscle as well that can protect our internal organs and tissues from trauma. Strength training, then, is a pillar and bulwark of our fitness training, and should not be neglected if it is safe for you to perform. It pays real benefits in daily life, too. Studies reported in journals of gerontology have reported that measured strength on the leg press machine correlated with greater capacity for activities of daily living among elderly women; and further, that active elderly women may outperform inactive elderly women a decade younger. And this applies just as well to us men!

St. Dominic (1170-1221) The Rosary Saint

Then he said to the disciple, "Behold, your mother."   *John 19:27*

Nothing seems tiresome or painful when you are working for a Master who pays well; who rewards even a cup of cold water given for love of Him.   *St. Dominic*

St. Dominic was educated under the tutelage of priestly uncle, so it was no surprise when he too became a priest. He felt called by God to start a new preaching order, which was called the Dominicans in his honor. At the time, there were several heresies spreading rapidly through the Church, and St. Dominic was praying devoutly to the Blessed Mother as to how to combat them. Mary suddenly appeared to St. Dominic and told him to pray her Psalter (an early form of the Rosary) in order to defeat the heresies. Dominic did as Our Lady asked, with near miraculous results. Some people mistakenly think that St. Dominic was the first person to ever be given a Rosary. Those who study the history of the Rosary know that the origins of the Blessed Mother's favorite prayer can be found well before St. Dominic's time. He certainly does deserve credit for spreading its devotion, however. Today, the Dominicans administer the Confraternity of the Most Holy Rosary. Anyone who pledges to pray one 15-decade Rosary each week can join. There are many blessings and benefits attached to membership in this group.

Dominic was a good friend of St. Francis of Assisi (Oct. 4) and both these holy men converted many hearts and minds through the teachings of their respective orders, both alive and well today.

Exercise: Learn more about the Confraternity of the Most Holy Rosary at www.Rosary-Center.org. If you are willing to commit just one hour a week to praying the Rosary (Glorious, Sorrowful and Joyful mysteries), consider joining this group. If you pray the Rosary while you exercise, you can fulfill your commitment with three 20-minute workouts each week, the minimum most experts recommend for cardiovascular health.

August 9

St. Teresia Benedicta of the Cross (1891-1942)

I am the way, and the truth, and the life.   *John 14:6*

One cannot desire freedom from the cross when one is especially chosen for the cross.   St. Teresia Benedicta of the Cross

As a gifted student who was raised in a religious tradition, embraced atheism in her teens, sought truth in philosophy, and was surprised to find it many years later in the writings of a great saint and Doctor of the Church, this is my (Kevin's) kind of saint! Edith Stein was the eleventh child of an Orthodox Jewish family. She rejected a belief in God in her teens and studied philosophy under the prestigious phenomenologist, Edmund Husserl, a thinker who would also influence Pope John Paul II. Her eyes were opened to the truth of Christ when she read the autobiography of St. Teresa of Avila (Oct. 15). Further, she would later translate, into German, the great *De Veritate* (On Truth) of St. Thomas Aquinas (Jan. 28) and declare herself a Thomist! She became a Discalced Carmelite nun in 1933, taking the name St. Teresia Benedicta of the Cross. As the Nazi menace grew in strength, her order transferred her from Germany to the Netherlands. On July 20, 1942, the Dutch Bishop's Conference issued a statement denouncing Nazi racism. Six days later, the Nazis began rounding up people of Jewish ancestry for their death camps. On August 9, 1942, St. Teresia would begin her new life with Christ after suffering martyrdom in a gas chamber at Auschwitz.

Exercise: Young Edith Stein learned things about the importance of the mind and unique personal, spiritual experience from Professor Husserl's phenomenological philosophy. When the mature Sister Teresia Benedicta embraced Thomism, she understood as well the truth that the human person is "hylomorphic," matter-and-form, body-and-soul unity. St. Thomas wrote that health is to the body as virtues are to the soul. St. Teresia embodied that ultimate godly fortitude that can sacrifice even the earthly body for the glory of God and the eventual reward of a glorified body in heaven.

St. Lawrence (100-158) Martyr

Beloved, do not be surprised that a trial by fire is occurring among you, as if something strange were happening to you. But rejoice to the extent that you share in the sufferings of Christ.   *1 Peter 4:12-13*

"Father, where are you going without your deacon?" asks St. Lawrence. "I am not leaving you, my son," answered the Pope. "In three days you will follow me."   *Pope Sixtus II*

St. Lawrence was one of seven deacons in Rome who were tasked with caring for the poor and needy. When some dissenters decided to kill Pope St. Sixtus II, Lawrence followed him, weeping with sorrow. The pope prophesized that Lawrence would die as a martyr three days later. Filled with joy, he prepared for his martyrdom. He gave what little money he had to the poor. A greedy Roman prefect thought that the Church was hiding treasures and he asked Lawrence to bring them to him. Lawrence promised to do so— in three days. On the day of his prophesized death, the saint brought all the poor, sick and needy to the prefect, declaring, "These are the great treasures of the Church." The prefect was furious and decided to have Lawrence executed by being roasted alive. According to legend, the saint cheerfully told his torturers, "Turn me over. I'm quite done on this side." He is such an important saint that he is mentioned by name each time we pray the First Eucharistic Prayer during Mass.

Exercise: The next time you hear the First Eucharistic Prayer during Mass, don't sigh and say, "Oh, the long one!" Instead, listen closely to the words of this prayer that you don't often hear. There are many great saints listed during Eucharistic Prayer I, and you're learning about quite a few of them in this book. If any are unfamiliar, look them up and read more about them.

We all like to barbecue, but certainly not as a form of torture. Do you know that grilled meat can contain carcinogens? To drastically reduce these cancer-causing substances, a simple solution is to marinate the meat before you cook it. Studies have also shown that adding garlic, rosemary, sage or olive oil to your meat can reduce carcinogens as well.

St. Philomena (c. 3ʳᵈ Century) Virgin and Martyr

Whatever you ask in my name, I will do it, that the Father may be glorified in the Son.
John 14:13

My children, Saint Philomena has great power with God, and she has, moreover, a kind heart; let us pray to her with confidence. Her virginity and generosity in embracing her heroic martyrdom have rendered her so agreeable to God that He will never refuse her anything that she asks for us.
St. John Vianney

St. Philomena is one of my (Peggy's) favorite saints because her story is fascinating, she has quite a personality, and her intercession is very powerful. Her remains, along with a vial of blood, were discovered in a Roman catacomb in 1802. Tiles sealing the tomb read, "Peace be with you, Philomena," and were inscribed with an anchor, arrows, a lance and a lily which meant that the young girl buried there was likely a virgin and a martyr. Her story has been told through private revelation. Her parents were Greek royalty and pagans but converted to Christianity and had their infant daughter, Philomena, baptized. She was taken to Rome when she was 13, and the cruel emperor Diocletian was captivated by her beauty. When she declared that she was a consecrated virgin and refused to marry him, he had her beaten and thrown in a dungeon for 37 days. When Philomena still refused his advances, Diocletian had an anchor tied around her and cast her into the Tiber River. Angels untied the anchor and carried her safely to shore. Next she was dragged through the streets, shot with arrows and thrown back in the dungeon to die. Again, a miracle occurred and she was healed of her wounds. She finally entered heaven as a martyr when she was beheaded.

Exercise: Do you have a patron saint? Some people are devoted to the saint who shares their name, others to their Confirmation saint, and some are devoted to a saint who is a patron for their career or hobby. If you aren't devoted to any particular saint, find one that interests you, learn more about him or her, and pray for that saint's intercession. Ask your patron saint to help you commit to a healthier lifestyle so that you can best fulfill your vocation on earth.

St. Clare of Assisi (1193-1253)
Foundress of the Poor Clares

Look, look on Jesus, poor and crucified, look on this Holy One, who for your love has died. — St. Clare of Assisi

When St. Clare's mother was pregnant, she heard a voice say that she would have a daughter who would bring God's light to the world. Indeed, Clare was a very beautiful and pious child. Although she was of royal blood, she was known to give her food away to the poor and go hungry herself. As a young woman, she met St. Francis of Assisi (Oct. 4). Clare longed to live a simple life and practice the virtues that the saint spoke about. She ran away from home and told St. Francis that she wanted to devote her life to God. Her beautiful long hair was cut off, she was given a scratchy habit to wear, and she was sent to live with the Benedictine nuns. Her family begged her to come home, but she explained that she was now devoted to serving God. Her younger sister joined her along with several other young women. St. Francis helped her to start a new order called the Poor Clares. When an army invaded her town, they planned to attack Clare's convent. She put the Blessed Sacrament in the window and calmly prayed for deliverance from the attackers, who ran away in fear. Clare spent the last 30 years of her life in sickness but was always cheerful and kind, completely devoted to prayer, penance, and serving the poor. Interestingly, she is the patron saint of television because near the end of her life, she was unable to attend Mass but was able to participate by watching a miraculous "broadcast" on the wall of her bedroom.

Exercise: Ask for St. Clare's intercession when you choose what to watch on TV and especially what you allow your children to watch. Unfortunately, there are many TV shows that do not portray Christian values. Try watching a channel that shows Catholic programs, like EWTN, or use your TV to improve your health by watching shows about fitness, nutrition, healthy cooking or an exercise program.

St. John Berchmans (1599-1621)

---

*Our true worth does not consist in what human beings think of us.
What we really are consists in what God knows us to be.*

St. John Berchmans

John Berchmans of Diest, Belgium is another saint who has left us with countless examples of piety and virtue despite few years on earth. His parish priest, Fr. Emmerick, knew from age seven, when the boy would willing arise early in the morning to serve more than one Mass, that the Lord would work wonders in his soul. At age nine, he spent hours each day at the bedside of his ailing mother, caring for her. He was cherished by his childhood friends for his affectionate kindness. When he lived with other boys in Fr. Emmerick's house, he willingly bore more than his own share of work, requesting the hardest chores. At age 17, John entered the novitiate of the Jesuits at Mechelen, and pursued further studies in philosophy at Antwerp and Rome. He was known for his total devotion to Mary, vowing to recite her Office daily, and also for his strict observance of the Jesuit Rules. Renowned as well for his powerful memory and depth of understanding, he was selected to take part in a philosophical discussion at the Greek College in Rome, then run by the learned Dominicans. He contracted a fever not long after and died. Within a year of his death, Duke Philip Aarschot would petition Pope Gregory XVI to start him on the path to sainthood.

Exercise: John Berchmans knew early on what God had in mind for him. How right he was to say, "If I do not become a saint when I'm young I shall never become one." What can we do to instill this kind of ardor in the youths in our lives? John was a proponent of what we call "house aerobics," – doing rigorous chores "with gusto" (an enthusiastic descriptor Kevin owes to Johnnette Benkovic). Do we instill in our children, grandchildren, or students, a sense of the value of hard physical and academic work? Are we teaching them that picking up after themselves shows respect for those with whom they live? If not, then it's time to get cracking! St. John Berchmans would approve.

St. Maximilian Kolbe (1894-1941) Martyr

God will give me freedom and peace from those who war against me, though there are many who oppose me.   *Psalms 55:19*

Whoever recognizes [Mary] as Queen and departs, as her knight, to conquer the world for her, will live, grow and flourish ever more abundantly. This applies to every soul, every association and every organization: religious institutes, nations, etc.   *St. Maximilian Kolbe*

Born Raymond Kolbe in Poland, the saint took the name Maximilian when he became a Franciscan as a teenager, later adding "Mary" to his name when he was ordained a priest. He loved the Blessed Mother dearly and started a group called the Militia of Mary Immaculate and a magazine called *The Knight of the Immaculata*. Still not convinced he was doing enough to spread devotion to Our Lady, he opened a center called "City of the Immaculate," where over 800 Franciscans lived, worked, and spread devotion to Mary. When the Nazis invaded Poland, Maximilian was arrested and sent to Auschwitz. When one of the prisoners escaped, the Nazis randomly chose ten men to torture and kill in order to discourage more escape attempts. One man, who was married with children, begged his captors for mercy, and St. Maximilian offered to take his place. The ten men were locked in a bunker without food or water and died a slow and horrible death. Maximilian preached to them, comforted them, and was the last to die.

Exercise: Today is my (Peggy's) wedding anniversary, and I am honored to share this date with a saint who is so devoted to the Blessed Mother. In her honor, pray Mary's favorite prayer today, the Rosary. Perhaps you can offer your prayer for the intention of the souls of all the people who were cruelly tortured and killed by the Nazis.

Since you spend more time in the sun this time of year, be sure to schedule a skin cancer check with a dermatologist. Skin cancer is not always obvious, so it is best to get regular skin checks, usually once a year. Tell your doctor about any suspicious lesions and be sure that he or she checks your scalp and between your fingers and toes.

The Assumption of the Blessed Virgin Mary (1ˢᵗ Century)

And a great portent appeared in heaven, a woman clothed with the sun, with the moon under her feet, and on her head a crown of twelve stars.   *Revelation 12:1*

From these proofs and authorities and from many others, it is manifest that the most blessed Mother of God has been assumed above the choirs of angels. And this we believe in every way to be true.   *St. Albert the Great*

The Fourth Commandment bids us to honor our father and our mother. Who could possibly honor His mother in a more glorious manner than He who came not to abolish the laws but to fulfill them? On August 1, 1950, Pope Pius XII defined as dogma what countless theologians of the East and West had declared throughout the centuries, and what countless artists, such as Rubens, had depicted with the utmost reverence and beauty—that the Holy Mother of God "was assumed body and soul into heavenly glory." The Assumption of the Blessed Virgin Mary is quite fittingly the highest of all of her feast days of honor within the Church, being her birthday in heaven, the ultimate crowning glory of her sinless life devoted to fulfilling God's divine plan for man's salvation.

Exercise: Note well the Church's recognition of the holy dignity of the human body. The very Mother of God was rewarded at the end of her life by joining God and the angels in heaven, not as a disembodied spirit, but in the fullness of body and soul. And we, too, can hope for the day in which we will experience the beatific vision of God within our own glorified bodies. All the more reason, then, to glorify God now with our bodies. And what better day is there, to honor Mary at the same time? Be sure to include some form of Rosary Workout today, being sure to include the Glorious Mysteries (and especially the fourth one!)

St. Rocco (c. 1340-1378)
Invoked for Contagious Diseases

O LORD, my God, I cried out to you and you healed me. *Psalm 30:2*

St. Rocco was marked as a holy man from birth, as evidenced by the red, cross-shaped birthmark on his chest. His parents, a French governor and his wife, died when Rocco was a young man. He gave away his inheritance and became a pilgrim. During his travels, he encountered many people stricken with the plague. Rocco found he was able to cure them through prayer and the Sign of the Cross, but eventually contracted the disease himself. Banished to a cave, he stayed alive through the assistance of a dog who brought him food each day. A curious nobleman followed the dog and discovered Rocco, bringing him to his castle where he eventually recovered. After a few more years of pilgrimage, Rocco returned to his hometown, only to be unrecognized, accused as a spy, and thrown in prison. Five years later, a jailer found him near death with a mysterious blue light emitting from his body. The jailer called the governor (the brother of Rocco's father) who demanded to know the prisoner's identity. When Rocco stated his name, his uncle demanded proof. Opening his robe, Rocco revealed the cross-shaped birthmark but died minutes later. Many miracles were worked through his intercession.

Exercise: Memorize a few aspirations. These are short prayers that can be said throughout the day. The more frequently you say them, the easier they will pop into your head. Examples are "Sacred Heart of Jesus, have mercy on us," "Jesus and Mary, I love you. Save souls!" or even simply, "Saint _____, pray for us." You can find many different aspirations online. You might even add these short prayers to your workouts. They are perfect to repeat while you're lifting weights or doing push-ups, sit-ups, etc.

St. Hyacinth (1185-1257)

Having so recently benefited from the long and happy pontificate of our first Polish pope, we sit well-poised today to honor the man who evangelized Poland and much of northeastern Europe. The learned priest and theological doctor, Hyacinth, born in Krakow, educated at Bologna and Paris, was so moved, while in Rome, by his encounter with the St. Dominic (Aug. 8), that he joined the Dominican order and returned to Krakow with St. Ceslaus (probably his brother) and two others, commencing to found and lead new Dominican convents there.

St. Hyacinth would later travel to evangelize and spread the Gospel to many countries to the north and east of Poland, in spite of the many dangers of the time. He, like his spiritual father St. Dominic, had a special devotion to Mary. The story is told that while in a church in Kiev, during a Tartar invasion, he grabbed the monstrance or ciborium containing the Blessed Sacrament to carry it to safety when he heard a female voice say in effect, "Take me, too!" He then was able to hoist onto his shoulders a massive alabaster statue of the Virgin Mary, far exceeding his normal strength, thus saving her image as well. St. Hyacinth received a warning on the eve of the Assumption (Aug. 15) that his death was near. He said Mass as a dying man on August 17, 1257, and on that date, this great Pole and Dominican began his life in heaven.

Exercise: The name Hyacinth may suggest, to some, the vain British sitcom character Hyacinth Bucket (she insists it's pronounced like "bouquet") in her show, "Keeping up Appearances." St. Hyacinth, however, was far more interested in truth! Let's bear this in mind in our training, too. The effects of training on our bodily appearance should be happy side effects and never our ultimate goal. We should focus more on developing function, like strength and endurance, than on how our bodies look to others.

St. Jane Frances de Chantal (1572-1641)
Patron Saint of In-Law Problems

"And how does this happen to me, that the mother of my Lord should come to me? Blessed are you who believed that what was spoken to you by the Lord would be fulfilled." Luke 1:43, 45

We should go to prayer with deep humility and an awareness of our nothingness. We must invoke the help of the Holy Spirit and that of our good angel, and then remain still in God's presence, full of faith that he is more in us than we are in ourselves. St. Jane Frances de Chantal

St. Jane was the daughter of a French nobleman who raised her as a single father when her mother died while she was still a baby. She was humble, hard-working, virtuous, and devoted to helping the poor and sick. Jane married a baron and bore seven children but became a widow when her husband died in a hunting accident. St. Jane forgave the man who killed her beloved husband and even adopted his son as her godson. She had a vision of the man who would be her spiritual director and who turned out to be St. Francis de Sales (Jan. 24). Under his guidance, she founded the Order of the Visitation of Our Lady. The women in her order were devoted to imitating the virtues of Mary as she visited her cousin Elizabeth. Jane founded 85 monasteries throughout France and Italy.

Exercise: In honor of St. Jane, meditate on the second joyful mystery, The Visitation. Read the story of Mary's visit to her cousin Elizabeth in Luke Chapter 1. Ask St. Jane to help you better comprehend this mystery and how it can be applied to your own life.

Improve your health and look 5 pounds lighter through better posture. Stand up tall, hold your head high, pull your shoulders back and down, and tuck your pelvis under. Stand sideways in front of a full-length mirror to make sure you're standing straight and tall. Regular exercise, especially strength training, can help improve posture.

St. John Eudes (1601-1680)

You, therefore, must be perfect, as your heavenly Father is perfect.
Matthew 5:48

Our wish, our object, our chief preoccupation must be to form Jesus in ourselves, to make his spirit, his devotion, his affections, his desires and his disposition live and reign there. All our religious exercises should be directed to this end. It is the work which God has given us to do unceasingly.
St. John Eudes

St. John Eudes led a long, active, and Christ-like life. He took a vow of chastity at 14, and commenced studies with the Jesuits, joined the Oratorian religious community, became a priest at 24, and went on two found two religious orders, the Congregation of Our Lady of Charity, who cared for reforming prostitutes, and the Congregation of Jesus and Mary (Eudist Fathers), dedicated to the spiritual and intellectual formation of secular priests and seminarians. St. John Eudes conducted over 100 parish missions. Known for his special dedication to the sacred hearts of Jesus and Mary, he composed the Mass and Office for the feast of the Holy Heart of Mary, first celebrated in 1648, and for the feast of the Sacred Heart of Jesus, first celebrated in 1672, and wrote the first book dedicated to the sacred hearts.

Exercise: Jesus has called us to perfect ourselves, the word "perfect" deriving from the Latin *perficere*, to make whole or complete. We must strive to perfect ourselves, body and soul. Try this simple workout sometime to build both strength and cardiovascular endurance. Do a chest press, a pull-down motion, and overhead press, a rowing motion, and a leg press, either in traditional HIT style (8-12 reps at 2 seconds up, 2 down), or in a super-slow fashion with a slightly lighter weight (4-5 reps at 10 seconds up, 10 seconds down). The kicker here is to take virtually no time for rest between each exercise. Once your heart rate is elevated in the first exercise, it will keep pumping away for the entire 10 or 12 minutes it takes to give all your major skeletal muscles an exercise in perfection!

St. Bernard of Clairvaux (1090-1153)
Doctor of the Church

Take my yoke upon you and learn from me, for I am meek and humble of heart; and you will find rest for your selves. For my yoke is easy, and my burden light.   *Matthew 11:29-30*

"My burden is light," said the blessed Redeemer, a light burden indeed, which carries him that bears it. I have looked through all nature for a resemblance of this, and seem to find a shadow of it in the wings of a bird, which are indeed borne by the creature, and yet support her flight towards heaven.   *St. Bernard of Clairvaux*

St. Bernard is considered one of the greatest saints of the twelfth century. At age 20, he decided to join a Benedictine monastery and was so persuasive that five of his brothers, his father, an uncle, and 30 friends joined him. The order grew quickly, and a new monastery was established, with Bernard as abbot. He is considered the second founder of the Cistercian order, reforming it to be more faithful to the rule of St. Benedict. He built several abbeys, and his holy example of heroic virtue resulted in a large increase in vocations to the order. His skills as an arbitrator were so well-known that he was called upon to reconcile a schism (division) in the Church at Rome. He was an advisor to kings, a counselor to the pope, a brilliant theologian, and an inspirational homilist, a writer, and a poet. St. Bernard was very devoted to the Blessed Mother, and is known as a great Marian scholar and a Doctor of the Church.

Exercise: St. Bernard is believed by some to have composed the Memorare. Work on memorizing this powerful prayer to Mary. I (Peggy) always recite it after I pray the Rosary: *"Remember, O most gracious Virgin Mary, that never was it known that anyone who fled to thy protection, implored thy help, or sought thy intercession was left unaided. Inspired with this confidence, I fly to thee, O Virgin of virgins, my Mother; to thee do I come; before thee I stand, sinful and sorrowful. O Mother of the Word Incarnate, despise not my petitions, but in thy mercy hear and answer me. Amen."* Think about your dental health today. Be sure to brush your teeth and floss regularly. It's important to keep your teeth and gums healthy. Get regular check-ups and x-rays so that you can prevent problems in the future.

August 21

St. Pope Pius X (1835-1914)

But as for you, teach what befits sound doctrine.   *Titus 2:1*

Instaurare omnia in Christo.   *St. Pope Pius X's Papal Motto*

Giuseppe Melchiorre Sarto was the humble son of a postman. Though immersed in the philosophical and theological wisdom of St. Thomas Aquinas (Jan. 28) and of Canon Law, when this long-serving pastor became Pope Pius X in 1903, he would never forget the needs of the common man and woman. Pope Pius X was a bold, plain-speaking, and outspoken champion of the perennial holy wisdom and practices of the Catholic Church. He would comprise the first one volume *Code of Canon Law*, encourage the resurgence of Gregorian chant, and openly combat against emerging Modernist errors, such as the indifferentism and relativism that Pope Benedict XVI continues to battle in our day. For his promotion of early Communion (at the attainment of seven, the "age of reason"), and of frequent Communion, he is known as, "The Pope of the Blessed Sacrament." His papal motto, drawing from Ephesians 1:10, means to renew all things in Christ. In 1951, this brave and holy defender of *orthodoxy* (literally, "straight doctrine") became the first pope to be canonized since St. Pope Pius V in 1712.

Exercise: St. Pope Pius X stood bold and upright in defense of the eternal truth, beauty, and goodness of the Church. I wonder today, how many parents even bother to tell their children to "stand up straight!" Even as my (Kevin's) sons have outgrown me in height, I have chided them at times for how much taller I sit in the pew! Slouching is a standard posture of our youth today, a natural result of too much sitting before electronic devices. I recall my dad preaching to me about the benefits of standing up straight. So, why not practice, as both a physical and spiritual exercise, standing, sitting, and kneeling straight? A simple method for doing so is to look straight ahead and stand, still, or kneel as "tall" as is comfortable.

Queenship of the Blessed Virgin Mary

The key to understanding Mary's Queenship is to recognize that she is a queen *mother*. The directive Jesus gave John at the foot of the cross was intended for us, too, "Behold your mother!" (Jn. 19:27). At Cana, Mary encapsulated Christian discipleship in her words to the stewards, "Do whatever He tells you" (Jn. 2:5). From the Cross, Jesus said the same, *but of her.* By identifying Mary as our Mother, Jesus affirmed her parental rights over us. Scripture says, "Obey your parents in the Lord, for this is right. 'Honor your father and mother that it may be well with you and that you may live long on the earth'" (Eph. 6:1-3). In effect, Jesus said from the Cross, "Do whatever *she* tells you." He could do this because in Mary we finally have a Mother who will communicate nothing but the will of God to her children. What does Mary ask of us? Even though Marian apparitions are matters of private revelation, those approved by the Church are vouchsafed as agreeing with the Faith entrusted by Jesus to the Apostles. In those approved apparitions, our Mother has asked us to pray the Rosary daily—just fifteen to twenty minutes out of a 1,440 minute day. I (Shane) pray it on my car ride to work. Mary made this request because it is impossible to "do whatever Jesus tells us" without assimilating His mysteries, His actions and teachings; and that only happens by *prayerfully* thinking on them. In the Rosary we join Mary in meditating on what the word of God (Scripture) tells us about the Word of God (Jesus). That is exactly how the Apostles spent the nine days prior to Pentecost!

Exercise: Can you guess the best day to begin praying the Rosary? Today. (In questions of faith, the answer is always "today," Heb. 3:7-4:7.) So pick up that Rosary as you head out the door to work today or as you exercise—see *The Rosary Workout* for a great way to use the Rosary in prayer and exercise. August 22nd is a perfect day to say it slowly, lovingly: Hail, holy Queen, Mother of Mercy.

St. Rose of Lima (1586-1617)

I am a rose of Sharon, a lily of the valleys.   Song of Solomon 2:1

Apart from the cross, there is no other ladder by which we may get to heaven.   St. Rose of Lima

Isabel de Flores, born in Lima, Peru, was one of 10 children born to her Spanish father and her mother of Incan ancestry. So beautiful as a child that she was known as "Rose," she would rub pepper and lye on her face and would roughen her hands with lime and hard labor so that men would not be tempted by her beauty, and so she could dedicate her whole self to Christ. Rose was profoundly moved by the model of St. Catherine of Siena (April 29), fasting thrice weekly, receiving daily the Blessed Sacrament, vowing a life of perpetual virginity, and joining the Third Order of the Dominicans, taking the name of Rose, at age 21. Sensing her call to work, as well as devotion, she helped her family by making and selling her own fine works of lace and embroidery, as well as flowers that she grew in the family garden. She would use a room in the house to treat sick children and the elderly, and in her last years lived a reclusive life in a little hut in the garden, inflicting severe self-mortifications and leaving only to receive the Blessed Sacrament. In 1671, she became the first canonized saint from the New World of the Americas.

Exercise: Not to say that a woman should mar her physical beauty in any way, but note how shocking it is in this day of a multi-billion dollar cosmetics industry to conceive that this saint would do so on purpose! We need not eschew the beauty of our bodily temples, but it bears repeating, that in order to glorify God, and not ourselves, and to develop the energy to serve our neighbors, rather than depleting our energy in overzealous training for a slim figure, both men and women should focus on function over form, on strength and endurance over appearance, and on feeling good over looking good. One way to do this is by recording and tracking workout progress. Tips on how to do that will be coming soon to a devotional entry near you!

St. Bartholomew (1ˢᵗ Century A.D.) Apostle

Scripture tells us next to nothing about the majority of the Apostles. Three of the Gospels call this Apostle by the name of Bartholomew, meaning "son of (bar) Talmai;" but John gives us his first name, Nathanael. The first thing John tells us about Nathanael is that he was not afraid to give his opinion. He may have done so a bit harshly, but Jesus saw past the rough edges, and praised him for his honesty (Jn. 1:47). True to form, once Nathanael recognized Whose presence he was in, he blurted out his confession of faith, "You are the Son of God!" (Jn. 1:49) and was a disciple from that point forward. After the events narrated in Acts 15, we are completely dependent upon tradition for how he exercised his ministry. It is said that he carried the Gospel as far as India and died a martyr in Armenia, after first being skinned alive. Once St. Bartholomew recognized the Truth about Jesus, he refused to compromise his speech – even when doing so would have spared him great physical pain. That called for a supernatural perseverance, without which none of us can be saved. Oh, we may not be called to physical martyrdom; but each of us has to take up our cross and die to ourselves *daily*. We have to witness to the truth about Jesus and the lifestyle to which He calls every human being. As the Master said, "whoever is ashamed of me and my words, of him will the Son of man be ashamed when he comes in his glory" (Lk. 9:26).

Exercise: Bartholomew reminds us of the perseverance each of us needs in lovingly speaking and living God's truth. Take a moment to think about your recent interactions with others. Did you live out your profession of faith in Jesus, or did you compromise by affirming this world's values? Ask God for perseverance in saying "only the good things" people need to hear, as opposed to the overly critical or lewd things that get a quick laugh. Ask God for perseverance in your strength and cardio training, too – one more push, one more minute than yesterday. Perseverance is a virtue that we want to permeate every facet of our lives, just as it did Jesus' and Bartholomew's.

St. Louis IX, King of France (1214-1270)

For thou dost meet him with goodly blessings; thou dost set a crown of fine gold upon his head.
Psalms 21:3

Rex Christianissimus (Most Christian King)
Title of the Medieval Kings of France

Some modern historians caricature the Christendom of the Middle Ages as a backward time when bookish men, bereft of worldly wisdom, debated amongst each other about the number of angels that could dance on the head of a pin. I'm more inclined to agree with the opinion of the triple-doctorate holder, James J. Walsh, M.D., Ph.D., L.L.D., who authored a book published in 1907 entitled *The Thirteenth: Greatest of Centuries.* For one thing, it boasted a saintly King of France, a devout champion of Christ who led two crusades, and befriended and supported at Paris such sublime Doctors of the Church as Sts. Albert the Great, Thomas Aquinas, and Bonaventure. What a loss the world felt in the decade between 1270 and 1280, when Louis, Albert, Thomas, and Bonaventure all would meet their Maker in paradise. So respected was this great leader that his image appears among those of great lawmakers that adorn both the U.S. House of Representatives, and the U.S. Supreme Court. He is the namesake of my own son's university of choice and the very city in which it resides – St. Louis University in St. Louis, Missouri. Would that any of the most powerful of modern, secular rulers could be such a saint in the making!

Exercise: At least during your first year of training, and also during times of intensified effort toward some fitness goal, we highly recommend that you record your training efforts in a journal. For your strength training, record the date, exercises, poundage, and repetitions. For cardiovascular training, record the date, exercise, time, and, depending on the activity, the distance, sequence of intervals if done, and, if a machine provides it, the number of calories burned.

St. Teresa of Jesus Jornet Ibars (1843-1897)

St. Teresa is one of those beautiful souls whose personal struggles gave her a deep appreciation for God's gift of the body. She put that body to use in giving thanks to Him. Teresa started her adult life working as a teacher; but shortly after the death of her father, she found herself homebound, suffering through a lengthy illness. Anyone who has abstained from friends and family for a couple of days while battling the flu should have a sense of how disconnected and useless Teresa felt during those months. When her health returned, the Holy Spirit inspired not only gratitude in Teresa, but also a burning desire to bring relief to other shut-ins, especially the elderly. With the financial help of her sister, Teresa opened a nursing home. A small group of women volunteered to assist her in caring for the elderly who came to live in the home. Teresa and her helpers went door-to-door throughout the community to ascertain and meet the needs of seniors – chores, donations of food and clothing, medicine. Within a year's time, Teresa and her companions had formed a religious congregation, the Little Sisters of the Abandoned Elderly. Other women felt inspired to join them, and the community and homes quickly opened in other Spanish cities – 50 in 25 years. The love the Holy Spirit gave Teresa for those ill and alone was spent lavishly during the cholera epidemic of 1897. Not willing to abandon their elderly in their greatest hour of need, 24 members of Teresa's community contracted and died from the illness. Although she herself did not contract cholera, the hours spent caring for the sick left Teresa physically exhausted. God called her Home in 1897.

Exercise: We live in a day and age when so few of us know the people who live around us. Why not go out for a walk today and be sure to greet the people you see out in their yards? If you see someone on your street that you haven't met, be sure to introduce yourself, "Hi, we haven't met yet; but I'm just a few doors down…" It may be the connection both you and your neighbor need. God has blessed you with the health to get out and about; put it to good use.

St. Joseph Calasanctius (1557-1648)

Open their eyes that they may turn from darkness to light, and from the power of Satan to God.
                                                            Acts 26:18

"My children," said the Curé of Ars, "I often think that most of the Christians who are lost are lost for want of instruction; they do not know their religion well." St. John Vianney, quoted in Butler's Lives of the Saints

Imagine a group of children roaming the streets of sixteenth century Aragon, Spain, seeking to find and kill the devil! And there is our 5-year-old, future saint, Joseph Calasanctius, leading them on their mission. Joseph would later obtain degrees in philosophy, law, and theology, and be ordained a priest at age 26. He felt drawn to Rome and was shaken by the poor living conditions and ignorance of the children of the poor. He proceeded to open "Pious Schools," establishing an order, the Piarists, which offered free education to up to 1,000 poor children at times. The schools spread to other European countries. Their studies integrated the secular and the religious, Latin and vernacular languages, academics as well as physical education. A true innovator, St. Joseph sought to anticipate and prevent mischievous behaviors rather than to harshly punish them, and would come to influence St. John Bosco (Jan. 31).

Exercise: OK, parents, we have two important jobs to do today. First, let's take at least 10 minutes to teach our children something about their faith, or Church history. Find a saint yet who might pique his or her interest? Why not share that story and talk a bit about that saint's life and lessons? Next, how about some home P.E.? What kind of physical exercise can you put in together today? Can you toss around a football, shoot some baskets, hop on your bicycles, or leash up Fido and take a vigorous walk through the neighborhood? Let St. Joseph Calasanctius (and the Curé of Ars as well) remind us that we need to talk and walk, and walk our talk with our children!

St. Augustine of Hippo (354-430) Bishop and Doctor

Augustine lived the parable of the Prodigal Son. His mother, St. Monica, raised him in the Faith, but by his "college years," Augustine had abandoned it to pursue paganism. While away from home studying rhetoric in Carthage, he became sexually promiscuous. He took a lover and eventually fathered an illegitimate son, Adeodatus. Augustine espoused the Manichaean religion, and then Neo-Platonism, before he encountered St. Ambrose of Milan. With St. Monica looking on, both Augustine and his son were baptized at the Easter Vigil of 387 A.D. The Holy Spirit works quickly, because within four short years, Augustine was ordained a priest, and in less than a decade, a bishop. In the story of his conversion, *Confessions,* Augustine prayed, "Late have I loved Thee." How easy it would have been for him to despair at the years he wasted and the mess he had made of his soul; but he knew that God gave him a new life in Baptism—a life that even if he fell from grace, he could recover in the Sacrament of Reconciliation. Augustine went on to lead the Church of Hippo, Africa, for 35 years, preaching sermons that we still study today and penning some 50 books. Augustine did not just come to an intellectual acceptance of Christianity. His lived experience showed that Christ Jesus really can "make all things new" (Rev. 21:5).

Exercise: We all have them: past actions and attitudes we regret. The audacious truth of Christianity, though, is that our past is but the smallest sliver of a life that will literally *never end.* Whatever damage you have done to your soul or body before is going to be redeemed; you are going to have a resurrected and perfected body and soul. The cooperation we start giving God now, the small steps we take toward reclaiming spiritual and physical health, are guaranteed to end in success! If you want true freedom from past regrets and a renewed outlook on what is possible, then make a decision today to receive the Sacrament of Reconciliation. Even if you aren't guilty of mortal sin, receive the grace to overcome the venial sins you keep fighting.

St. John the Baptist (1ˢᵗ Century)

He must increase, but I must decrease.   *John 3:30*

Prepare Ye the Way of the Lord.   *Song title from the musical "Godspell"*

St. Luke tells us that the extremely young John the Baptist makes his presence known even within the womb. When Blessed Mary came to visit her pregnant cousin Elizabeth, the yet unborn John leaped for joy at the voice of she who bore his cousin and Lord within her womb. John would live a harsh, disciplined, and ascetic life in the desert, feeding on locusts and wild honey, all the while preparing and making straight the path for the Messiah by baptizing the faithful with water. When this greatest of God's prophets beheld the Christ who could baptize with the Holy Spirit, he declared himself unfit to even untie the thong of His sandals.

The Baptist would later speak out with boldness against King Herod's incestuous and adulterous marriage to Herodias, wife of the king's living brother. After her infamous dance for the king's entertainment, he promised young Salome anything she wanted. After consulting with her mother Herodias, that which she desired and received was St. John's head on a platter.

Exercise: John gave up his comforts, prestige, freedom, and even his head to live the will of God unflinchingly. He decreased, so that Christ could increase. What can we do today to decrease the self, in the imitation of the humble prophet? Here's a suggestion. Sometime today, take a long walk of at least 20 minutes, preferably in a safe, but secluded area, like a wooded walking path or along a country road (or if not possible, even on a treadmill). All the while, repeat to yourself these words of profound simplicity, attributed to the ancient Egyptian Desert Fathers: the Jesus prayer: *"Lord Jesus Christ, have mercy on me, a sinner."* When you return home, let your next meal be simply water, bread (substituting for locusts!) and honey.

St. Jeanne Jugan (1792-1879)

St. Jeanne received the gift of baptism on the very day of her birth. In retrospect, it seems that the Lord was preparing her for the difficult childhood that lay ahead. It was the period of the French Revolution and France was in chaos. Four of her seven siblings died as infants and her father passed away when she was only four. That said, one can imagine that Jeanne became used to hard work at an early age. She also made a habit of praying the Rosary. During her twenties, she took a job as an assistant nurse at the local hospital, and in her thirties as a house servant. As with her early reception of baptism, these fields of employment were preparation for the next stage in her journey. The people of Jeanne's town were in dire straits: 40% were unemployed, many dispossessed of their homes. When Jeanne laid eyes on one woman, not just homeless but also blind, the charity Christ had nurtured in her heart erupted. Jeanne brought the woman back to her apartment and placed her in her own bed. Sloughing off false pride, Jeanne took to begging in the streets to raise money for the needy. She rented an apartment where she was able to care for 12 senior citizens and eventually a rundown convent where she gave housing to 40 seniors. Other women were inspired by her example, and Jeanne found herself, now in her fifties, the founder of a new religious community, the Little Sisters of the Poor. Her sisters and their houses spread from Europe to Africa, America, and Asia.

Exercise: Jeanne's service to the Lord went in stages, each one consisting of the grace and experiences she would need to face the next. There is an important lesson to be learned here for physical conditioning. Do not be deterred by the fact that you are unable to run a 5-K, or bench press a hundred pounds. If you are faithful to your 20 minute walk, you will soon find yourself capable of a 30 minute walk, and then a 40 minute walk. In time you might want to try jogging a short distance. Faithfully practice the HIT method of weight lifting, starting with the maximum weight you can bench press 12 times today, and you will be surprised at how the number starts to creep up.

St. Raymund Nonnatus (1204-1240)

Christ Jesus, who gave himself as a ransom for all...　　　*1 Timothy 2:5-6*

We reckon seven corporal almsdeeds ... which are expressed in the following verse: "To visit, to quench, to feed, to ransom, clothe, harbor or bury."　　　*St. Thomas Aquinas*

St. Thomas Aquinas wrote his monumental *Summa Theologica* in the same thirteenth century in which St. Raymund Nonnatus lived and died. Thomas included "to ransom the captive" in his list of the seven corporal works of mercy in which we act through charity to tend to the bodily needs of our neighbors. (For a modern rendering of the corporal and spiritual works of mercy, see paragraph number 2447 of the *Catechism of the Catholic Church*.) Unfortunately, in their day, there were plenty of captive slaves in need of ransoming. Enter St. Raymund. His mother died during his birth, and he was delivered by Caesarian section. Indeed, the name "nonnatus" means "not born." But he was born all right, and countless people were glad that he was. He entered the Order of Our Lady of Mercy, and a few years later he was sent with a sizeable sum of money to the Barbary Coast of Algiers to set ransomed Christian slaves free. When the money was exhausted, he modeled Christ Himself by ransoming himself to free yet more captives. For his successful conversion of some of his Muslim jailers, he was tortured and even had his lips pierced and sealed with a lock. He, himself, was later ransomed by his own Order, and he was made a Cardinal before his death.

Exercise: Go to the *Catechism of the Catholic Church*'s section on love for the poor and read paragraphs 2443-2449. Go also to the *Summa Theologica*, Second Part of the Second Part, and read Question 32 on Almsdeeds (easily accessible online). Reflect upon how each of these great saints we are reading about excel in the charity they each express through their corporal or spiritual acts of mercy tend to their neighbor's bodily temples and the souls within. Which act of mercy will you perform today?

September 1

St. Anna, Prophetess (84 B.C. - ? A.D.)

She did not depart from the temple, worshiping with fasting and prayer night and day.   *Luke 2:37*

We encounter Anna in that powerful scene of Jesus' presentation in the Temple (Lk. 2:22-40). A widow for over sixty years, Anna's life was completely devoted to worshiping God and interceding for the needs of her people. Her simple life of prayer, a union of body (fasting) and spirit (worship), earned her *the appreciation of God*. He came to meet her in the flesh, allowed her to gaze upon His infant face, and then to act as the first prophet of the New Testament era. Through Anna the Lord gives us a concrete manifestation of the beatitude, "Blessed are the pure in heart, for they shall see God" (Mt. 5:8). Anna's ability to be so focused upon God that she could fast (at least to some degree) *daily* might seem unattainable to the majority of us, at least at the present moment. Personally, I (Shane) have an ongoing battle with the urge to overeat. I have yet to graduate to fasting (other than during Lent), but the Lord has allowed me to make some headway this past year: Each day I ask Jesus to share His temperance with me and then I do my best to take in no more than two thousand calories. I of course have special days where I relax this rule, holidays and birthdays; but it is a discipline that I always go right back to, and the Lord has given me success with it. As of this writing, this small change, combined with exercise, has allowed me to shed 52 extra pounds I had been carrying around, and in only eight months time.

Exercise: If you aren't in the habit, keep track of your calories as you go through the day. If your calories go over 2000 for most men of average height and weight, or about 1500-1700 for most women of average height and weight, then you might want to do a little planning tonight as to how you can bring that number down a little tomorrow. (Two or three low-fat yogurts for lunch—approximately three hundred calories—is a trick I use.) Step by step, you and I are going to graduate to fasting one day. "Jesus, please share your temperance with us."

St. Stephen, King of Hungary (975-1038)

And Stephen, full of grace and power, did great wonders and signs among the people.
Acts 6:8

My dearest son, if you desire to honor the royal crown, I advise, I counsel, I urge you above all things to maintain the Catholic and Apostolic faith with such diligence and care that you may be an example for all those placed under you by God, and that all the clergy may rightly call you a man of true Christian profession.
St. Stephen in a letter to his son, St. Emeric

When baptized by St. Adlabert, young Vajk, son of Crown Prince Geza of Hungary, aptly chose the name of Stephen, for he too would work great wonders in the name of God. He would establish, under Pope Sylvester II, 11 Episcopal sees, converting Hungary from paganism to the Catholic Church. He would establish a monastery in Jerusalem and hospices for pilgrims as far away as Constantinople. He established just laws, fought only defensive wars, and was never defeated. Fascinating details of his story persist into modern times. His incorrupt right hand remains a most sacred relic, displayed in the Basilica of St. Stephen in Budapest. The holy crown that Pope Sylvester II had placed upon his head was placed in the safekeeping of the U.S. government in 1945, and was stored in Fort Knox, Kentucky, until returned by President Jimmy Carter in 1978. Stephen and his Queen Giselle also raised a saintly, and later, sainted son Emeric, but they were to bear his tragic death in a hunting accident. St. Stephen was particularly devoted to Blessed Mary, and died on August 15, 1038 on the Feast of the Assumption.

Exercise: Speaking of Hungary, today I (Kevin) will provide a tip to keep you from getting *too* hungry (sorry). I have rediscovered recently that the use of protein blender drinks and candy bar substitutes has worked wondrously to help restore dietary temperance, removing all desire for sweets and deserts. This topic is so important that I'll lay it out in detail in exercises for September 3rd and 4th, as well.

St. Pope Gregory the Great (540-604)

Thou dost cause the grass to grow for the cattle, and plants for man to cultivate, that he may bring forth food from the earth. Psalms 104:14

Quia qui divina sapient videlicet suprahomines sunt. (Those who have wisdom of divine things are, so to say, supermen.)
St. Pope Gregory the Great

This former monk was a pope of nearly undisputed greatness for oh so many reasons. He was canonized virtually immediately after death, is recognized as a saint in churches separated from the Catholic Church, and was even praised by John Calvin. He also gave the English their name. When he inquired about a group from Britain who'd arrived in Rome, he remarked that they were as beautiful as angels. They came to be known in Europe as Angles, from which we derive Anglo-Saxons, Anglican, England, English, etc. There are two ways in which this great saint has impacted me (Kevin) within the last two months as I've written. Having written a book refuting atheism that featured the concept of the "superman" as a recurring theme, I was stunned to discover that Pope Gregory beat Nietzsche to the punch by about 1,500 years, being the first to use the term "supermen" in Western literature. His "supermen," however, far from rejecting God, were "super" because they immersed themselves in God's wisdom. Hence, the saints we are honoring are the true Supermen (and Wonder Women!) Secondly, I've recently acquired the weekly habit of attending a traditional Latin Mass every Saturday morning. My first was a High Mass, featuring *Gregorian* chant, and he also instituted that form of the Mass.

Exercise: I've (Kevin) found that sweet or salty snacks, even fruits or nuts, tend to increase my appetite. I had almost perfect dietary temperance in my teen years because I believed naively that "health foods" would force my muscles to grow. Now I see they can have a real role to play. I'll explain and provide some recipes tomorrow.

September 4

St. Rose of Viterbo (1235-1252)

God may perhaps grant that they will repent and come to know the truth.
                                                      2 Timothy 2:25

Prayer reveals to souls the vanity of earthly goods and pleasures. It fills them with light, strength and consolation; and gives them a foretaste of the calm bliss of our heavenly home.   *St. Rose of Viterbo*

Rose was born to a poor family in Viterbo, Italy, and was known for her piety, even as a toddler who often tended to toddle toward the altar at Mass! By the age of 10, the Blessed Mother instructed her to join the Third Order of the Franciscans, and she took to the streets preaching repentance and defending the pope at a time when the papacy was being oppressed by Fredric II, Holy Roman Emperor. Her family was even exiled from the town for a time for her preaching, but they would return soon after the death of the emperor and Pope Innocent IV's triumphant return to Rome. At 15, St. Rose was denied entrance to the Poor Clare's for lack of a dowry, but she foretold that she would be admitted after her death. She died at 17, and her corpse was later buried at the Poor Clare's convent, St. Mary of the Roses. Each year to this day her incorrupt body is carried through the streets of Viterbo. She was long believed to have died of tuberculosis, but on June 11, 2010, a team of scientists was allowed to examine her corpse and deduced the most likely cause was a heart defect.

Exercise: You too may find that various high-protein candy bars substitutes and protein powders (whey is recommended) may be just what it takes to eliminate the desire for excess snacks between meals or while relaxing, reading, or watching TV in the evening. Here is a favorite simple guy's recipe. 1). In a blender, thoroughly frappe 1 cup crushed ice, 1 cup 1% or skim milk, and 1 scoop protein powder of whatever flavor you choose. 2). Drink. (Add a tablespoon of peanut butter or substitute ½ cup fresh or frozen fruit of your choice for ½ cup of the ice if you want to get fancy.)

September 5

Blessed Mother Teresa of Calcutta (1910-1997)

What an amazing time for you and I to have lived—to have seen the life of one of the great saints! Born in Albania, Gonxha Agnes Bojaxhiu joined the Institute of the Blessed Virgin Mary at age 18 and took the name Sr. Mary Teresa in honor of St. Thérèse of Lisieux (Oct. 1). Almost immediately, she was sent to Calcutta, India, to teach in one of the order's schools for girls. She held the position for 20 years before being made the school's principal. It was during that same period that she took final vows and became known as Mother Teresa. Two weeks after turning 36, on a crowded train ride from Calcutta to Darjeeling, she experienced an intense call from Jesus: "Come be My light." She was to leave her life of teaching to take up the task of carrying Him to the poor. For two years, her religious superiors discerned the call she had received before granting permission for her to minister to the poor and dying in Calcutta's slums. What started as a one-woman-mission quickly grew as Teresa was joined by former students. By 1950, the Missionaries of Charity was formally established as an independent religious community. In 1979, she won the Nobel Peace Prize, and by 1984 had founded four other religious communities! Her work inspired countless thousands, even outside the bounds of Christianity, to volunteer their time, expertise, and energy to assisting the poor and marginalized both at home and abroad. It wasn't until after her death in 1997 that the world discovered the painful "dark night of the soul" she lived with for 50 years. Despite the darkness she felt inside, Mother Teresa continually placed herself in the hands of Jesus, receiving Him in the Eucharist each morning.

Exercise: God gives us the gift of health and strength for the purpose of serving our brothers and sisters. In the spirit of Mother Teresa, embrace the performance of some small act today in a spirit of great love: take your child to the park, offer to cut your elderly neighbor's grass, or take whatever opportunity presents itself. Little tasks, done with great love—that was how Mother Theresa affected the world.

St. Eleutherius of Spoleto (died 585)

I f St. Eleutherius' story was good enough to make the cut in St. Pope Gregory the Great's book of saints, then it's good enough for this one! St. Eleutherius was abbot of the monastery of St. Mark's, near Spoleto. His friend, the monastic pope, St. Gregory the Great (Sept. 3) had invited him to Rome. One Easter eve, Pope Gregory had been unable to participate in the Lenten fast because of an illness. He asked Eleutherius to join him in prayer for his health at St. Andrew's Church. Eleutherius raised his mind and heart to God with tears and supplications, asking for his friend's health, so that he might partake in the penitential suffering he desired. Upon leaving St. Andrew's, Pope Gregory felt a resurgence of strength within his breast and was able to resume his fast. Eleutherius would die around 585 at a monastery in Rome.

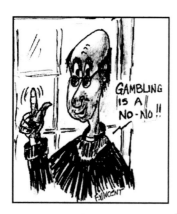

Your mind and body will get you through this world—your soul will carry you beyond, so why gamble on any of it?

Exercise: Here is a simple way to combine prayer with training for a resurgence of strength of your own, using a version of what we will call "contraction hold training." If you have access to machines with separate weight stacks for each arm, like some pull-down, row, biceps curl, or triceps extension machines, perform a normal repetition with both arms, then hold your right arm in the completely contracted end position while you lower the weight with the left arm and perform a complete repetition with the left arm alone. Then, hold the left arm in the contracted position and complete a rep with the right. Alternate until exhaustion; this should come a few repetitions sooner than normal if using your regular weight. To combine prayer, silently say one Jesus Prayer, (see Aug. 29) during each repetition.

Blessed Frederick Ozanam (1813-1853)

Like us and most of our readers, Frederick worked toward holiness by attending to his family and work. Faith had not always come easy to him, though. As a teenager in the aftermath of the French Revolution, his exposure to copious amounts of anti-Catholic literature seeded doubts about the Faith. They were eventually overcome during long walking discussions with one of the priests at his college. By the time Frederick left to study law at Paris' Sorbonne, he was well-equipped to defend the Faith. He put together a discussion group made up of Christians, atheists, and agnostics who gave speeches and publically debated the burning topics of the day. It was during one such meeting that his discipleship was challenged to make a leap forward. An atheist attending the group took him to task over how Frederick talked a great deal about the virtues of Christian Faith but didn't have any impressive actions to back up his claims of its salvific power. Rather than becoming defensive and offering an excuse, Frederick recognized his deficiency and set about correcting it. He and a friend ventured into the slums of Paris and started giving whatever assistance they could to residents. It was the beginning of a ministry known the world over, the St. Vincent de Paul Society. As a lawyer and then a professor of literature, Frederick made time to work for the good of the poor. Once married, his wife Amelie joined him in this beautiful work.

Exercise: We human beings are a composite of body and spirit. Blessed Frederick Ozanam understood that ministering to people's minds and souls while neglecting their physical needs was a cheap counterfeit of Christian love. So here you are doing your spiritual reading and reflection, loving and tending to your soul as God wishes. Now take that next step, literally, and go out for one of those long walks that Blessed Frederick reaped so much good from, and mull over what clothing and goods you are able to take to the St. Vincent de Paul Society.

St. Corbinian (670-730)

Like a roaring lion or a charging bear is a wicked leader over a poor people.
Proverbs 28:15

Those who with God's help have welcomed Christ's call and freely responded to it are urged on by love of Christ to proclaim the Good News everywhere in the world. Catechism of the Catholic Church, paragraph 3

St. Corbinian bears close connections to both the very earliest and the very latest proclaimers of Christ on earth. Like St. John the Baptist (Aug. 29), he spoke out against a ruler who had married his brother's wife, and a symbol of one of his legendary deeds adorns the papal coat of arms of Pope Benedict XVI. Corbinian was born in Frankish territory and would live for 14 years as a hermit in Chartres near the Church of St. Germain. His peace was frequently disturbed by students and other seekers of his counsel. His devotion to St. Peter prompted him to make a pilgrimage to Rome. Legend has it that on his way there, a bear killed his pack mule, whereupon Corbinian obliged the bear to carry the pack the rest of the way to Rome before it returned to its forests. At Rome, the pope encouraged him to evangelize Bavaria as the Bishop of Friesling. There he encountered Duke Grimoald, who had married a woman named Biltrudis against Church law. While the Duke was repentant, Biltrudis sought Corbinian's death. He left in exile and returned by invitation of the new ruler after Grimoald's death and Biltrudis' abduction by invaders.

Exercise: St. Corbinian's bear can be seen in the right upper portion of Pope Benedict XVI's papal coat of arms. The bear symbolizes the Bishop of Friesling himself (Pope Benedict having been named St. Corbinian's successor as Archbishop of Friesling-Munich in 1977), and the pack is the burden of his bishopric.

Today, invite the Holy Spirit to help you accept God's grace to tame the savage, bear-like impulses to sin so that your energy can, instead, be given to your call spread the Gospel of Christ to your family and neighbors by your actions and your deeds.

St. Peter Claver (1580-1654)

Born in Spain, Peter relocated to South America while just a novice with the Jesuits and remained there the rest of his life. He took up residence in Cartagena, Columbia—the center of the slave trade in the New World. The atrocities he saw perpetrated upon the Africans brought there for sale tore his heart. God's will became clear. When he was ordained, he wrote the following vow in the registry immediately after his name, "the slave of the Africans forever." During Peter's 40 years of ministry, he baptized 300,000 African slaves. He went out to meet ships, pulling alongside them in a small boat. He brought food down into the hold for the captives and tended their wounds. Once the slaves were moved from the ships to the fenced-in yards, Peter went among them with more food and medicine. He tried to learn as many of the African dialects as possible and passed along this knowledge to others who served as catechists. Peter's commitment to the well-being of the African slaves did not endear him to many of his fellow Europeans. He was outspoken and made sure that the few rights afforded slaves were not violated. When he preached parish missions, instead of staying with wealthy members of the parish, he would ask to be taken to the slaves' quarters and would sleep alongside them. (Talk about preaching a sermon without ever saying a word!) Peter reached out to others on the fringe of society as well. He made frequent visits to hospitals and met with those who had been condemned to death, reconciling them to God.

Exercise: Peter's example invites us to examine how we look upon our neighbors. You have worked these past months to bring balance to your soul and body. Do you ever catch yourself looking down upon others who have not yet made this same commitment? Ask the Lord for His eyes and heart for your neighbor. God infinitely loves every person he has created, and they have an innate dignity that we are called to respect. To grow in Jesus' image as Peter did, decide on a small act of kindness that you can perform for the person who most frustrates you. Perform it as a manifestation of God's love for them.

September 10

St. Nicholas of Tolentino (1246-1306)

For my flesh is food indeed, and my blood is drink indeed.   *John 6:55*

How can I be said to fast, when every morning at the altar I receive my God?   *St. Nicholas of Tolentino*

Nicholas was born in answer to his mother's prayers to St. Nicholas of Myra. He was to be a most devout and studious child and became an Augustinian hermit at age 18. He lived in monasteries where he served as a model of the monastic lifestyle in striving for holy perfection. At age 25, he was ordained a priest. He heard the voice of angels repeating, "To Tolentino," and moved there in 1274. For more than 30 years, until his death, he would preach on the streets and tend to the poor and the sick of that Italian city. Once, when very ill, he received a vision of Mother Mary, St. Augustine, and St. Monica, and was instructed to eat a bread roll dipped in water. He ate it, was cured, and used it to cure others. To this day, "St. Nicholas Rolls" may be obtained at his shrine.

Exercise: Bread has been the staff of life since time immemorial, but in our carbohydrate conscious age, it has sometimes taken a bad rap. Whole grain breads that have not been stripped of their fiber and vitamins are a very fine source of food energy, fiber, and B-vitamins. Whole grain rolls can be just as good, as well. The problems tend to come in when we slather our bread or rolls with toppings. In honor of St. Nicholas of Tolentino, why not have some whole-grain bread and rolls today, and eat them plain as a most simple means of light fasting? And even better yet; is it possible to get to Mass today to receive the bread of life?

St. Jean-Gabriel Perboyre (1802-1840)

Born just after the French Revolution, Jean knew what level of commitment accepting the call to the priesthood entailed. He entered a seminary for the Congregation of the Missions. From the start, Jean had a tremendous desire to serve in the missions and take the Gospel to China. Before this desire was realized, he was first assigned to several years of teaching in the seminary. When sent to the missions in 1835, his commitment to reaching the Chinese people was total. He learned the language, shaved his head except for a long pigtail, grew a mustache, and mastered the chopsticks. He began visiting and strengthening small Christian communities. He ministered to street children by feeding, sheltering, and catechizing them. He was tireless in his mission. Even while communicating Jesus' light to so many others, interiorly Jean experienced a "dark night," much like Blessed Mother Teresa (Sept. 5). Four years into his ministry to the Chinese, authorities renewed their persecution of Christians. When Jean's whereabouts were revealed by a frightened catechumen, he was quickly arrested. He underwent three trials and more than 20 tortuous interrogations. Throughout, he refused to renounce his faith or divulge the names of any other Christians. The parallels between Jean's martyrdom and Jesus' passion are striking: one of Jean's catechumens was forced to spit upon him and strike him. He was led out to the place of execution among condemned criminals, stripped of a purple robe, and tied to a stake in the form of the cross before finally being strangled. Jean stepped from this world into Paradise on this date in 1840.

Exercise: Jean's complete dedication, even in the midst of interior "darkness," calls us to reflect again upon our commitment to spiritual and physical health. We should not the desire to compromise to reside within us. Vices gluttony and laziness are unwelcome in our temple. If to repent, then do so right now; God's mercy is infinit

St. Guy of Anderlecht (950-1012)
"Poor Man of Anderlecht"

Blessed are the poor in spirit, for theirs is the kingdom of heaven.
Matthew 3:3

The Church's love of the poor...is a part of her constant tradition.
Catechism of the Catholic Church, paragraph 2443

One of the great wonders and joys of the communion of saints is that we join in it with men and women of all ages and nationalities, with thinkers and doers, with sublime theologians, dynamic Apostles, holy popes and just kings, and also with peasant farmers, home makers, seamstresses, and church janitors. Today's great Belgian saint was born to a very poor family of farmers. His devotion is often displayed in portraits of St. Guy taking time from plowing to pray, while a generous angel plows for him! Later, much like St. Andre Bessette (Jan. 6), he obtained great joy as a church sacristan, and though very poor himself, was beloved for his generosity to those who were poorer still. At one point, a merchant, either seeking to help or perhaps to defraud the uneducated young man, lured Guy away from his church on a business venture. The business' ship sank and Guy had been replaced at his church in the meantime. He undertook a pilgrimage to Rome and Jerusalem, guiding other pilgrims along the way and returning to Belgium to a devout and austere life in penance for his bout of greed.

Exercise: What things in this world pull you away from the love of Christ and compassion for the poor? The next time your heart is set on a tempting, but unnecessary purchase of some kind, could you write out a check instead to a charitable apostolate? And here is an idea for a miniature physical and spiritual pilgrimage: Memorize the Stations of the Cross and mentally associate them with 14 specific locations throughout the course of a walking route of at least a mile or so. When you arrive at each location, meditate upon that station until you arrive at the next.

September 13

St. John Chrysostom (c. 347-407) Bishop and Doctor

Chrysostom wasn't John's last name, but is a Greek word meaning "Golden mouth." Schooled as an orator prior to his conversion at age 20, he has gone down in history as one of Christianity's greatest preachers. John's initial fame as a speaker came from his 12 years of preaching while in Antioch, one of the ancient centers of the Faith. Constantinople was the capitol of the Roman Empire and when its bishop died, Emperor Arcadius insisted that John be installed there as its bishop. Arcadius quickly regretted his decision when John turned his considerable rhetorical skill to calling for repentance among both clergy and laity (royal court included). The emperor had him banished, but recalled the very next day following threats of rioting and an ominously-timed earthquake! A second exile followed, though. When the Empress Eudoxia had a statue of herself constructed in silver and placed down the way from the cathedral, John spoke out against the dancing and lewd behavior that accompanied it. He was exiled first to Armenia and then even further, to the shores of the Black Sea. Forced to walk the distance in poor weather, John died along the way. The toll the trip took on him was likely exacerbated by ascetical practices earlier in life. When first baptized, John spent six years in the desert, living in a cave. He consistently forced himself to go without sleep for days at a time, resulting in kidney damage and life-long gastro-intestinal problems.

Exercise: Pursuing virtue means walking a fine line, not going to extremes in our spiritual exercises or muscular/cardiovascular training. We see in St. John's life what happens when we take our physical disciplines further than we are meant—we damage God's temple. We must strike a balance between challenging ourselves to make spiritual and physical progress, and doing so at the appropriate pace—one that gives us time to mentally process and recover our physical strength. If you have exercised for the past few days then perhaps you should allow your body to recuperate today. St. John, pray for us that we may proceed with true wisdom.

St. Notburga of Eben (1265-1313)

Through love be servants of one another.   *Galatians 5:13*

God comes to the aid of the poor and rebukes those who turn away from them.   *Catechism of the Catholic Church, paragraph 2443*

St. Notburga of Eben, an Austrian peasant maiden, house servant, and farm worker, was, like her Belgian counterpart of two centuries prior, (St. Guy of Anderlecht, Sept. 12), rich in humility and in generosity to those more poor than she. A cook in the house of Count Henry of Rothenburg in the Tyrol Mountain region of Austria, Notburga would give the excess food to the poor, until after the death of Henry's mother, when Henry's wife, the Countess Otillia, found out and ordered that the scraps be fed to the hogs instead of the poor. Notburga then cut back her on her own food intake to share with the poor, but was fired when Otillia caught her doing so. Notburga then took work as a field hand, with the stipulation that she be free to go to church on Sundays. After Otillia had died and his land encountered many misfortunes, Count Henry invited Notburga back to his castle, where she would serve as housekeeper for the rest of her life. Legend has it that before her death, she asked that her corpse be laid in a wagon pulled by two oxen, and that she be buried wherever they stopped. The oxen stopped, and she was buried, in front of the chapel of St. Rupert in Eben.

Exercise: Perhaps we may glean two lessons today from St. Notburga's life of generosity and humble, hard work. Are there any unnecessary extravagances in your own diet? Could perhaps the money for one pricey coffee drink per week be set aside in a jar and the money distributed to a food bank before this Christmas? And what a perfect day for a "house aerobics" session. Why not set a timer for 30 minutes or an hour, put some good Christian music into your CD player or some kind of listening device, and cook or clean with gusto today in honor of St. Notburga?

September 15

Our Lady of Sorrows

I imagine Simeon's prophecy had to always lurk in the back of our Lady's mind. "What will happen to Jesus? When?" For the next several days, her heart must have skipped a beat every time her baby cried. Did she think the sword had arrived when they fled to Egypt, or when Jesus went missing for three days? Those were but the briefest foretastes of what Mary endured when she gazed up at Him from beneath the Cross. There she saw her Son – the flesh He took from her ripped, the blood He took from her flowing out of wounds too numerous for her to count. Someone reading this has looked upon his or her own child at the point of death and knows Mary's pain, that feeling of impotence at her inability to help Him. The majority of us beg to never be visited with that aspect of the Cross; even beginning to contemplate it makes us shudder. Mary was the first to live the mystery of redemptive suffering, to share the pain of Jesus so as to bring good to the Mystical Body (Col. 1:24). The mystery is continued in you and me, whenever a section of the Cross is pressed upon our shoulders.

Exercise: You may have heard of "making reparation" for our sins not just to Jesus, but to Mary. It may have sounded strange, but once we reflect on how our sins became manifest in the sufferings inflicted upon Jesus, we understand that those same sins caused His Mother's heart to be pierced. When Jesus told His Church, in the person of St. John, to "Behold your Mother," implicit within it was the call to comfort her. And it is simple to do – when we love Jesus, we bring healing to the heart of Mary. Sr. Lucia of Fatima communicated a method for doing this, the First Saturday Devotion: On the first Saturday of five consecutive months, go to Confession, receive the Eucharist, pray five decades of the Rosary, and meditate on the Mysteries of the Rosary for 15 minutes. (I should add that those two elements are ideal to do while getting your cardio, offering any discomfort to the Father, in union with Jesus) Why, you could take a brief walk right now . . . over to the calendar, to schedule October's First Saturday Devotion.

St. Cyprian (died 258)

Behold, how good and pleasant it is when brothers dwell in unity!
Psalms 133:1

You cannot have God for your Father if you do not have the Church for your mother.... God is one and Christ is one, and his Church is one; one is the faith, and one is the people cemented together by harmony into the strong unity of a body. St. Cyprian

Cyprian was a rich, successful lawyer and orator in northern Africa during tumultuous times for the declining Roman Empire and the persecuted, yet growing Catholic Church. He was converted as an adult through the ministrations of the aging priest Caecilianus, who entrusted his wife and family to Cyprian's care upon his death. Cyprian would take a vow of chastity before his baptism, distribute his great wealth and property to the poor, and soon become a priest and the bishop of Carthage. His first book as a Christian compared the emptiness of worldly success to the true joy experienced in union with Christ and his Church. One issue in which he played a central role was that of how to bring back to the Church persons who had denied Christ under threat and torture; Cyprian insisting that genuine penance must precede return to the fold. Cyprian learned in August 258, that Pope Sixtus and four deacons were martyred by the Romans under the edict of Emperor Valerian. As a Catholic bishop, Cyprian too would be exiled and then martyred on the 16th of December of that same year. He insisted that his beheading occur in Carthage, surrounded by his flock.

Exercise: Bodily exercise is important, indeed, and hopefully you are now establishing many good habits for tending your bodily temple, but today let us reflect on the extent that we are tending to that body of Christ which is the Church. How often are we making it to the doors of our own parish or to the countless other church doors waiting to open to us during our travels? And how about our frequency in availing ourselves of the Sacrament of Penance, making amends for our slights and transgressions against our Holy Mother?

St. Robert Bellarmine (1542-1621) Cardinal and Doctor

Small in stature but massive in intellect and spirit, St. Robert was a great force in the Counter-Reformation. The lectures he gave at the Roman College to address the doctrinal errors of the Protestant Reformers were gathered into a book, *De Controversiis*—a book of such logical force that university chairs were founded in Protestant England and Germany for the express purpose of making a response! Robert went on to act as theologian for two popes, work on revisions to the Vulgate, weigh in on the Thomist and Molinist dispute over free will, and defend the Church against King James I of England's theory of royal supremacy. Robert oversaw the composition of two catechisms and was an attentive and proactive shepherd to Capua, which he served as an archbishop. He was even involved in the early stages of the "Galileo affair," recommending prudence and leniency. St. Robert's brilliance was complemented by the virtue of charity. When the poor were ill-clad, Robert went so far as to give them the tapestries off his walls! He acted as provincial to the Jesuits' Naples province and had the privilege of acting as St. Aloysius Gonzaga's confessor prior to the young saint's death at 23.

Exercise: It takes incredibly strong shoulders to bear responsibilities such as St. Robert's. I propose that you honor St. Robert today by putting in some work on your physical shoulders. Upper body strength is a great asset in performing charitable deeds for family and friends—from moving furniture and performing home maintenance to picking up and carrying crying toddlers. If you haven't done so already, work a lateral raise (or shoulder fly) into your HIT routine: You can perform this exercise with free weights; remember to select a dumbbell weight that you can lift with good form, at least nine times. Hold the weights at the side of the body and, while keeping your arms nearly straight with the elbows slightly bent and unlocked, raise your arms up to the sides so that your body forms a T-shape. Then bring the weights back down to your sides.

St. Joseph Cupertino (1603-1633) Patron Saint of Pilots

Clearly, what God wants above all is our will which we received as a free gift from God in creation and possess as though our own. When a man trains himself to acts of virtue, it is with the help of grace from God from whom all good things come that he does this. The will is what man has as his unique possession.   St. Joseph Cupertino

I (Peggy) am fond of St. Joseph Cupertino because he is the patron saint of pilots. I was an Air Force instructor pilot for nine years, and my husband was also an Air Force pilot. St. Joseph kept us safe in the air. Although he was not a pilot, Joseph frequently levitated during prayer and was known as "The Flying Saint." Unfortunately, many people viewed his levitation as a circus stunt and would gather to watch the saint fly around while deeply absorbed in prayer, making him uncomfortable. Joseph wanted to be a monk but found it difficult to find the right order. One refused to take him because he was too stupid. Another kicked him out because he broke everything. He was finally allowed to be a stable boy for a Franciscan order. He won them over with his sweetness, hard work, and purity, and he was eventually ordained a priest. Joseph was frequently transferred to different monasteries because he would fly around during Mass, meals and other inappropriate times, distracting the other monks and priests. He was eventually confined to a small room and adjacent chapel but never complained, continuing to grow in humility and holiness until his death. Interestingly, during the investigation for his cause for canonization, over 70 people were found to levitate through his intercession. His life is the topic of a DVD called *The Reluctant Saint.*

Exercise: St. Joseph needed some time to find his vocation in life. If you struggle with your vocation or find your pray routine difficult, ask for St. Joseph's guidance. You might not be able to fly or levitate, but you can get off the ground and improve bone and muscle health with plyometric training. A simple exercise is to bend your knees, swing your arms up and jump as high as you can. Land as softly as possible with knees bent, and repeat 8-10 times. This is a somewhat advanced exercise, so do not attempt if you have injuries or do not exercise regularly.

September 19

St. Januarius (died c. 305) Bishop and Martyr

What records we have of Januarius' life were not written until long after the fact. What appears certain is that he was the Bishop of Benevento, Italy, and was martyred during the persecution instigated by the Roman Emperor Diocletian. Legend holds that he was ordained a priest at just 15, and raised to the office of bishop in his early 20s. It goes on to say that he and his deacon, Festus, were taken into custody while visiting an imprisoned deacon. It would seem that the authorities' first attempt at execution did not meet with success; stories say that Januarius emerged from a furnace and/or the bear-filled Flavian Amphitheatre in Pozzuoli unscathed. This bishop was finally silenced through decapitation; or so his persecutors thought. It seems that Januarius' relics are still testifying to God's glory some 1,700 years later! His relics were transferred to Naples shortly after death and a series of ever more elaborate sanctuaries constructed for them, with the city's cathedral being their resting place since the 14th century. Twice a year—on the first Sunday in May, and *today*, his feast—the Archbishop of Naples brings a sealed ampoule of Januarius' blood before the congregation. He tilts it upside down to show its solidity, and then the whole congregation begins to pray. Eventually the blood becomes liquid before the congregation's eyes. The first written record of the event comes from 1389. The few times that the miracle did not occur turned out to be years of tragedy for the city—like in 1980, when an earthquake claimed the lives of almost 3,000 people across southern Italy.

Exercise: So Januarius' blood is most likely flowing freely today (think positive), but what about your own? For the past 80 years, cardiovascular disease has been the leading cause of death in the U.S. How do we fight it? You've got it—diet and exercise. One thing you can do to improve your diet is to monitor your daily cholesterol intake. For a healthy person, the American Heart Association recommends no more than 300mg/day; and for a person with heart disease, 200mg. So check those food labels today, and see how you fare.

September 20

St. Eustachius and Companions

For much of his life, St. Eustachius was a practicing pagan, and his original name before converting to Christianity was Placidus. Before his conversion, St. Eustachius served as a colonel and commander-in-chief in the Roman army. He was a wealthy and influential man, and although he was not yet a Christian, he gave generously to the poor. One day, after a victorious battle against the Persians, St. Eustachius went on a hunting trip that would change his life. It started out ordinarily enough – he caught sight of a deer and pursued it unsuccessfully for quite a while. But when he finally caught up to the deer, it was standing still on a hilltop, a glowing crucifix between its horns. As he stared at this wonder, a voice spoke to him, "I am the Christ whom you honor without knowing it; the alms you give to the poor have reached Me." St. Eustachius fell off his horse in amazement and awe, just as St. Paul had done. After this experience of grace, St. Eustachius was baptized, took his Christian name, and led his wife and two sons into the ChSurch with him. After his conversion, St. Eustachius was separated from his family, and he also lost all of his material possessions. Despite the hardships that he faced, he continued working hard and staying faithful to the Church. Eventually, after fifteen years of separation, he and his family were reunited. However, their happiness was short-lived, as the new Roman Emperor, Adrian, tried to force him to worship his pagan gods. When St. Eustachius, along with his family, refused to adhere to his command, they were roasted to death in a brazen bull.

Exercise: Are you a hunter? If you strengthen your calves and thighs through regular exercise, it will be easier to trudge through that snow the next time that you're after game, or to climb up that hill. Do a stair step exercise today, alternating your legs as you step onto, and then off, the step. If you are fairly fit, try doing this exercise for about 10 minutes a day. As you exercise, reflect on St. Eustachius' life, especially focusing on his ability to persevere through difficult times and on his role as a father helping his family find God.

September 21

St. Matthew (1ˢᵗ Century A.D.) Apostle and Evangelist

I t takes an exceptional person to walk away from a lucrative career and uproot their entire life when the Lord calls. That is what Matthew did. He threw a magnificent party so that his friends could meet Jesus, and then he and the Master hit the road. Was it hard for Matthew to make that change? Was there an interior struggle? His Gospel does not tell us. It does, however, reveal the mindset to which grace brought him: Matthew's Gospel speaks time and again of the "*kingdom* of heaven." The earth and everything on it belongs to the Lord. We are not our own. Our bodies, minds, homes, families, goods, etc., all belong to the King, and are given to us on loan, to invest wisely (Mt. 25:13-20). At the moment of death everything reverts to the Lord. What we have used to love the Lord, hidden in the least of His brothers and sisters, will merit us an eternal reward (Mt. 25:31-46). What we have selfishly kept to ourselves will weigh us down and prevent us from entering God's embrace. "For what will it profit a man if he gains the whole world and forfeits his life?" (Mt. 16:26). Looking at his life and earthly goods with an eye to eternity gave Matthew the freedom to follow the Lord wherever He led. Matthew crisscrossed the Holy Land, endured persecutions, and finally sat down to commit an account of our Lord's life to writing.

Exercise: Material goods. They can sure cause us a great deal of stress. The Lord calls us to make use of them, not become consumed with acquiring or holding onto them. Detachment is important in the spiritual life. A good way to begin practicing detachment is to thank the Lord for everything He has given you. The health and skills you make use of to earn a living come from Him. The very atoms of your body are held in existence by nothing but His will. He allows you to make use of all these. Visualize yourself, and all of the goods with which you have been entrusted, resting in the Father's hands. Now, ask the Holy Spirit to cement this truth in your mind. Return to that image throughout the day, and spend some time reflecting on Matthew 6:31-33.

September 22

St. Thomas of Villanova (1448-1555)

But above all these things have charity, which is the bond of perfection.
Colossians 3:14

Charity is not just giving, rather removing the need of those who receive charity and liberating them from it when possible.
St. Thomas of Villanova

St. Thomas of Villanova was the embodiment of Christ-like charity in sixteenth century Spain. It is even reported that as a child, he sometimes went around naked, having given his clothing to the poor! As a man, he would join the Augustinian order, becoming a priest, the Archbishop of Valencia, and a counselor and confessor to Holy Roman Emperor Charles V. So simple and beautiful were his sermons, that Charles would exclaim, "The Monsignor can move even the stones!" He was charitable to the poor in his diocese to the extent that two-thirds of the episcopal revenues went out in alms. He made sure, for one example, that no poor maiden lacked a dowry on her wedding day. Here, today, in the United States, Villanova University in Pennsylvania is one of the institutions that bear his holy name.

Exercise: Please notice this generous saint's wisdom concerning charitable giving. Though he would, and did, gladly give the shirt off his back (and more!) to fill the needs of his neighbor, he also sought to help enable his neighbors to fill their own needs – and the needs of their neighbors! So here is a simple lesson in strength training that we might impart to help others become more self-sufficient in tending to their own fitness needs, and I (Kevin) will develop this over the course of my next few entries. The very motions of our limbs and torsos involve pushing and pulling, kind of like giving and taking. Certain sets of muscles are involved in pushing, and their complementary partners are involved in pulling. By using this simple concept, it is easy to construct a variety of brief workouts that thoroughly train the body. I'll provide examples on September 24.

September 23

St. Pio of Pietrelcina (1887-1968)

Padre Pio, or Fancesco Forgione, was born into a family of profound faith. Their daily spiritual diet consisted of the Mass and Rosary, garnished with joyful celebrations of the saints. When Francesco entered the Capuchin novitiate at age 16, he took the name Pio in honor of Pope St. Pius V, his hometown's patron. Pio was ordained a priest at 23, but because of poor health, he spent the first six years of his priesthood living the Capuchin rule in his family home instead of the monastery. When we think of Padre Pio, it is natural for our minds to go to the supernatural phenomena: ecstasies, levitation, healings, the reading of penitents' souls, bi-location, and the stigmata. He received the wounds of Jesus only a month after ordination, during a vision of Jesus and Mary, and retained them for 50 years. Although the mystical phenomena drew crowds to him, they were never Pio's focus. In fact, he tried to keep many things secret; but the Lord frustrated his attempts. Rather than the miraculous, which drew the crowds to him, Pio's life was centered upon even more powerful acts of God: Mass and the hearing of confessions. Pio was a spiritual director to thousands over the course of his life. As beloved as he was, Padre Pio was no stranger to suffering. Not only did he suffer from recurrent illness and the physical pain that accompanied the stigmata, but Pio also endured false accusations being made against him to the Congregation for the Doctrine of the Faith. During the lengthy investigation, he was barred from hearing confessions or doing any spiritual direction.

Exercise: Even though he was surrounded by supernatural favors and besieged by crowds, Padre Pio consistently exemplified humility. His eyes and heart were so fixed upon Jesus that he seemed barely fazed by adulation and suffering. As we notice positive changes to our physique, we need to stay clear about our motivation. It's always nice to receive a compliment, but our true motivation is to be the person God created us to be—not "more" than we were created to be (because of excess weight), nor less (by becoming fixated on outward appearance).

St. Gerard Sagredo (980-1046)

The Lord stood by me and gave me strength to proclaim the word fully, that all the Gentiles might hear it.   *2 Timothy 4:17*

The martyr bears witness to Christ who died and rose, to whom he is united by charity. He bears witness to the truth of faith and of Christian doctrine.   *Catechism of the Catholic Church, paragraph 2473*

Today's saint was a Benedictine abbot of the monastery of San Giorgio Maggiore Island off Venice. (Readers are encouraged to view photos of this magnificent church as it stands today, completely filling the island.) Anyway, during a pilgrimage to Palestine, he stopped to meet St. King Stephen of Hungary (Sept. 2) who persuaded him to stay and convert the pagan Magyars. He became the first bishop of Csanad and was tutor to the young prince and later saint, Emeric. St. Emeric would precede his father in death. King Stephen died in 1038 and some pagan forces regrouped. In 1046, St. Gerard and some colleagues were martyred by pagan soldiers. Some reports describe a lance to the heart; others say that he was rolled down a steep hill in a wagon or a spiked barrel. Gellert Hill in Budapest is named after a variant of his name. He is considered the Apostle of Hungary and the first Venetian martyr.

Exercise: Let's continue the entry from September 22 to learn some simple ways to craft workouts to build our strength with the simple, "push and pull" concept. In pushing movements, the muscles involved in pushing contract, while the muscles involved in pulling are relaxed and stretched, and vice-versa. A simple, upper body, push-pull combination is the chest press and the row. If done seated in machines, they are almost mirror image movements. The chest press works the pectorals (chest muscles), front deltoids (shoulders), and triceps (back of the arms), while the row works the latissimus dorsi (upper back), rear deltoids, biceps, and forearms. (Stay tuned for more entries.)

September 25

St. Sergius (c. 1314-1392) Priest and Abbot

In any and all circumstances I have learned the secret of facing plenty and hunger, abundance and want. I can do all things in him who strengthens me.   *Philippians 4:12-13*

Forget Joseph Stalin, this is Russia's true iron man — and patron saint. Sergius was born into a noble family, but lost it all at age 15 when their principality was taken over by a rival noble. The family relocated to the outskirts of Moscow, where they worked the land as peasants. Rather than devote himself to regaining material possessions, both Sergius and his brother Stephen felt called to the life of hermits in the forest. Authentic holiness has a beauty completely independent of socio-economic circumstance, and Sergius quickly found himself surrounded by disciples. Together they set to work cutting down trees, hauling lumber, and constructing Holy Trinity Monastery. Communal religious life had disappeared from Russia during the Tartar invasion, and it was Sergius and his monks who were responsible for its restoration. Although he would rather have lived as a simple member of the community, the saint reluctantly accepted ordination and appointment as abbot of Holy Trinity. His wisdom was sought not only in religious matters but in secular matters, too. Prince Dimitri Donskoi sought both his advice and intercession for his plans to unite the Russian nobility and to liberate their country from the Tartans. He attributed the resultant victory to Sergius' prayers.

Exercise: Sergius reminds us of how easy it is to get caught up in the creature comforts of life, and forget that we can exist without them. Today, why not resolve to go without the use of one? Walk the kids to school instead of driving; or if you need to drive, keep the radio turned off and have more conversation or family prayer. Here's a challenging one: leave the television off for the entire day. (All right, maybe that's one to aspire to!) Whatever comfort you decide to go without, make each time it comes to mind an opportunity to pray for your religious community, your local parish. Ask the Holy Spirit if there is a role He would like you to take up as a greeter, lector, choir member, or office volunteer.

September 26

Sts. Cosmos and Damian (died 303)

Is there no balm in Gilead? Is there no physician here? *Jeremiah 8:22*

Life and physical health are precious gifts entrusted to us by God. We must take reasonable care of them, taking into account the needs of others and the common good.

Catechism of the Catholic Church, paragraph 2288

Sts. Cosmos and Damian were twin physicians from Arabia who donated their services without pay; hence their nickname of "The Moneyless." So well-known were they for their mastery of the science of medicine and for their charitable acts of healing, that they came to the attention of the Roman authorities and were tormented and martyred by beheading on September 27, 303. They are patron saints for pharmacists, physicians, and surgeons.

Exercise: Let's continue with examples for crafting workouts on the simple principles of pushing and pulling. Here are some additional, simple push-pull pairings for your perusal: Overhead Press/Pull-down, Incline Press/Pullover, Biceps Curls/Triceps Extensions, Lateral Raises/Bent Over Dumbbell Flys, Wrist Curls/Reverse Wrist Curls, Squats, Leg Extensions, or Leg Press/Leg Curls, Abdominal Crunches/Low back machine, hyperextensions, or dead-lifts.

Whole body workouts of 6-8 exercises can easily be crafted by choosing one or two push/pull combinations involving the upper body, one for the torso, and one or two for the legs. For example: Press/Pull-down, Biceps/Triceps, Abdominal/Low Back, or Leg Press/Leg Curl. In the last entry on this subject (Sept. 28), I'll (Kevin) explain how to lay out push/pull workouts focused on specific body parts. For now, let's pray to Sts. Cosmos and Damian for their intercession for our health and for the health of our families.

St. Vincent De Paul (1580-1660)

You have met saints of all different stripes in this book, but few have had lives as colorful as St. Vincent. Born to a family of French peasants, he went on to attend college and then additional theological studies prior to his ordination in 1600. Vincent's reversals of fortune, however, were just beginning. Five years after his ordination, while traveling by ship from Marseilles, he was taken captive by pirates and sold into slavery in Algeria! Within two years time, though, his master converted from Islam to Catholicism, and he and Vincent fled the country. Vincent's first stop in Europe was Rome, but he was quickly dispatched from there to France, where he became chaplain to the queen. It was during this time that he first became known for his service to the poor and his skill as a preacher. Vincent went from service to the queen to acting as a tutor in the house of Count de Gondi. De Gondi was "general of the galleys," responsible for all the convicted criminals put to work rowing French ships. The condition of these prisoners was horrible, and Vincent used his service to de Gondi as a means of becoming chaplain to the prisoners and obtaining medical care for them. The French bishops also made use of Vincent and his congregation in implementing Trent's call to establish new and effective seminaries. At one point, he was directing a third of the seminaries in France. Working to relieve the dire needs of the poor is what Vincent is most well-known for today. He inspired the wealthy to make exceedingly generous gifts to the poor. He physically visited the poor and began sheltered workshops. For this purpose, he and St. Louise de Marillac founded the Daughters of Charity, now an international society of apostolic life.

Exercise: Today we want to imitate both Vincent's simplicity and service to the poor. Select just one closet in your residence. Go through it and take out any items that do not fit you or you have not worn in a while. Promptly place them in a bag and set them by the door so that you can drop them at the St. Vincent de Paul Society.

St. Wenceslas (903-929)

You have condemned, you have killed the righteous man; he does not resist you.
James 5:6

There must be on supreme virtue essentially distinct from every other virtue, which directs all the virtues to the common good; and this virtue is legal justice.
St. Thomas Aquinas (ST, II-II, Q. 58, a.6)

Today's saint is the namesake of the beloved Christmas carol about "Good King Wenceslas." He was born to the Christian Duke of Bohemia and his pagan wife Drahomina. He was educated in the faith by his devout grandmother, Ludmilla. After the death of his father, his mother grabbed power and proceeded to administer unjust and cruel laws. Young Wenceslas was able to gain a large portion of the land and be declared king by Emperor Otto. He administered just laws and built up the Church, while actively practicing personal virtue. He had a special devotion to the Blessed Sacrament and personally cultivated the wheat and grapes that would be used at the daily Mass. His own brother, Boleslas, who had invited him to celebrate the feast of Sts. Cosmos and Damian (Sept. 26), slew him with a sword on the doorsteps of the church. St. Wenceslas served as a model for just kings throughout the Middle Ages, and is a revered patron of Czechoslovakia to this day.

Exercise: Today, let's do justice to some specific "push/pull" strength routines for particular body parts. For a focused chest and back workout, try chest presses followed by pull-downs and then inclined presses or some kind of chest flying motion followed by some kind of row. For arms, try barbell curls followed by dips and a machine or dumbbell curl followed by a triceps extension. For legs, try squats followed by lighter, near stiff-legged dead-lifts, and then leg extensions followed by leg curls. For the midsection, try sit-ups or crunches followed by hyperextensions or good mornings, then twists followed by dumbbell side bends. (I'll conclude the explanation on September 30.)

Sts. Michael, Gabriel, Raphael - Archangels

Isn't it surprising that although Scripture records over 200 appearances of angels, we're told the names of only three? It alerts us to the importance of the angels we celebrate today. Why are they called *arch*angels? St. Thomas Aquinas responded that, even though there are mightier spiritual creatures such as the cherubim and seraphim, archangels are the highest ranking among God's messengers (*Angelos* in Greek) to men. Among the archangels, Michael is regarded as the head, the one who led the angelic army in victory over Satan (Rev. 12:7-9). His name, *Mica-El* in Hebrew, means "Who is like God?" It is the perfect rejoinder to Satan's rebellious cry. Michael is the protector of the Israelite nation (Dan. 12:1) and the Church, the new Israel (Gal. 6:16; Dan. 12:1-3). Gabriel's name means "Power of God." He was entrusted with the most important announcement in the history of the world, the Incarnation. Gabriel was also sent to announce John the Baptist's conception and birth to parents long considered barren. Gabriel appears in the Old Testament too, delivering prophetic words and interpretation to Daniel the prophet (Dan. 8:16-26; 9:21-27). It is common to identify Gabriel as both the angel who spoke to St. Joseph in dreams and the angel sent to strengthen Jesus in Gethsemane. Raphael, or "God heals," is known to us from the Book of Tobit, one of the seven deuterocanonical works of Scripture. Among the truths taught by the book is the healing and protective ministry God has entrusted to this archangel. Raphael, disguised as a human being, leads young Tobias to his future bride and gives the young man the wisdom he needs to both deliver his bride from a demon and restore sight to his blind father. Tradition identifies Raphael as the angel who went down to the pool of Bethesda to give the waters healing properties.

Exercise: In the HIT-spirit of "working smarter, not harder," invoke these powerful friends' intercessions for each difficulty that arises today.

St. Jerome (341-420)

Be not among winebibbers, or among gluttonous eaters of meat; for the drunkard and the glutton will come to poverty, and drowsiness will clothe a man with rags.   *Proverbs 23:20-21*

A fat stomach never breeds fine thoughts.   *St. Jerome*

S t. Jerome was one of the four great Latin Fathers of the Church—along with Sts. Ambrose (Dec. 7th), Augustine (Aug. 28th), and Gregory the Great (Sept. 3rd)—and was the author of the *Vulgate*, the monumental translation of the Bible into Latin.

St. Jerome was certainly no mincer of words. As you might glean from the quotation above, he called them as he saw them! Perhaps it is fitting that in the Middle Ages he is sometimes depicted with a lion, deriving from a story that the fearless saint had removed a thorn from a lion's paw. His figure looms so large, I'll stop his story here and leave you to countless other sources to learn about this great saint through his own writings and the writings of others.

Exercise: Concluding the "push/pull" strength exercises that started on September 22, note that if you choose a particular four exercise routine to focus on chest and back, or arms, or the midsection, or legs, then do only one or a few other exercises for other parts of the body that day, if you do whole body workouts. For example, if you do the chest/back combo, then do an abdominal exercise and a leg exercise that day. If you work out several days per week, doing only a few body parts at a time, your workout may be complete after only the four exercise push/pull cycle. Oh, note that St. Jerome may have been exaggerating a bit in the quotation above. The Church has been blessed with wonderful thoughts of some men of girth who followed Jerome (e.g., St. Thomas Aquinas and G. K. Chesterton). We'll talk a bit on October 3rd about the difference between girth and gluttony!

St. Thérèse of Lisieux, Doctor of the Church (1873-1897)

*For me to love You, Jesus, as You love me, I would have to borrow
Your own love and then only would I be at rest.*   *St. Thérèse of Lisieux*

At first glance the 24 year old Thérèse might seem quite the contradiction—one of only 33 Doctors in the Church's 2,000 year history, she spoke of how "learned" books gave her a headache; she is co-patron of the foreign missions, and yet spent her entire adult life cloistered behind convent walls! The eyes of faith however, recognize that the Lord and His Church have made a profound statement in bestowing these titles on Thérèse. They are the recognition that her "Little Way" is a brilliant encapsulation of the Gospel, making sainthood accessible to all. Thérèse came to the realization, quite early on, that the only way she could become a saint was for Jesus to make her one. She made it her aim not to pursue some "great work" for the Lord, but to simply follow through on the small tasks assigned to her with exuberant love. Thérèse is a Doctor of the Church because she taught the deep Truth of the Gospel, which God the Son became incarnate in Mary, *and continues to take flesh in us,* turning even our simplest human activities into divine expressions of Love. Living out that truth is transformation, salvation! Thérèse's lot was not to proclaim the Good News on the shores of Japan the way her co-patron St. Francis Xavier did, but to pray and call down the grace that not only make the missions successful, but without which they would not even be possible.

Exercise: Begin each day by re-consecrating yourself to the Lord—offering your whole self and every little thing you do, or that will be done to you, up to the Father in union with Jesus. St. Paul referred to it as our "spiritual worship. . . to present [our] bodies as a living sacrifice, holy and acceptable to God" (Rom. 12:1). St. Thérèse had a way of uniting body and soul and extending her act of consecration through every minute of the day, even into her sleep: In her *Act of Oblation to Merciful Love* she prayed, "O my Beloved, I desire at every beat of my heart to renew this Oblation an infinite number of times." *Now,* who wants to do some cardio?

October 2

The Guardian Angels

On today's feast I (Shane) am reminded of a story told by my college roommate. When he and his sister were young, their parents were on staff with Campus Crusade for Christ. Money was very tight, and so the young family was living in a rented home in a less desirable section of town. The back door of the home opened from the laundry room onto an alley. One Saturday night in late summer, while their father was away, their mom was doing laundry. She had opened the back door, allowing the air to circulate through the mesh of the storm door. Around 10 p.m., the mother heard laughter outside from the alley. As she made her way to the door to see what was going on, it suddenly started to open. Two men, obviously drunk, began to make their way inside; they had seen her from the alley and thought she could use some company. Before the mother could do a thing, the two men's eyes became transfixed on something behind her and their faces took on an expression of abject terror. They turned tail and bolted back into the alley. When the mother turned around to see what was behind her, all she saw were her two small children playing. When her husband arrived home and she shared the event with him, the only explanation they could come to was that the two men had been allowed to "see" the angels standing guard over my young roommate and his sister. (For a similar story, see 2 Kings 6:8-17). The angels who guard us are not plump cherubs. They are spiritual beings of such terrifying power that Scripture often shows human beings falling down as if dead when they manifest themselves; and yet, they are our constant companions. There is no persecution or pain frightening enough to drive them from our sides.

Exercise: Ask the Holy Spirit to make you more aware of the action of your Guardian Angel. Thank your angel. Today would be a great day to begin incorporating an old prayer into the start of each new day, "Angel of God, my guardian dear. . ." Invoke the Archangels' intercession too.

St. Gerard of Brogne (died 959)

Put on then, as God's chosen ones, holy and beloved, compassion, kindness, lowliness, meekness, and patience... Colossians 3:12

Every man is naturally every man's friend by a certain general love.
St. Thomas Aquinas (ST, II-II, Q.114, a.1)

Noble-born St. Gerard of Brogne near Namur, northern France (modern-day Belgium), was a soldier turned church builder, priest, hermit, abbot, and founder of 18 monasteries. When called to reform abbeys of the region, he replaced lax clerics and canons with devout monks. This great restorer and builder of Benedictine abbeys spent many years living in a small cell that he built next to his monastery as a means of self-mortification. Though an ascetic and a reformer, St. Gerard was widely known and loved for his interpersonal sensitivity and warm, kind demeanor.

Exercise: Christ did not tell us to *respond* or *react* to others as we would have them respond or react to us, but rather to actively *do!* We need to train ourselves to be attentive to the needs of those around us, and to build the energy within ourselves to do what it takes to serve them. For this reason, I (Kevin) feel obliged to plug a favorite modern book, *The Hidden Power of Kindness* (Sophia) by Fr. Lawrence Lovasik. (At least it's not one of mine!) Among the easiest ways to exercise kindness is by a kindly look, smile, and nod of acknowledgement both to friends and strangers. And back now to St. Jerome and fat stomachs! God has graced each one of us with unique personalities and also unique bodies, but bodies do indeed, by nature, gravitate towards thinness, muscularity, or corpulence. We can all perfect our own natures to some degree, but should always exercise kindness toward those who tend to be skinnier or fatter than the current ideals (even if he or she happens to be you—or me!)

St. Francis of Assisi (1181-1226)

As I (Shane) share in *The God Who is Love*, the year following my conversion at age thirteen was spent attending a non-denominational church. It was beneficial for me in many ways, but I also picked up the church's objections to a wide range of Catholic beliefs. When I took a trip to Assisi the next year, I was transformed. As soon as our bus came within city limits, a peace settled over me. That was how Jesus struck up a friendship between Francis and me.

St. Francis. When you hear that name—even though at least ten other canonized saints bear it—isn't it the man from Assisi who springs to mind? A wealthy soldier and playboy, he walked away from it when Jesus beckoned. The Lord spoke to him from a crucifix: "Rebuild my Church." Francis then took to rebuilding dilapidated buildings. Even though never ordained, he founded the Order of Friars Minor, an order that has given many priests and bishops, and even four popes, to the world. Francis' love and holiness were legendary—kissing lepers or diving into thorn bushes before tolerating a lustful thought. His love of nature and her Creator found expression in the famous *Canticle of the Sun*. Unarmed, he followed the Crusaders in hopes of converting warring sultans. He constructed the first nativity scene and was one of the first advocates of Eucharistic Adoration. At the end of his life, Jesus bestowed the stigmata upon Francis.

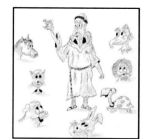

Exercise: First the spiritual: Spend a few minutes gazing upon a crucifix. Look at each of the wounds our Lord received out of love for you. Now express your love to Christ. Now the physical: Cut the grass and get a jump on mulching those early falling leaves. If the yard is already ship-shape then take a stroll around the neighborhood and try to see the world through Francis' eyes. (They were filled with both wonder and thanksgiving.)

Blessed Bartolo Longo (1841-1926)

Realize how far you have fallen. Repent, and do the works you did at first.   Revelation 2:5a

My only desire is to see Mary who saved me and who will save me from the clutches of Satan.   Final words of Blessed Bartolo Longo

Few conversion stories are as dramatic as that of the Italian Blessed whom we remember today. Bartolo Longo was raised in a faithful Catholic family, and remained devoted to Christ until his college years. During those years, like many, he drifted from the faith. His indifference to Christianity quickly morphed into hostility toward Christ Himself. This shift became more dramatic as Bartolo became involved, and eventually obsessed, with the occult, even going so far as to become a satanic priest who demonstrated publicly against the Church.

Fortunately, Bartolo's family and friends never considered him a lost cause, and through the help of some devoted Catholics, he was brought back to the faith and became a Dominican tertiary. He took his shame at the injuries he had caused to Jesus and used it as a way to invigorate himself in advancement of the cause of Christ, building orphanages, schools, and other charitable institutions; even a Church! While never fully being able to avoid demonic attacks (often in the form of public slander) during his lifetime, this man who started well and fell hard has now been officially recognized as one of the holy men and women of the Catholic Church.

Exercise: Is there some goal that you once committed yourself to, but have now abandoned? Reflect on some of your previous plans for exercise and spiritual growth, and think about which ones might be worth revisiting. Think about your reasons for giving up on those goals, and pray for discernment about which ones God might be asking you to take back up again.

October 6

Blessed Maria Ana Mogas Fontcuberta (1827-1886)

When one reads of Maria Fontcuberta's childhood, it is hard to imagine, from a human standpoint, how she grew into a positive, joy-filled Spanish sister. She lost her father when only seven, and her mother when 14. She was blessed to spend the rest of her adolescence in the care of her maternal aunt, a widow without children. Her aunt, a member of high society in Barcelona, was able to offer her a plethora of rich experiences, from education to charitable work. As wonderful as the life of a young socialite could be, though, Maria had already glimpsed the "one thing necessary" for her life. In love with the Eucharist and the Blessed Mother since her first communion, Maria discerned that her life lay in a religious vocation. The Lord arranged for her path to cross that of two Capuchin nuns who had been given permission to live outside their convent for a time for the purpose of establishing an institute that would educate children. Maria was drawn by the Franciscan spirit – the love of humility and the simplicity of life – and joined their endeavor. Her heart, exposed to the pain of such loss during childhood, was especially sensitive to children and their needs. The local bishop entrusted them with a school near Barcelona. Within a short time, the two nuns returned to their Capuchin community and Maria found herself in the role of a young Mother to a religious institute. Her final years were spent overseeing one of the institute's schools in Madrid.

Exercise: Blessed Maria was able to weather the storms of childhood and find fulfillment in life because she recognized who was needed at the core of her person. You can give your physical "core," your stomach muscles, some attention today, too, by performing 15 crunches: Lie down on your back with your knees bent and hands either across your chest or behind your head. While flattening your lower back against the floor, tighten your abdominal muscles and exhale as you bring your shoulder blades up off the floor. Keep your neck straight, but avoid tensing the neck muscles too much; you want the abdominals to do the work. Hold the contraction for 2-3 seconds.

St. Dubtach (died 513) Archbishop of Armagh, Ireland

He will feed his flock like a shepherd...   *Isaiah 40:11*

Compassionate pastor and inspired teacher of Armagh's flock, O Hierarch Dubtach, thou art a model of piety for both the pastors and the laity of Christ's holy Church. Intercede with Christ our God that we may be given grace to emulate thee in bringing others to Him that we all may be saved.   Troparion of St. Dubtach Hierarch, Tone 1

Today Cardinal Sean Brady is the 115th Archbishop of Armagh, comprised of 61 parishes in northern Ireland. The first bishop of that Holy See was none other than St. Patrick (March 17), and the sixth, from 497-513 was St. Dubtach, our saint of the day. Armagh was the seat of an explosion of Irish saints and scholars in the 5th and 6th centuries A.D. Christian Ireland was built upon a monastic foundation, and many of its early bishops were abbots as well. Thereby, these shepherd-like pastors indeed modeled piety by their fervent, personal devotion to Christ. Further, they certainly brought others to him, as witnessed by the rapid and enduring legacy of the Catholic faith within the Emerald Isle, and beyond it, through the great Irish missionaries, like St. Columba of Iona (June 9).

Exercise: What is your national background? Note well how the Catholic Church so clearly bears its "four marks" of the Nicene Creed as one, holy, catholic, and apostolic. Catholic means "universal" and we see how every land can claim its own great saints and blessed in Christ. Of course, we are all called to be saints. We must not forget Christ's call to "be perfect" (Matthew 5:48). What are we doing to bring honor to our own land by spreading the good news of Christ to those with whom we live? How can we take the inspiration we glean from so many great saints and run with it to those whose lives intersect with our own? Let's think about that today and act upon it.

St. John Leonardi (1541-1609)

St. John was born into a middle-class family in the region of Lucca, Italy, shortly after the Protestant Reformation. As a young man, he deepened his spiritual life through participation in a lay confraternity. His family arranged an apprenticeship for him with a pharmacist, but John eventually left to pursue seminary studies. He was ordained a diocesan priest in 1572, on the heels of the Council of Trent. His great desire was to see the council's teachings reach the men and women in the pew and effect a grassroots transformation. A few young men started seeking spiritual direction from him after they were inspired by his preaching and his work in the hospitals and prisons. John rented the church of Santa Maria della Rosa as a headquarters for his little group, which he came to recognize as the beginnings of a new religious order. John lived to see his community approved as a congregation, but it did not receive recognition as a religious community, the Clerks Regular of the Mother of God, until 1621, during the pontificate of Gregory XV. Solid catechesis was integral to the Catholic Counter-Reformation; and John and his congregation were instrumental in forming the Confraternity of Christian Doctrine. The confraternity's goal was the equipping of the laity for teaching the faith. John published a doctrinal compendium that was used well into the 19th century.

Exercise: One of Pope John Paul II's tremendous gifts to the Church was the 1994 *Catechism of the Catholic Church*, the first universal catechism in over 500 years. Soaked in Scriptural references and the insights of the saints, it elucidates four key areas of Christian Faith: Creed (core beliefs), Liturgy, Morality, and Prayer. If you are unfamiliar with it, then please go online today and read the first few paragraphs. If there is a question you have always wondered about, do a quick Google search for it in the Catechism. If you are already own a copy, then ask yourself if you could fit reading just one page of it a day into your schedule.

St. Louis Bertrand (1526-1581) Apostle of South America

Little children, let us not love in word or speech but in deed and in truth.
1 John 3:18

For words without works never have power to touch or change hearts.
St. Louis Bertrand

St. Louis Bertrand is a man after my (Kevin's) own heart and mind in his love of St. Thomas Aquinas's *Summa Theologica*. What this Dominican lacked in intellectual prowess and theological acumen of his own, he filled by his immersion and memorization of wisdom within the *Summa*. Building on Sts. John's and Louis' quotations above, for example, one of my favorite quotes from the *Summa* is this one: "Now the love of neighbors requires that not only should we be our neighbor's well-wishers, but also his well-doers." We all have different personalities, and Louis was noted to be lacking in humor, but full of piety and gentleness. He was ordained in Valencia by Archbishop Thomas Villanova (Sept. 22), and at 36, he journeyed to Panama, Columbia, and many islands of the Caribbean. Though he spoke only Spanish, he was reportedly blessed with the gift of tongues and won thousands of souls to Christ.

Exercise: Note well how St. Louis compensated for weaknesses in his nature through his own efforts in cooperation with God's graces. His lack of a sense of humor was countered by his earnest kindness. His lack of theological creativity was countered by his immersion in the works of the greatest theologian who came before him. His lack of knowledge of the languages of the Native Americans was countered by the Holy Spirit's gift of tongues. What are we doing to compensate for our own spiritual and physical weaknesses? "Grace perfects nature." Let's ask ourselves today, are we open to God's grace, and willing to do our part? Then, let's pick out, pray about, and work on one thing today.

St. Francis Borgia (1510-1572)

God's grace is astounding. If it can instill humility in a duke related to an emperor, king, and pope; you can rest assured that it can do the same for you. Francis, a member of the Spanish royal court since age 18, succeeded his father as Duke of Gandia at age 33. Never abusing his position, Francis was the consummate Christian gentleman. He took Eleanor de Castro as his bride while a young man and the two welcomed eight children into the world. For 20 years, the couple lived a life of love, united to the Eucharist. When Eleanor died, Francis heard a new call—to bestow his dukedom upon his eldest son and join the newly founded Jesuit Order. As a Jesuit, Francis' humility reached new heights. The former duke, so used to servants, was made to sweep the kitchen and serve meals to his fellow religious. If he dropped anything, he had to kneel and petition those at table to pardon his ineptness. When he did so without the least hesitation, his superiors recognized it as an indication of his stewardship, that the eyes of Francis' heart were not fixed upon what "felt best" for himself, but rather upon obedience to God's will. Francis had imagined a life of quiet reflection among the Jesuits, but his superiors put the administrative talents he had honed during public life to work for the good of the order. He founded a number of Jesuit colleges in Spain before being selected as Superior General of the order.

Exercise: In honor of St. Francis, who knelt in humility before so many, we're going to do some lunges today. After warming up, you will need about a 10 foot space in front of you. With back straight and eyes looking forward, bring your hips back slightly. Bend from the waist as you extend one foot in front of you at a 90-degree angle; your knee should be over (not farther than) your toes. Bring your back leg down toward the floor, also at a 90-degree angle. It should not touch the floor, but come within about an inch of it. Straighten up and repeat, beginning with the other leg coming forward. Do not overdo this exercise; no more than 10 this first time! And don't forget to bend those knees in prayer before you rest that sweaty brow.

St. Mary Soledad (1826-1887)

For the sake of Christ, then, I am content with weaknesses, insults, hardships, persecutions, and calamities; for when I am weak, then I am strong.   *1 Corinthians 12:10*

Children, live together in peace and harmony.   *St. Mary Soledad*

Bibiana Antonia Emanuela was the second of five children in the family of a shopkeeper in Madrid. Devout from early childhood, she sought to join the Dominicans in her youth. When unable, either due to poor health or a long waiting list, she was led, in 1848, to found a new order of sisters tending to the sick. Taking the name of Mary Soledad (*soledad* being the Spanish word for "desolate, " and a name associated with Mary of the Seven Sorrows), she took charge of the Handmaids of Mary serving the sick. She would travel to Africa and die in Cuba. She would endure many trials, struggles, criticisms, and setbacks, even being deposed as superior of her order for a time. Indeed, one of her spiritual daughters would say, "Mother Mary is like an anvil. She is constantly taking a beating." Still, she would receive support even from the Queen of Spain herself, and would be reinstated. By the time of her death, 46 houses of Handmaids were serving the sick and the poor around the world. Her words quoted above were advice to her order at the time of her death.

Exercise: Will you be content if you suffer criticism for your attempts to tend to your bodily temple? Will you bear it with equanimity when your temperance fails and you overindulge, when your fortitude falters and you've missed a workout, when despite your prudent workout planning, you find that you've strained a muscle, sprained an ankle, or developed a case of the flu? Let's think today about St. Mary Soledad and pray that she bless us with her anvil-like strength, patience, and ultimate perseverance.

October 12

Sts. Felix, Cyprian, and Companions (5ᵗʰ Century)

The bishops Felix and Cyprian and almost five thousand members of their African flocks were persecuted by the Vandal king, Hunneric, an Arian. This entire mass of Christians was put on a death march into the Sahara Desert. Hunneric's army kept them moving at the point of a spear. Those who collapsed were dragged behind the soldiers' horses. Those who survived into the desert were finally starved to death.

We Christians living in the United States can scarcely imagine enduring physical violence for confessing the Faith. But we are living in a time when continuing to articulate certain moral truths may cause us to be labeled as intolerant, bigoted, or "haters." Natural Law holds that proper human behavior, including sexual behavior, is not subject to personal whims or urges; but is governed by "laws" discernible by logical observation. According to both Natural Law and Jewish and Christian Revelation, behaviors such as abortion, same-sex marriage, and euthanasia are inherently wrong. The Western world is in the midst of rewriting its morality, exchanging moral absolutes for subjectivity. We Christians understand that each compromise is a rejection of the One Who came into the world to testify to the Truth (Jn. 18:37). We must endure in professing our Faith in all its fullness, no matter what the earthly cost is.

Exercise: Try and extend your cardio workout anywhere from one to five additional minutes today. Throughout your exercise, rotate between the Jesus Prayer (*"Lord Jesus Christ, Son of the Living God, have mercy upon me a sinner"*) and petitioning God for both the grace of final perseverance (Mt. 24:12-13) and wisdom in your speech (Lk. 12:11).

October 13

St. Edward the Confessor (1003-1066)

Many who were paralyzed or lame were healed.   *Acts 8:7*

"The most pious Edward."   *Lennox in Shakespeare's MacBeth, Act 3, Scene VI*

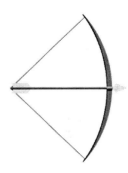

Due to a Danish invasion of Britain, Edward, young son of King Ethelred II and Emma, daughter of the Duke of Normandy, remained in exile in Normandy for 27 years before he ascended the throne to become a most just and "pious" king at age 40. Indeed, he would become a patron saint of kings. Edward was known for his love of hunting and falconry, but even more so for his purity, piety, and kindness. He would greet beggars and lepers at the palace gate and many reported healing at his touch. He attended daily Mass, built the Church throughout England, and strengthened its bonds with Rome. The greatest work of architecture of his reign was construction of the stone abbey at Westminster.

Exercise: The greatest abbeys, churches, cathedrals, and basilicas throughout Europe, like Rome, were not built in a day! Some were begun by young workers who would die of old age, never having seen the completion of their work while on earth. Many of these great temples to God would stand for hundreds of years, only to be renovated or rebuilt, usually on even grander scales. (Such is the case for Westminster Abbey, now an Anglican church famous for its royal coronations and royal weddings. It was built by Henry III, a devotee of St. Edward, in 1245, with construction continuing until 1517.) So too, is the building of our bodily temples a project for a lifetime. Thankfully, there are so many enjoyable ways to train our bodies. Wonderful new equipment like strength and cardio machines is developed all the time. If you adopt the fitness lifestyle, we pray you'll have many exciting years ahead of you to craft your own temple *ad majorem gloriam Dei.*

St. Pope Callistus I (Papacy c. 218-223)

When history begins its story of Callistus, he was a slave to Carpophorus, a Christian and banker serving in the household of Caesar. Callistus was entrusted with money by his master and used it to start a bank serving the Christian community. When Callistus made poor investments and lost all of the funds, he went on the run. His master had him captured and, to make a rather convoluted story short, Callistus found himself sentenced to work in the mines of Sardinia. However, the emperor's mistress was sympathetic to the Christians and interceded to have all those sentenced to Sardinia freed. Callistus returned to Rome, but Pope St. Victor thought it best that he stay clear of the city, and sent him to Antium with a monthly stipend. Once Zephyrinus succeeded Victor as pope, Callistus was recalled and put in charge of a Church cemetery. He was quickly ordained Zephyrinus' archdeacon and, upon Zephyrinus' death some eighteen years later, his papal successor. Callistus' mercy toward repentant sinners earned him harsh criticism from St. Hippolytus and Tertullian. He did not require penance of pagan converts for sins committed before baptism, and following sufficient penance, he allowed those guilty of fornication and adultery to return to the Eucharist. Callistus also insisted that, even though it was forbidden under Roman law, there was nothing inherently wrong with a noblewoman marrying a low-born man, or even a slave. In all of the actions for which he was criticized, Callistus did nothing more than make use of the keys entrusted to Peter and his successors to loose the Church error and bind it to truth (Mt. 16:17-19).

Exercise: Our popes will always have their harsh critics, and sometimes a pope's sinful personal behavior deserves it. Regardless, however, the office of Pope deserves our constant respect and the men who hold it our prayers. Pray for the Holy Father today, that God give him wisdom and courage to speak His Truth in love. Pray that the Holy Father be constantly united to the Sacred Heart and not fall into temptation.

St. Teresa of Avila (1515-1582)

Like pillars of gold on a base of silver, so are beautiful feet with a steadfast heart.   *Sirach 26:18*

Accustom yourself continually to make many acts of love, for they enkindle and melt the soul.   *St. Teresa of Avila*

Young Teresa of Avila, Spain, had it all—brains, beauty, and bravado—but she devoted it all to Christ, and thereby, to us. We saw how St. Benedicta of the Cross (Edith Stein, Aug. 9) was converted to Christ by reading Teresa's autobiography. St. Thérèse of Lisieux (Oct. 1) would bear her name, join the Carmelite order Teresa had reformed, and later join her as one of three female Doctors of the Church, along with St. Catherine of Siena (April 29). Another great mystic and church doctor, St. John of the Cross (Dec. 14) was her friend and collaborator. Her order of Carmelite nuns were known as "discalced," (literally "shoeless," hence our "feet" quotation!) and she worked as an untiring administrator and an unwavering model of virtue to make the order grow in numbers and in holiness. Her *Interior Castle* is a beautiful and accessible classic that describes seven spiritual "mansions" with the interior spiritual castle that lead to ultimate union with God.

Exercise: For anyone who trains the body, the feet will eventually make their presence known and demand their proper care! Never lift weights while "discalced," as plates could be dropped accidentally upon unsuspecting toes. Also, take the time to buy proper, well-fitting shoes for running and walking, and replace them when they become worn. Consider sweat-wicking socks for hot summer runs, lest unsightly pain blisters arise in protest. If you have access to soft grassy areas or a nice beach, consider walking and running discalced (OK, barefoot) at times. I (Kevin) did this during a vacation trip to Myrtle Beach last summer and found a pleasant soreness in muscles of the shins that weren't used to do the extra stabilization work.

St. Margaret Mary Alacoque (1647-1690)
Saint of the Sacred Heart Devotion

The sacred heart of Christ is an inexhaustible fountain and its sole desire is to pour itself out into the hearts of the humble so as to free them and prepare them to lead lives according to his good pleasure.
St. Margaret Mary Alacoque

Today's saint is especially dear to me because I am named after her. I go by Peggy, which is a nickname for Margaret. (Both names mean "pearl.") Like my namesake saint, I am devoted to the Sacred Heart of Jesus. Margaret Mary was saintly even as a child, and made a vow of perpetual virginity at the age of four. She spent much time praying in front of the Blessed Sacrament and received frequent visions of Jesus, usually as the Crucified Christ. Her father's death drove her family into poverty, and Margaret became ill and bedridden for several years. She joined the Order of the Visitation at age 24, but was considered clumsy and very ordinary by her fellow sisters. This perception changed quickly when Jesus appeared to her and told her to spread devotion to His Sacred Heart and its treasures of mercy. In a series of visions, she was given instructions for the Sacred Heart devotion and the promises to those who devote nine consecutive First Fridays to honoring the Sacred Heart of Jesus and receiving Communion. St. Margaret Mary died at age 43, and her last words were, "I need nothing but God, and to lose myself in the heart of Jesus."

Exercise: Learn more about the First Fridays devotion and the promises attached to it at www.SacredHeartDevotion.com. Check your calendar and the Friday Mass schedule at your parish, and set a goal to receive Communion on nine consecutive First Fridays. If this is not possible, try to go to Mass on Fridays when you are able and pray the Litany of the Sacred Heart (easily found online) on First Fridays. On Fridays, many people relax their healthy eating and exercise habits. While you're praying to the Sacred Heart, ask for the strength to be disciplined with your weekend meals and workouts.

St. John the Dwarf (c. 339-405)

I f your unofficial surname is "The Dwarf," chances are that you already have at least one strike against you when it comes to being introduced to others. St. John, who from his youth lived in a home burrowed into the desert floor of Skete, started off his hermit's life with a reputation for digging himself holes in more than one sense. Though committed to Christ, he was known not only for being short in stature, but short in temper as well. And while significantly pre-Napoleonic, his younger years were marked by what we might call a "Napoleon Complex," wherein his insecurities in regard to his size led to a certain odd conceit and overcompensation when it came to his dealings with others. Fortunately, St. John was able to overcome those insecurities, and although he never hit a physical growth spurt, he hit enough of a spiritual one to move past his own self-centered views about his body. His youthful pride melted into a time-tested humility, and by the end of his days, he was revered by many for his extraordinary holiness.

Exercise: Dissatisfaction with our physical appearance is an almost universal phenomenon. Because we don't have the "body of a god," we can sometimes be blinded to the fact that each of us is made in the image of God. The cultural pressure to be physically perfect can squash our sense of self worth, and cause us to become overly defensive or awkwardly vocal about what we feel are our physical flaws. St. John teaches us that our bodies aren't the only things that make up our persons; that even if we can't perfect our physical structures, we are still called to strive for spiritual perfection. How many times per day do you make insecure jokes about your height, weight, skin, or some other aspect of your physical appearance with which you're not comfortable? How often do you get defensive when you don't feel like you compare well physically with others? How many of these comments about yourself are born of a desire for improvement, versus a desire for approval? How can appreciating the physical challenges of others increase your appreciation for the unique way you've been created?

October 18

St. Luke, Evangelist (1ᵉ Century A.D.)

E very Christian owes a tremendous debt to Luke. Think of how diminished the New Testament would be without his infancy narrative. There would be no Annunciation, Visitation to Elizabeth, Nativity, Presentation in the Temple, or Jesus being found there at age twelve. We could not read the parables of the Good Samaritan or Lazarus and Dives, nor the stories of Jesus appearing on the road to Emmaus and ascending to heaven from Bethany. And where would our knowledge of the early Church be without Luke's Acts of the Apostles? Luke after all, was one of the Apostle Paul's traveling companions, giving us first-hand testimony. So greatly is Luke known for his evangelical activity, that we often forget that he was a doctor as well. We catch glimpses of it in the interest he takes in describing Jesus' healing miracles and the way he communicates Jesus' compassion and mercy. It goes without saying that Luke put his medical skills to work in tending to God's people. It no doubt meant a great deal to the early Church; Scripture minces no words when it comes to the role of the physician: *"Hold the physician in honor, for he is essential to you, and God it was who established his profession. . . My son, when you are ill, delay not, but pray to God, who will heal you. . .Cleanse your heart of every sin. . . Then give the doctor his place lest he leave; for you need him too. . . he too beseeches God that his diagnosis may be correct and his treatment bring about a cure. He who is a sinner toward his Maker will be defiant toward the doctor" (Sir.38:1-15).*

Exercise: Many of us tend to avoid the doctor, as if the very act of not hearing his diagnosis means there isn't a problem. The Lord gave us doctors for a reason, and not to make use of them is downright foolish. Avoiding doctors may also be a sinful lack of responsibility for our bodily temples, and that goes for physical ailments as well as psychological. Maybe you feel fine but you have been putting off blood work, a colonoscopy, or a mammogram. Time to take the bull by the horns by picking up that phone and making an appointment. (Hmm... could it be more than a coincidence that Luke's symbol is the ox?)

October 19

St. Peter of Alcantara (1499-1562)

A man without self-control is like a city broken into and left without walls.
Proverbs 25:28

We talk of reforming others without reforming ourselves.
St. Peter of Alcantara

Peter of Alcantara guarded his own interior city of God with unparalleled self-control. He left home at 16 and joined the Discalced Franciscans. A careful observer of their rules, he became known for his inspired preaching and his manual on prayer. At age 40, however, he aspired to a new level of self-control and denial, initiating the first convent of the "Strict Observance." It was said that the friars' cells looked more like graves than living spaces. His own cell was only 4½ feet long, without even the room to lie down flat. Peter wore a sackcloth and coat and he traveled barefoot. Among those who profited most from his holy spiritual direction was St. Teresa of Avila (Oct. 15). Peter experienced mystical ecstasies and died while kneeling in prayer on October, 18, 1562.

Exercise: How about two quick suggestions for building temperance, that virtue of self-control? We'll consider one today and the second during tomorrow's exercise. First, build the habit of doing at least one small good thing every day that you would really rather not do, or normally wouldn't bother or think to do. It might be best to do this early in the morning, so it is not forgotten. Can't think of one? How about making your spouse a cup of coffee or tea or clearing and washing his or her dinner plates? Or perhaps, inspired by St. Peter of Alcantara himself, do this: Find one of your favorite prayers in Latin. Spend five minutes of your prayer time each morning on your knees, learning and memorizing it. Once you know it, pray it each morning and consider adding another – *In nomine Patris, et Filii, et Spiritus Sancti....Pater noster, qui es in coelis: sanctificem nomen tuum....Ave Maria, gratia plenae, dominus tecum....Gloria Patri, et Filio, et Spiritu Sancto, sicut erat in principio et nunc, et semper, et in saecula saeculorum. Amen.*

St. Acca (660-740)

Behold, you are beautiful, my love; behold, you are beautiful; your eyes are doves.   Song of Solomon 1:15

The Church attaches great importance to Jesus' presence at the wedding at Cana. She sees in it the confirmation of the goodness of marriage and the proclamation that thenceforth marriage will be an efficacious sign of Christ's presence.

Catechism of the Catholic Church, paragraph 1613

Today is my (Kevin's) anniversary and my co-authors allowed me to have this day in the devotional; hence the quotation from King Solomon's song to his lovely bride.

Now, as for St. Acca, this bishop of Hexham was a great patron of learning and also of sacred music. His library was of use to Venerable Bede, historian and Doctor of the Church. Acca encouraged Bede to write a commentary on St. Luke's Gospel, to provide a simpler, briefer alternative to that of St. Ambrose (Dec. 7). I can't help but note that St. Albert the Great (Nov. 15) would also later be known for his famous commentary on the same Gospel of the holy physician. St. Aelred (Jan. 12) would write of the life of St. Acca.

Exercise: Spouses are both privileged and obliged to see the beauty within each other's souls, and to help each other and their families achieve eternal bliss in heaven. They can also do a lot to help each other tend their bodily temples. Is there some form of exercise you can do with your spouse, if even a walk or some gardening? Can you help each other in the pursuit of healthy diets, neither leading the other into temptation? Why don't you talk this over today and pray about it too, perhaps on a stroll through the park or the neighborhood?

St. Ursula (died about 451)

Put not your trust in princes, in a son of man, in whom there is no help.   *Psalms 146:3*

Strive with all your might to remain as you are called by God and to seek and desire all the ways and means necessary to persevere and make progress to the very end. *St. Angela Merici, Foundress of the Ursulines*

Many legends and romances have accrued to the name of St. Ursula and her 10, or 11, or even 11,000 virgin martyr companions. The basic story is that this Romano-British princess sought to forestall an arranged marriage to a pagan governor and set sail with a group of maiden companions on a pilgrimage throughout Europe to Rome. On the way back home, in Cologne, Germany, Ursula and her companions were set upon by a horde of Huns, refused to submit or recant their faith, and were tortured and martyred in various cruel ways. There is a Church of St. Ursula in Cologne with an ancient stone inscription noting the martyrdom there of a group of virgins, and St. Ursula's legends have had a wide-ranging and lasting impact. Christopher Columbus named the Virgin Islands after St. Ursula and her companions. When I (Kevin) did neuropsychological research with several groups of generous nuns, the first subject who, after several trials, recited back to me a list of 15 words I'd called out, and in their exact order, it was an 89-year-old sister, who wore the Ursuline habit! For almost 500 years, the Ursulines have provided quality Catholic education to young girls.

Exercise: Though our intellectual soul is spiritual, it exercises its functions in unison with the body, through our senses and our brains. If we are to tend our temples, we must train our brains and minds, as well as our hearts and our muscles! We must give ourselves mental, as well as physical and spiritual exercise. So, at least every now and then, let's crack open a challenging theological book or test our mettle on memorizing important facts of the Catechism. I think the daughters of St. Ursula would approve.

Blessed Pope John Paul II (1920-2005) The Athlete Pope

Born Karl Wojtyla in Poland, the future pope was a talented athlete. He played football, soccer, and volleyball and was an avid cyclist, skier, swimmer, runner, kayaker, and hiker. He needed the endurance during his 26-year papacy, the second longest in history. As pope, he often hiked in the Alps and encouraged exercise and sports. He spoke 13 languages and traveled the world, visiting 129 countries. He is considered to be one of the most influential world leaders of the twentieth century and is credited with helping to end communism in his native Poland as well as the rest of Europe. The pope reached out to people of all faiths, improving the Church's relations with Jews, Muslims, Buddhists, Eastern Orthodox Catholics, and Protestants. He greatly valued the example of holy men and women, beatifying 1,340 people, canonizing 483 saints, and declaring St. Thérèse of Lisieux a Doctor of the Church. John Paul dearly loved young people and established World Youth Day to bring young Catholics from around the world together for prayer and fellowship. He was also deeply devoted to the Blessed Mother and the Rosary. He credited Mary with deflecting the bullet that nearly cost him his life during an assassination attempt. He forgave his gunman and visited him in prison. Pope John Paul II died on April 2, 2005 and was beatified on May 1, 2011.

Exercise: JP II enjoyed the combination of exercise and prayer, especially in the beauty of nature. Today, find 20 minutes to exercise outside. Since it takes just 20 minutes to pray a Rosary, combine the two. Try something new with a Rosary Circuit Workout. Warm up with the opening prayers, then walk, jog, jump rope, etc. while you pray the first decade. During the second decade, do slow body weight squats. Walk (or do another cardio exercise) during the third decade. For the fourth decade, step up and down on a low bench or step. Finish the Rosary by going back to your cardio exercise, then cool down and stretch. For more Rosary workout ideas, visit www.RosaryWorkout.com.

St. John of Capistrano (1385-1456) The Soldier Saint

My son, eat honey, for it is good, and the drippings of the honey-comb are sweet to your taste. Know that wisdom is such to your soul...
Proverbs 24:13

Those who are called to the table of the Lord must glow with the brightness that comes from the good example of a praiseworthy and blameless life. They must completely remove from their lives the filth and uncleanness of vice. Their upright lives must make them like the salt of the earth for themselves and for the rest of mankind. The brightness of their wisdom must make them like the light of the world that brings light to others.
St. John of Capistrano

St. John of Capistrano obtained both the wisdom of the world and the wisdom of God. A jurist and Governor of Perugia, he was sent by the King of Naples as an ambassador to broker peace with Malatesta, was imprisoned for a time, and his heart was converted to Christ. He became a Franciscan in 1416, on the feast of St. Francis of Assisi (Oct. 4). He was strongly influenced by St. Bernardine of Siena (May 20), shared with him a powerful devotion to the Holy Name of Jesus, and became an unusually successful preacher north of Italy in lands like Germany, Poland, and Hungary.

Shortly after Constantinople and the Christian Byzantine Empire had fallen to the Turks in 1453, St. John himself, at age 70, led a wing of the Christian army against the Turks at the battle of Belgrade.

Exercise: First, let's pray for today's solider/saints, for the brave men and women who put their lives on the line for our freedom and safety. Next, let's ask ourselves what good can we do with that freedom and safety today? What are we doing to make ourselves worthy of God's banquet? Are we striving to grow in the wisdom of God with scriptural and theological reading? Are we translating our wisdom into action as modeled by the words and deeds of St. John of Capistrano?

St. Anthony Mary Claret

Anthony was born near Barcelona, to a family involved in the manufacturing of wool goods. He was apprenticed to a weaver from the time he was 12 until age 20. Throughout that time he also studied Latin and French, which was excellent preparation for his future life in the Church. He discerned a call to the priesthood while in his early 20s and was ordained after six years of study. Initially attracted to the Jesuit's and Carthusian's missionary impetus, Anthony instead decided to devote himself to the evangelization of his home province of Catalonia. His missionary inspired him to found the Congregation of the Missionary Sons of the Immaculate Heart of Mary. He also founded a publishing house, the Religious Library, in Barcelona. He republished and gave away Catholic classics—over 4.5 million books and 3.5 million pamphlets! The pope appointed Anthony Archbishop of Santiago, Cuba, a chair that had been vacant for 14 years. Anthony proved a strong leader. He reformed the seminary, challenged his clergy to live more disciplined lives, validated 9,000 marriages, and gave missions in the parish churches, preaching thousands of sermons. Anthony bore his share of the Cross too; his calls to repentance angered many. There were at least 15 unsuccessful attempts to kill him, and his face was cut open by a man enraged at the conversion of his mistress following one of Anthony's sermons. Anthony returned to Spain in 1857, and became chaplain to Queen Isabella II. When revolution broke out in 1868, he followed the queen into exile in France. He was preparing to participate in Vatican Council I when he died in 1870.

Exercise: If we are sincerely trying to live like Jesus, then we will experience opposition, both internally because of our sin, and externally because of a fallen world. The challenge is to immerse ourselves deeper in the Lord when these things happen, instead of seeking relief in sinful habits such as overeating or escapism. Use each frustration that arises today as a reminder to pray, "Jesus, unite my entire life to Yours and make it a gift to the Father."

Sts. Crispin and Crispinian (died 286)

Better off is a poor man who is well and strong in constitution than a rich man who is severely afflicted in body.   *Sirach 30:14*

If thou shouldst acknowledge and love Christ thou wouldst give not only all the treasures of this life, but even the glory of thy crown itself in order through the exercise of compassion to win eternal life.
Sts. Crispin and Crispinian

These noble-born Romans, likely brothers, gave up their worldly wealth and honor to spread the Gospel of Christ to the people of Gaul at Soissons. They heeded the instruction of their model St. Paul: "If anyone will not work, let him not eat." (2 Thessalonians 3:10). As St. Paul supported his missionary work by making tents, Sts. Crispin and Crispinian preached by day and made shoes by night. They won over many by their impassioned pleas for Christ, and by their simple, caring ways. Since they lived during the time of the Christian persecutions of the Roman Emperor Diocletian, they were eventually led before his co-emperor, Maximianus. The quotation above is part of their reported reply to the judge of their fate on earth, before the sword brought these martyrs to heaven.

Exercise: These ancient saints are wonderful models of the virtues of humility, simplicity, charity, fortitude, and good old-fashioned hard work! Though nobly born, they did not hesitate to tend to the needs of men's feet, as well as their souls. Today, or the next day we work, let's find some small way to tend to the needs of our co-workers, employees, supervisors, or customers in body and perhaps in soul. Let's recognize the potential for physical exercise at work, if only a walk up and down the stairs or around the block. More importantly, let's recognize the inherent human dignity in every manner of honest work. Sts. Crispin and Crispinian showed how to make the work of a humble shoemaker infinitely more glorious and efficacious than that of an emperor!

Blessed Damian dei Fulcheri (c. 1395-1484)

D amian, a Dominican and life-long resident of Italy, was known as a holy man in a rather unholy time. Like many of our saints, his early life was marked by trauma. A mentally-ill man abducted the infant Damian from his home. Like any Catholic parents terrified for their child's safety, his mother and father begged the Blessed Mother to intercede for his safe return. Search parties were launched. The one that finally located Damian said that they were drawn to search that particular spot by an unusual light that quickly dissipated. Our saint entered the Dominicans as a young man and became known for his preaching, by which God moved many hearts to conversion. Given Damian's eventful infancy and the "Blessed" in front of his name, it is natural to expect exciting tales from his adult life, but they are not there. He passed through the world and into eternal life without any fanfare, a simple priest who had gone about his work day in and day out. His consistent, humble witness was remembered and made his tomb a place of pilgrimage. It wasn't long before stories of miracles started to accumulate. Damian's life speaks to us today, passing through our daily and yearly routines of work and/or ministry, quietly performing our duties. Like Damian, we manifest Jesus' 30 years in Nazareth, His "hidden years." On the outside, we may not stand out from the crowd in the least, but God is molding us into ever more faithful dwelling places for Himself. Our goal, like Damian's, is to receive His seal of approval when our "hidden years" give way to the life of glory.

Exercise: Continue with the virtuous habits you have worked to form over these past ten months. Is today a cardio day? Then ask Jesus to share His perseverance with you and do your cardio. Are you due for a HIT session? Then get lifting. Have you started praying the Rosary daily? Grab those beads. Go to work and put in an honest day's labor. Visit with your co-workers. Have dinner with your family and enjoy their company. Eternal life begins now.

October 27

St. Frumentius (died about 383) Apostle of Ethiopia

Stay with me, and be to me a father and a priest...   *Judges 17:10*

Abuna; Abba Salama.   *Titles of St. Frumentius*

When early in the fourth century a skirmish broke out between a ship of Phoenician merchants and natives of the north coast of Ethiopia, all of the Phoenicians were killed with the exception of two young brothers, Frumentius and Edesius. They were taken to King Axum, and he took them under his wing, making Edesius his royal cupbearer and Frumentius his trusted treasurer and secretary of state. St. Frumentius encouraged visiting merchants to publicly practice the Christian faith, and he won over many native Ethiopians to Christ. When he petitioned St. Athanasius (May 2) to send them a bishop, the saint decided that Frumentius himself was the ideal candidate. The people loved their Apostle, St. Frumentius, calling him Abuna (Father) and Abba Salama (Father of Peace).

Exercise: Fathers are called to be priests, kings, and prophets within their own households, and a very fatherly thing indeed is to help one's children grow in physical and spiritual fitness (though mothers certainly have their own role here as well). What healthy thing can you do today to 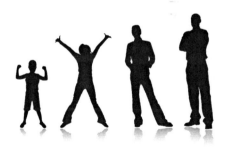 teach your children to tend their bodily temples? Can you shoot some hoops, toss around a football, go for a walk or a bike ride, praying for a fruitful time together before you start, and finishing by crafting a healthy meal together? What will it be? And can you make it a weekly routine?

Sts. Simon and Jude (1ˢᵗ Century) Apostles

There is a tradition that says these two Apostles met martyrdom together in Beirut. St. Simon is said to have been sawed in half, and St. Jude to have been clubbed to death.

Today's first saint, Simon, was the only member of the Twelve described as a Zealot in Luke's Gospel and Acts of the Apostles. It gave rise to the common understanding that Simon belonged to the Zealots, a party that advocated armed rebellion against Rome. This belief is called into question by a number of today's scholars who observe that the term we translate as "Zealot" was also frequently used in N.T. times to describe someone especially zealous in following Jewish law, such as a Pharisee. Simon is said to have evangelized in Samaria, Egypt, and Persia.

When one looks closely at the lists of the Apostles, one will notice that Matthew and Mark do not list the Jude spoken of by Luke and John, but instead have the name Thaddeus. Because of this it has become common to refer to today's second saint as Jude Thaddeus. (It also serves to distinguish him from Judas Iscariot.) Some Catholic writers identify him as the writer of the Epistle of Jude, a blood relative of Jesus. In art, it is common to see Jude holding an image of Jesus' face. This stems from the legend that, after the Resurrection, Jude was sent to heal King Abgar of Edessa, to whom Jesus had previously sent an image of His face. He is also said to have evangelized in Samaria, Syria, and Libya.

Exercise: Sts. Simon and Jude heard Jesus teach that once He, the Bridegroom, was taken from the earth, His followers would fast (Mt. 9:15); and they did exactly that. Taking them as your example, cut one meal in half today and unite your sacrifice with prayer for the success of evangelists, especially those in the Middle East where Simon and Jude ended their lives as martyrs.

October 29

St. Narcissus (99-216)

Remember Jesus Christ, risen from the dead...   *2 Timothy 2:8*

And the third day He rose again, according to the Scriptures, and ascended into heaven.   *From the Nicene Creed*

This Narcissus was certainly no man to fall in love with his own reflection in a pool like the self-absorbed youth of Greek mythology! Christian bishops of Jerusalem were not known for their long tenures, and Narcissus became the thirtieth of the line around the age of 80. In 195, he co-presided over a council in Caesarea that determined that Easter would be commemorated on a Sunday and not with the Jewish Passover. Narcissus suffered intrigue from members of his own diocese and exiled himself to the desert for a time, only to return to Jerusalem and reign as bishop, some said, until his natural death at 116!

Exercise: Tending our physical temples is not going to make us live forever—at least not on earth in these earthly bodies! We can look forward with faith and hope, though, to eternal life and joy with God in our future glorified bodies. For those who might enjoy pondering St. Thomas Aquinas' thoughts on those glorified bodies, I direct you to Questions 80-96 in the Supplement to the *Summa Theologica*, complete with such intriguing titles as "Of the Integrity of the Bodies in the Resurrection," and "Of the Agility of the Bodies of the Blessed."

If you've joined us in our daily quest to build integrity and agility in our earthly temples, you may be all the more prepared to enjoy the glorious bodies that await us. I don't know about you, but I'll be curious to see what Sts. Narcissus and Thomas look like in their glorified physiques!

October 30

St. Alphonsus Rodriguez (1533-1617)

All of us will probably find St. Alphonsus easy to relate to, because there doesn't seem to be a struggle he didn't face. He was sent away at age 12 to be schooled by the Jesuits but had to return two short years later when his father died. He helped his mother to run the family business, the buying and selling of wool. Alphonsus took over the company when he was just 23. A few years after that, he fell in love and married Maria Suarez, but they experienced tremendous heartache—the loss of two children within their first two years together. Maria died in childbirth the following year. Alphonsus lost both their surviving son and his own mother a short time later. The emotional toll and heavy taxation crippled his business, and he had to sell it off. If not for the comfort and spiritual direction of Jesuit priests, he probably would have been lost to grief and depression. Instead he entered into a deep and profound relationship with God.

Alphonsus was almost 35 when he applied for entry into the Jesuit community in Sergovia, Spain, but was refused because of his lack of education. He wasn't discouraged, though; he actually re-enrolled in grammar school and applied to the Jesuits of Valencia, Spain two years later. He was initially turned down by them too, but their provincial made an exception and allowed Alphonsus entry to the community as a lay brother. Within a few months he was transferred to the Jesuit college on the island of Majorca, where he served as doorkeeper for the next 40 years. It was not until after St. Alphonsus' death that his journals were discovered and his comrades truly began to grasp the depth of his spiritual life and the mystical graces with which he had been favored.

Exercise: Humbly standing at that door day after day required that Alphonsus have a sturdy pair of legs. You can strengthen your own, and raise your heartbeat in the process, by performing some more lunges. You can consult Oct. 10 for proper form. Try to add a few more repetitions today.

St. Wolfgang of Regensburg (934-994)

Let us rejoice and exult and give him the glory, for the marriage of the Lamb has come, and his Bride has made herself ready; it was granted her to be clothed with fine linen bright and pure – for the fine linen is the righteous deeds of the saints.   *Revelation 19:8*

This feast is glorious, because it manifests exteriorly, the hidden life of Christ. The greatness and perfection of the saints is entirely the work of His spirit dwelling in them.

Jean-Jacques Olier, Founder of the Society of St. Sulpice

Perhaps it is fitting that the saint gracing the date we celebrate in modern America as Halloween is named Wolfgang. Further, a famous painting from nineteenth century German artist, Schwind, depicts the legend of St. Wolfgang in his full Episcopal garb as bishop, forcing a hideous devil to help him build a church. Halloween is not truly for ghouls, however, but like every day is a day that the Lord has made, and it is truly a hallowed evening that precedes that great day of All Saints we'll celebrate tomorrow. St. Wolfgang was made Bishop of Regensburg (Ratisbon) in 972, as would St. Albert the Great (Nov. 15) almost three centuries later. He was sent by Emperor Otto II to bring Christ to the Magyar people of Pannonia, would serve as tutor to Emperor Henry II, would restore many monasteries, and retire in his last years to live as a hermit.

Exercise: The saints serve as models and sources of inspiration for the many different ways they used their diverse talents and situations in the common cause for Christ. There are also many successful people in the fitness world which can inspire us by their innovations in ways to tend the temple. For the exercise for November 2nd, I will provide an example of a technique I (Kevin) have gleaned from one of my strength trainer mentors, the late former Mr. Universe, Mike Mentzer (who interestingly, like my other fitness mentor, Mr. Over 40 USA Clarence Bass, was born on St. Albert's feast day!)

Feast of All Saints

I looked, and behold, a great multitude...from all tribes and peoples and tongues, standing before the throne and before the Lamb, clothed in white robes...   *Revelation 7:9*

The Church Triumphant, what an image! What kind of service do they offer to God? They "bring golden bowls full of incense, which are the prayers of the [earthly] saints," that they and the angels then offer up to God (Rev. 5:8, 8:3-4). A key part of their ministry is praying for us! They have been where we are, and they know what kind of struggles we face. They are participating in Jesus' own high priestly ministry: "For we have not a high priest who is unable to sympathize with our weaknesses, but one who in every respect has been tempted as we are, yet without sin" (Heb. 4:15). The twelfth chapter of the Epistle to the Hebrews is a fantastic place to turn on All Saints Day. It reminds us that whenever we approach God, we draw near to the saints in heaven too, "angels in festal gathering" and "the spirits of just men made perfect" (Heb. 12:19-24). Even when far from our conscious minds, they continue to surround us as a "great cloud of witnesses" (Heb. 12:1), cheering us toward the finish line and interceding for our needs. The saints know that we are a composite of body and soul, and that we are called to honor God in both. They want to see us pray, speak, act, eat, and rest the way God intended, so don't ever feel that there is any need for which you cannot ask for intercession!

Exercise: Start to work on your own litany of saints. When I (Shane) drive my kids to school each morning we have a list of favorite saints we call out, following each name with "Pray for us!" If you are struggling with overeating call upon someone like St. John the Baptist. (A guy content living on locusts and honey is a fantastic prayer partner when you're tempted by that fifth piece of pizza.) I would also encourage you to get into the habit of bringing *all of heaven* to bear on your needs throughout the day. It's as easy as praying, "I ask all of you angels and saints around God's throne to intercede for. . ."

All Souls Day

But the souls of the righteous are in the hand of God, and no torment will ever touch them. In the eyes of the foolish they seemed to have died, and their departure was thought to be an affliction, and their going from us to be their destruction; but they are at peace.

Wisdom 3:1-3

As for certain lesser faults, we must believe that, before the Final Judgment, there is purifying fire. He who is truth says that whoever utters blasphemy against the Holy Spirit will be pardoned neither in this age nor in the age to come. From this sentence we can understand that certain offenses can be forgiven in this age, but certain others in the age to come.

Catechism of the Catholic Church, paragraph 1031

Many Christians who would never think of walking into the house of a friend with muddy galoshes think it unfounded that we might need to wash up our souls a bit before entering one of the mansions Christ's Father has prepared for us. Today the Church remembers and prays for the souls in purgatory, undergoing the arduous, cleansing purification that will prepare them for the eternal bliss of the beatific vision of God in heaven. Let us remember today to offer up prayers for the legions of souls who have left the world before us with stains of venial sin.

Exercise: Today I will remember my muscular mentor, Mike Mentzer, by introducing you briefly to his most intense strength-building technique (*a method only for those who are already very fit*). In this variant of omni-contraction (all contraction) training, select maximum poundage for a single repetition (do only with machines, for safety). After the positive repetition, perform a negative very slowly, holding the weight for brief, 3-second pauses on the way down, near the top, near the middle, and near the bottom. Slightly decrease the weight so you can do another repetition the same way. Finally, reduce slightly more and do a final, third repetition. Your muscles will feel the cleansing, growth-producing fire!

St. Martin de Porres (1579-1639)

Martin was born in Lima, Peru, the illegitimate son of a Spanish conquistador and a freed African slave. Both he and his younger sister grew up in poverty. Beginning at age ten, Martin was apprenticed with a barber/surgeon. Around this same age he started spending hours of his night in prayer. By the time he was fifteen, he had discerned a call to the religious life and entered the Dominican Convent of the Rosary as a servant. His obvious holiness forced his superiors to discard the restriction that barred African-Americans from becoming friars.

Reports of the miracles started to abound. Because of Martin's prior education, he was placed over the convent's infirmary. When sections of his monastery were cordoned off due to illness, brothers reported Martin somehow coming to them despite the sealed doors. He also offered medical attention to Lima's poor, sometimes effecting healing by something as simple as dispensing a glass of water. Martin was also devoted to the care of the city's slave population, some of whom reported being miraculously visited and encouraged by Martin when first captured *in Africa!* The young friar was a force for good throughout Lima; he distributed food to some 160 people daily and oversaw an orphanage and school for street children. When he died all of Lima turned out to pay their respects.

Exercise: The source of Martin's miraculous life is not hard to guess. It was the hours spent in prayer. A story is told of how when a fire broke out overnight in the chapel where Martin was praying before the Blessed Sacrament, he was so absorbed in contemplation that he was oblivious to his fellow Dominicans' efforts to extinguish the fire. St. Martin found his hunger for acceptance, competence, and even food satisfied at the table of the Eucharist. It is said that the gentle Martin could not bring himself to eat the meat of animals and chose to live as a vegetarian. Remember this great saint today by foregoing a large portion of meat for an extra helping of vegetables. Soy beans, lentils, and kidney beans are all good sources of protein.

St. Charles Borromeo (1538-1594)

Before you speak, learn, and before you fall ill, take care of your health.   *Sirach 18:19*

Be sure that you first preach by the way you live. If you do not, people will notice that you say one thing, but live otherwise, and your words will bring only cynical laughter and a derisive shake of the head.   *St. Charles Borromeo*

Not long after some within Christendom had rent Christ's Church asunder in the name of Reformation, a young man arose, born to a powerful family, nephew to Pope Pius IV, elevated through the ranks at incredible speed and was made a cardinal at age 22. The favored son of a Medici would prove just the medicine the Church and its people needed for healing. Though privileged by birth, Charles Borromeo would go through school on the most meager of stipends from his father and overcome a serious speech impairment as a child. He led the Church through crisis in his youth as a great leader of the Counter-Reformation, becoming one of Italy's most successful bishops as Archbishop of Milan, and was an overseer of the famous *Catechism of the Council of Trent*. A gifted administrator who impacted the world, he was known and loved for his acts of interpersonal charity, like stopping at the roadside to teach a poor man to pray the Our Father and Hail Mary, and refusing to leave plague-stricken Milan. Essentially worn out by his ceaseless activity, Charles died at age 46, his last words being "*Ecce venio,*" "Behold, I come."

Exercise: Who knows better the extent to which we live what we preach (or "walk our talk") than our own immediate families? Here is a suggestion for today or tomorrow. Arise early in the morning and after spiritual reading and prayer time, set a timer for 20-30 minutes and quietly perform a little "house aerobics" workout that will surprise and please your spouse. Clean out the refrigerator, or do all the dishes or laundry, or tidy and dust his or her study or special room. Don't mention it to him or her, and prepare a nice breakfast when he or she gets up.

Blessed Guido Maria Conforti (1865-1928)

Blessed Guido entered Parma, Italy's seminary, when he was seventeen years old. Not long after his arrival, he read a biography of St. Francis Xavier (Dec. 3) and became enamored with the missionary vocation. He wrote to both the Jesuits and Salesians with the hope of becoming a missionary, but only met with frustration. Guido went on to be ordained a diocesan priest, with a new dream of serving in a local parish. Instead his bishop assigned him to be a seminary professor. He was next made the seminary's vice rector and then his diocese's vicar of clergy. In time he came to see the building blocks God was moving into place.

While working at the seminary, Guido met fourteen young men with a hunger for the missions. He was able to establish a missionary seminary for them under the patronage of Francis Xavier. In the years that followed, not only was Guido elevated to the office of bishop, but he also saw his Xaverian Missionaries re-evangelize their native Italy and proclaim the Gospel in China.

Meeting with frustration and disappointments in our attempts to serve the Lord can be confusing. "Lord, I am trying to do this for You. Why won't you make the road smooth?" As with Blessed Guido, the Lord allows difficulties to strengthen us in our resolve to serve. Guido's frustrated efforts in joining the Jesuits and Salesians were God's way of starting an entirely new missionary congregation!

Exercise: Ask the Holy Spirit to show you a time in your own life when He used a difficulty to set you on a path to blessing. Throughout the rest of your day, each time your plans are frustrated (and you know they will be), turn to the Lord and say, "I don't understand, but I know You love me. Whatever you are working out here, thank You." That's praying like a saint!

St. Leonard (died 559)

But at night an angel of the Lord opened the prison doors and brought them out...   *Acts 5:19*

Punishment has the primary aim of redressing the disorder introduced by the offense. When it is willingly accepted by the guilty party, it assumes the value of expiation.
Catechism of the Catholic Church, paragraph 2266

Many legends and romances have accrued to the story of this great sixth century saint. A noble of the court of Clovis I, the first Catholic King of a united France, Leonard was converted with the king by St. Remigius, Bishop of Reims. He left the court and received permission from the king to release any prisoners he found ready and worthy of liberation. With a grant of land from the king—the king gave him all the land he could cover on the back of his donkey during a day of prayer—he built a monastery within a vast wooded land, employing many holy former prisoners to clear the land and do other good works.

Exercise: We saw, in St. Joseph Cafasso (June 23), one other example of the many saints whose hearts did not neglect persons in prisons. God's mercy extends to every person who accepts it, and freedom may come when the prisoner has paid his rightful dues. Of course, he or she may also do God's work while imprisoned. Prisons are known as physical training grounds, since many are equipped with weight rooms and the prisoners generally have plenty of time to train their bodies. How much more important, though, is the training of their souls to move toward Christ. I (Kevin) happened to do my first college teaching of psychology at a prison. Let us pray today, in honor of St. Leonard, for all incarcerated men and women, those who serve at our jails and prisons, and for those Christ-like souls who perform prison ministry.

St. Didachus (1400-1463)

Today we celebrate one of our Franciscan saints. During Didachus' early years he sought spiritual direction from a priest of the Third Order Franciscans and lived as a hermit. In the hope of making further spiritual progress, he became a lay brother in the Franciscan convent in Castille, Spain. Didachus did make great gains in prayer and became renowned for the insights he gained during meditation. As sparse as his formal education was, it did not stop the order's theologians from seeking him out for conversation. Didachus eventually accepted an assignment as a missionary brother to the Canary Islands, off the northwest coast of Africa. He was instrumental in bringing a large number of pagans to conversion. He augmented his prayer, acts of kindness, and evangelization with extreme penances.

When he returned to Rome for the canonization of St. Bernadine of Siena, an epidemic struck the convent in which he stayed. God used it as an opportunity to work many miracles through Didachus' hands, miraculously multiplying supplies and healing the sick over whom Didachus made the Sign of the Cross.

Exercise: We trace the Sign of the Cross over ourselves at the beginning and end of every prayer, but do we stop to appreciate its significance? Each time we make it, we proclaim the Gospel: Through Baptism we have been empowered to enter the life of the Triune God with our entire mind (touch forehead), heart (touch chest), and strength (touch both shoulders). God's grace allows us to fulfill Israel's *Shema*, which Jesus identified as the Greatest Commandment (Mt. 22:37-38). Today, each time you make the Sign of the Cross, do so slowly and deliberately, renewing your consecration as God's Temple, the dwelling place of the Father, Son, and Spirit. Make the Sign of the Cross over the doors of your home and your space at work, dedicating all that happens there to the Lord your God.

The Feast of the Holy Relics

And as a man was being buried, lo, a marauding band was seen and the man was cast into the grave of Elisha; and as soon as the man touched the bones of Elisha, he revived, and stood on his feet.

2 Kings 13:21

Nevertheless, it does concern the deceased what is done with his body: both that he may live in memory of man whose respect he forfeits if he remains without burial, and as regards a man's fondness for his own body while he was yet living, a fondness which kindly persons should imitate after his death.

St. Thomas Aquinas (ST, II-II, Q.2. a.2)

What a paradox that many modern souls who view the veneration of holy saints' bodies, bone fragments, or other articles as something archaic and bizarre will go to great lengths to obtain simply the autographs of men and women who excel in hitting little balls into holes, knocking bigger ones over fences, or swishing bigger ones still from the three-point line! There is nothing wrong with honoring excellence, and there is no higher excellence than living one's life in a Christ-like manner! Though I (Kevin) will tell this tale in full in an upcoming book *(Three Irish Saints)*, I'll just note for now, that through the generosity of a devout Catholic lady, as I write these words today, a relic of St. Brigid of Ireland (Feb. 1) sits upon my desk. Veneration of relics of the saints goes back very early in the Church's history and remains a beautiful way to honor the very bodily temples of the saints, and to inspire us to emulate their sanctity.

Exercise: For a mild physical workout and a powerful spiritual one, before the week is out, visit the gravesite of a loved one and pray for, and to, him or her. Then take 20 minutes or more for a leisurely walk through the cemetery, reading the names and inscriptions, picturing these people's lives on earth, their deeds, and their families. Remember the Church triumphant in heaven, as well as the Church suffering in purgatory, and ask yourself, as a member of the Church militant on earth, what you can do to help win souls to Christ's kingdom.

Dedication of St. John Lateran

Most Holy Lateran Church, of all the churches in the city and the world, the mother and head.   Inscription on the façade of St. John Lateran

Today's feast crystallizes the intent of this book – to recognize ourselves, both individually and corporately, as the Temple of God and to live our lives accordingly. The Archbasilica of St. John Lateran is considered the mother church of the entire world. It was first dedicated on this date in 324 A.D., by Pope Sylvester I, and has been the Basilica of the Bishop of Rome ever since. The adjoining palace was the papal residence for 1,000 years and the basilica was the location for five ecumenical councils. Additionally, it houses reliquaries containing the skulls of Peter and Paul. The readings for today's feast are also a theological treasure trove. In the first reading we hear Ezekiel prophesy to the exiles of Judah about the new Temple that God would build (47:1-2, 8-9, 12). Living water would flow from it, renewing the land. The second reading comes from Paul (1 Cor. 3:9-13, 16-17). Paul reminds us that we, the Church, are the prophesied Temple; the Holy Spirit, the Living Water, dwells in us. Because of that we must be careful how we build upon the grace given to us in Baptism – we have to build with lasting materials, virtues. This theme is continued in the reading from John's Gospel (2:13-22), where Jesus cleanses the Temple. We are told that Jesus actions flowed from his "zeal" for God's House. He cleanses us because of His great love for us. He has made us members of His very Body, the ultimate earthly dwelling of the Divinity.

Exercise: The best way to honor today's feast is to tend your temple as scheduled – cardio, HIT, or rest. Feed your body the good things it needs and feed your soul through minutes alone with the Lord. If you want to do something further, then by all means make a visit to the Lord in the Eucharist. Kneel before Him in your parish church or its adoration chapel.

St. Andrew Avellino (1521-1608)

A false witness will not go unpunished, and he who utters lies will perish.   *Proverbs 19:9*

CHRISTIAN SOUL! If you seek to reach the loftiest peak of perfection, and to unite yourself so intimately with God that you become one with spirit with Him, you must first know the true nature and perfection of spirituality in order to succeed in the most sublime undertaking that can be experienced or imagined.
Lorenzo Scupoli, "The Spiritual Combat"

Aptly named Lancelloto, this great saint was known in his youth for his handsome appearance, but despite the attention he garnered from young ladies, he was devoted to chastity for Christ, and would become a priest at 26. A skillful civic and canon lawyer, he once committed perjury on behalf of a friend. His heart was convicted with penance when he read the verse from Proverbs quoted above (also see Proverbs 19:5). He would join the order of the Theatines, take the name Andrew in honor of love for the cross (see entry for Nov. 30th), and do great service to the Church. He would be called upon for assistance by St. Charles Borromeo (Nov. 4), and among his disciples would be Lorenzo Scupoli, author of the enduring spiritual classic, *The Spiritual Combat*. He died at 89, soon after a suffering a massive stroke while saying Mass, and is a patron of stroke victims.

Exercise: We find from time to time a mention of the saints' great physical beauty (e.g., Sts. Brigid, Teresa, Rose of Lima, Tutilo, Andrew Avellino), as well as some who were noted to be homely or scarred (e.g., Sts. Tekakwitha and Charles Borromeo). Have you ever noticed how a face you initially find attractive may lose some of its luster when you see that it crowns an uncharitable soul? On the contrary, do not the loving eyes and the caring smile of the most homely faces bring true joy to our hearts over time? Remember well, there is nothing wrong with enhancing our physical appearance though fitness training, as long as we remember that beauty of soul far outstrips beauty of body.

St. Martin of Tours (c. 316-397) Bishop

The son of a tribune in Rome's Imperial Horse Guard, St. Martin seemed destined for military service. He first felt drawn to Christianity when he was 10 years old, and much to his parents' disappointment, sought catechetical instruction. He was required to join the cavalry at 15. While stationed at Amiens on guard duty, Martin's life took a turn when he was approached by a beggar. Filled with compassion for the man, Martin cut his military cloak in two and gave the man half. That night in a dream he saw Jesus clothed in the cloak and praising Martin's charity before the angels. After the dream Martin sought release from the army; his conscience would no longer allow him to take up arms in the emperor's often unjust military campaigns, and he became baptized. After his baptism, he was off in search of St. Hilary of Poitiers (Jan. 14). St. Hilary's holiness was well known, and Martin desired him for a spiritual director. When St. Hilary was amenable to the idea, Martin took up residence in the nearby wilderness and remained there for the next 10 years. Because much of the province was still pagan, Martin would make preaching excursions to neighboring towns. Others, drawn by his preaching and example, followed him to the wilderness. Without intending to, Martin became the founder of Gaul's first monastery. When their bishop died, the people of Tours requested Martin as their new prelate several times, but he refused. They finally resorted to luring him into the city under false pretenses and making him bishop through popular acclaim. He accepted ordination but insisted on establishing a new monastery outside the city walls.

Exercise: St. Martin understood that silence was often necessary to discern the Holy Spirit's inspirations. Cutting back our food intake to 2,000 calories a day (see "calories" in glossary) is good for our health, but when it comes to prayer, we are meant to *feast* every day! Join me today in taking ten minutes to find a quiet place and, as the Psalms say, "taste and see the goodness of the Lord."

St. Cummian Fada (591-662)

Health and soundness are better than all gold, and a robust body than riches.   *Sirach 30:15*

You can scarcely excuse yourselves for knowingly rejecting the observances of the Universal Church.   *St. Cummian Fada*

Deriving, (Kevin speaking), from a long maternal line of Munstermen (of the southwestern province of Ireland), I'm pleased today to introduce this son of the King of West Munster. Called "Fada," meaning "the Tall," for his height, he also attained the heights of learning, as is shown in an extant Paschal letter, in which he quotes from the Latin Vulgate, cites canon law, as well as Church Fathers like Sts. Augustine, Jerome, Cyprian, and Gregory the Great. He would become head of the famous Clonfert monastery and later found a monastery that came to be called Kilcummin in his honor. Along with St. Brendan (May 16), he was counted among the foster-children of St. Ita, "The Brigid of Munster." This learned abbot was a great defender of the one, holy, catholic, and apostolic Church, advising his Irish brethren that if all else failed; they should take their disputes to Rome.

Exercise: How rich is the communion of saints in all kinds of physical temples too; from the thin, to the heavy, to the muscle-laden; from the frail to the robust, from the youthful to the aged; and today, we will ponder the long and the short of them. Matt introduced us to the colorful St. John the Dwarf (Oct. 17), and today we meet St. Cummian the Tall. Pay attention to the next Olympics, Senior Olympics, or Special Olympics, and you will see athletes of all shapes, sizes, ages, colors, and heights as well. As long as we are not burdened with a disease that prevents physical training, regardless of our natural physique or stature, we can all work to make our bodies more healthy and sound. Indeed, even if you are confined to a bed, you can pray for the health of your loved ones, and perhaps even read about and study the principles of health and fitness, and share with them your wisdom.

November 13

St. Frances Xavier Cabrini (1850-1917)

Mother Cabrini is one of those people who grew in strength as the years passed. She entered the world with such a low birth weight that she was immediately rushed to the parish church for Baptism. As a young woman, her application to the convent was rejected twice due to insufficient health. Frances looked for opportunities to serve the Lord's people as a layperson. Impressed by her work straightening out a poorly run orphanage, her bishop suggested that she begin her own religious institute. Her father had regaled her early in life with the missionary adventures of St. Francis Xavier, and she earned her teaching certificate under the tutelage of the Daughters of the Sacred Heart. Given her inspirations, it was very natural to call her order the Missionary Sisters of the Sacred Heart. The name proved providential because she and her sisters were invited to go to New York as missionaries to the marginalized population of Italian immigrants. During her life, Mother Cabrini made the arduous journey back and forth across the Atlantic a number of times, tending to her religious daughters in the U.S. and Europe. The woman thought too physically weak for religious life laid brick, nursed, taught, went door-to-door raising money, and administered an order booming in vocations from its beginning.

Exercise: If you have been performing the recommended HIT exercises in this devotional, then you have already learned from experience that your level of strength can still increase in adulthood. Remember the principles we shared at the beginning of the book: When you are able to perform 12 repetitions of an exercise slowly, with good form, then in your next session attempt to increase the weight by a couple of pounds. If you can perform 8 or 9 repetitions, with good form, at the new weight, then continue working with it in subsequent sessions – trying to add a repetition or perform the movement more slowly until you are ready for another increase.

St. Lawrence O'Toole (1128-1180)

But they who wait for the LORD shall renew their strength, they shall mount up with wings like eagles, they shall run and not be weary, they shall walk and not faint.
Isaiah 40:31-32

The individual bishops are the visible source and foundation of unity in their own particular Churches.
Catechism of the Catholic Church, paragraph 886

This son of an Irish chieftain was taken hostage around age 10 by Dermod Mac Murchad, King of Leinster in eastern Ireland, and spent years under harsh conditions with barely enough to eat. His father was later able to transfer his care to the Bishop of Glendalough. Lawrence would become the abbot of the Monastery of St. Kevin (June 3) at Glendalough, and would later receive unanimous election as Archbishop of Dublin, receiving votes from Irish High King Rory O'Connor and even from his former captor King Dermod Mac Murchad (now married to Lawrence's sister). Dublin at this time in its history was ruled by Danes and Norwegians, but St. Lawrence won them over too, especially by his pastoral zeal when Dublin was hit by a famine. A devout and holy man, he was also a promoter of Gregorian chant.

Exercise: Reminded by St. Lawrence's love for Gregorian chant, today I (Kevin) will recommend an exercise I've done many times. Plug an electronic listening device into your ears, put on some Gregorian chant, head out the front door, and run without weariness or walk (preferably without fainting.) The slow reverent chants work so well for a slower paced workout. This will work just as well on the treadmill, bike, or even doing the house or yard chores. Better yet, if you're musically inclined, take the time to learn some chants and provide your own reverent music!

St. Albert the Great (1200-1280)

A man's wisdom makes his face shine...   *Ecclesiastes 8:1*

St. Albert can fittingly be called the miracle and wonder of our time.
Ulric of Strasbourg

I (Kevin) am pretty sure that if I could write only one complete biography in my lifetime, it would be of St. Albert the Great. (Well, actually, I'm more than pretty sure. I've written only one complete biography so far, and its title is *St. Albert the Great: Champion of Faith and Reason*.) My space is so limited here that I'll simply list a few of his deeds, roles, and titles: Professor and Holder of the Dominican Chair of Theology at the University of Paris, Dominican Provincial of Germany, Bishop of Ratisbon, Preacher of the Cross for the Deliverance of Holy Places, papal lecturer in theology and papal peacemaker, originator of the plan of studies for the Dominicans, establisher of convents and monasteries, author of approximately 130 works of anthropology, astronomy, botany, chemistry, dentistry, geology, Mariology, medicine, philosophy, physics, psychology, Scripture, theology, zoology (and more), teacher and mentor of St. Thomas Aquinas (Jan. 28), Patron Saint of Science, and Universal Doctor of the Catholic Church.

Exercise: Judging from the quotation from Ecclesiastes, St. Albert's face must have glowed like few others! But there is another reason why his cheeks may well have been ruddy. Though raised with reluctance for about two years to the Episcopal dignity of bishop, in order to reform a troubled diocese, St. Albert never forsook his Dominican vow of poverty. He earned himself the nickname of "Bishop Boots," for his rough and simple boots — and those boots were made for walking! Dominicans walked all over Europe; in fact, Albert fined two "lazy" priors to several days of only bread and water for traveling on horseback or in a carriage. The Dominicans are also known for the rosary. Let's plan a Rosary Workout walk today in honor of Great Saint Albert.

St. Gertrude the Great (1579-1639)

O nly a precious few out of our thousands of recognized saints have been designated "Great." Gertrude's *Spiritual Exercises* and the first-person account of her mystical experiences included in the Helfta Dominican's *Herald of Divine Love* continues to instruct the faithful today. Saints and spiritual writers the caliber of Francis de Sales and Teresa of Avila identified her as an inspiration. Gertrude went to live in the Dominican Monastery of St. Mary in Helfta, Saxony, when she was only five years old. She had most likely been orphaned. St. Mechtilde (see Feb. 26th) looked after the children sent to the monastery for education, and the two struck up a friendship that spanned a lifetime. Gertrude's keen mind allowed her to excel in the study of philosophy and Latin literature, but she abandoned both at the age of 26. She was already a committed disciple and had taken religious vows, but the Lord Jesus burst into her life in a new way at that age – inviting her in a vision to take His hand and allow him to lift her over the sinfulness that continued to hold them apart. Gertrude's thirst for Him became insatiable. She sought to know the Beloved through Scripture, the writings of the Church Fathers, and the great theologians who came after them. The Lord showered His Love upon her through a host of mystical experiences, many focused upon the Heart of Jesus.

Exercise: Jesus chose Gertrude to begin calling the Church to deeper reflection upon His Sacred Heart, opened for us on the Cross (Jn. 19:34-37). Jesus made her recognize how He offered His own Heart to the Father, His own prayer, in union with ours, perfecting our offering. Did you follow the exercise recommendation on Oct. 8, to read a page or two from the *Catechism of the Catholic Church*? St. Gertrude had a keen mind when it came to philosophy and the literary classics, but she prized the study of the Faith above all. Open up the incredible gift God has entrusted to you and read at least one more page of the catechism before you call it a day.

St. Hugh of Lincoln (1135-1200)

I know all the birds of the air...   *Psalms 50:11*

Animals are God's creatures. He surrounds them with his providential care. By their mere existence they bless him and give him glory. Thus men owe them kindness.

Catechism of the Catholic Church, paragraph 2416

After the death of Hugh's mother when he was only eight, Hugh accompanied his father to a priory near Grenoble in southeastern France. Hugh thrived in the monastic lifestyle, was made a deacon at age 19, was named prior of another nearby monastery, and then entered the Grand Chartreuse, chief monastery of the Carthusians. (If you've seen the moving 2005 silent film *Into the Silence,* that is where it was filmed.) He progressed through the ranks there, was eventually made prior of the first Carthusian monastery in England at Witham, and in 1186, Hugh became the Bishop of Lincoln. He was devoted to education of the young and care for the sick. His emblem includes a beautiful white swan, the fabled Swan of Stowe, which befriended the saint, following him everywhere and guarding him while he slept!

Exercise: Notice how many saints were known for their loving care of animals, and even for their animal friends; St. Francis (Oct. 4) at the forefront and others too, like St. Kevin (June 3) and his otter, and even St. Albert (Nov. 15), who was known in his youth as the only person who could lead at will the fabled White Horse of Lauingen. We are to care for animals, though the Catechism (2418) reminds us that though we may love animals, we "should not direct to them the affection due only to persons." So, perhaps after prayers this would be a great day to walk the swan, or at least the dog.

St. Rose Philippine Duchesne (1769-1852)

I feel that I am a worn out instrument, a useless walking stick that is fit only to be hidden in a dark corner.   St. Rose Philippine Duchesne

D o your noble resolutions seem to end in frustration? Fearing all those interruptions that pop up around the holidays? Meet your new patron. Born into French society, Philippine had a lifelong desire to be a missionary in the New World. Something always seemed to get in the way, though: When she first joined a religious order, it was dispersed by the French Revolution. She found herself tending to the needs of fugitive priests and the imprisoned instead of the souls of Native Americans. Once confirmed, it was another 14 years before she received permission to join the missions; and when she arrived in the New World, her bishop sent her not to the Native Americans but French settlers, to establish schools for their children. When she finally made it, at age 72, to the Potawatomi tribe, she was too infirm to help with manual labor; and with no mastery of the native language, she was unable to teach the children. Instead she practiced small acts of love; *and she prayed.* The Potawatomi named her "Woman-Who-Prays-Always."

Exercise: If your workout efforts aren't yielding results as quickly as you had hoped, or your workout schedule has had a few interruptions, don't become discouraged. You are working on a temple meant for eternity. Some of these "interruptions" are God's invitations, other building projects to which He wants you to contribute. The schools Philippine founded while "waiting" to work with the Potawatomi helped lay the groundwork for Catholic education throughout the U.S.; almost a 150 years later I (Shane) attended her canonization as a representative of Duchesne High School! Make a list of brief, alternative workouts you can do when interruptions arise. Set a timer and climb the basement steps for 10 minutes; or how about 20 minutes of "free stepping" on the *Wii-Fit* while you watch the evening news? Doing what you can, when you can, is the way to long-term results; take it from *Saint* Rose Philippine Duchesne.

St. Agnes of Assisi (1197-1253)

Agnes was the younger sister of St. Clare (St. Francis' dear associate). When Clare left home to follow Francis, 15 year-old Agnes set off after her just two weeks later. Their father, a count, sent relatives and armed men to retrieve Agnes, but as soon as St. Clare hit her knees in prayer, Agnes' body became so heavy that the entire group of men was unable to lift her. Her enraged uncle raised his arm to strike her but it fell limp to his side, momentarily paralyzed. As a result, Agnes was at her sister's side for the founding of the Order of the Poor Ladies, or Poor Clares. Their mother and sister Beatrice later joined them.

Agnes was Clare's constant support in upholding the order's commitment to imitate Jesus in His poverty. Francis dispatched Agnes to begin and then act as abbess to a convent in Monticello. She went on to establish Poor Clare convents in Venice, Padua, and Mantua. She was at her sister's side in her final earthly moments and, ever the faithful disciple, followed Clare from the life of poverty to glory only three short months later.

Exercise: Clare could not have achieved all she did without the God-given support of Agnes. Touch base with your training partner(s) and prayer partner(s) today. (It's great when they can be one and the same!) Just hearing from you will be an encouragement to them and vice versa.

St. Felix of Valois (1127-1212)

And the Holy Spirit descended upon him in bodily from, as a dove, and a voice came from heaven, "Thou art my beloved Son, with thee I am well pleased." *Luke 3:22*

*Christians are baptized in the **name** of the Father and of the Son and of the Holy Spirit; not in their **names**, for there is only one God, the almighty Father, his only Son, and the Holy Spirit: the Most Holy Trinity.* *The Catechism of the Catholic Church, 233*

Felix of Valois renounced his worldly goods and retired to the forest to live a hermit's life of prayer. He was later joined by St. John of Matha, who proposed they found an order dedicated to ransoming the Christians held captive during the Crusades. They would found the Order of the Holy Trinity for the Ransom of Captives in 1198, and it would become known for the cross of red and blue on its emblem. As the order grew, its mission expanded to include care of the sick in hospitals, education, and evangelization. Trinitarians are still found around the world, leading lives of contemplation and active ministry, placing special emphasis all the while on the mystery of the Holy Trinity.

Exercise: Hopefully each day now we are striving to honor the Holy Trinity through the proper care of our bodily temples, ransoming our bodies from the captivities of gluttony and inactivity. There are actually three main physical components of the proper training of the body: 1) strength training, 2) cardiovascular endurance training, and 3) a healthy, nutritious daily diet. On which will you give special emphasis today? Here is a suggestion. Perhaps Thanksgiving looms around the corner. Why not give thanks to the Trinity, your hosts, and your family, by trying a very small portion of food from every dish they provide you, savoring each bite, and not going back for seconds, or thirds!

St. Pope Gelasius I (Papacy 492-496)

When Pope Gelasius shepherded the Church, the political capitol of the Roman Empire had shifted from Rome to Constantinople. As a result, the Patriarch of Constantinople felt that he, and not the pope, should be recognized as head of the churches of the East. The emperor, residing in Constantinople, thought it a grand idea – but Gelasius, not so much. Like a worthy successor to Peter, Gelasius took a rock-like stand and enunciated the age-old truth: Jesus gave the Church its structure and no one – no emperor, no patriarch, not even a pope – had the authority to change it. Jesus ordained Peter to the office of Prime Minister in his Kingdom, the one to whom all the other Apostles were to look. Wherever Peter went, he took his office with him. When he settled in Rome he was that local church's "overseer," or bishop. The offices of Prime Minister and Bishop of Rome were fused in the person of Peter. Those who have gone on to succeed him as Bishop of Rome have likewise succeeded him as Prime Minister of Jesus' Church. Gelasius' stand helped maintain the unity of the Church for another 500 years before the definitive break between East and West occurred.

Exercise: We live in the aftermath of many other breaks in the unity of the Church. When tensions rise, people on both sides have been guilty of sinful conduct. Humility is lacking in the ones who refuse to give up their personal interpretations of Truth for that of Christ's Body and choose to separate themselves; and is lacking when shepherds have responded in a condescending manner, instead of with love. If you find yourself disagreeing with somebody today, before a word leaves your mouth, recall how you are meant to speak the Truth in love. Ask yourself, "Is this a matter of God's Truth, or opinion?" If opinion, then express yours respectfully. Is there a middle position that could allow you to both move forward, or is this a matter that you can actually let slide? If you find yourself disagreeing on a matter of doctrinal or moral Truth on which Jesus and the Church have definitively spoken, then what words and tone of voice will you need to proclaim the Truth with the most success of it being heard?

Sts. Philemon and Apphia (1ˢᵗ Century AD)
Patrons of Employers and Altar Societies

Philemon and Apphia were a married couple who lived in Colossae (now ruins in modern Turkey) during the New Testament days. They were a generous couple and allowed their home to be used for church services. It was a time well before church structures had been built and early Catholics relied on people like Philemon and Apphia to open their homes for group worship and prayer. It is likely that when the Christians of Colossae first read Paul's Letter to the Colossians, it was at the home of Philemon and Apphia. Paul felt a certain closeness to this couple. In his Letter to Philemon (which was actually a letter written to three people: Philemon, Apphia, and Archippus who was probably their son), Paul requested a room to be prepared for him, for he had hopes to visit the couple. Philemon and Apphia were also some of the earliest Catholics to contemplate the validity of slavery. They owned a slave named Onesimus who ran away from their home. Paul encouraged the couple to forgive Onesimus and to even consider freeing him from his slavery. Tradition tells that they honored this request. Sadly, Philemon and Apphia were martyred; the couple was stoned to death for their Christian practices and beliefs during the persecutions of Emperor Nero (A.D. 54-68).

Exercise: The feast of Saints Philemon and Apphia hovers closely to the feast of Christ the King, the last Sunday of Ordinary Time. Because this couple was so generous with their home, maybe you could commemorate their feast by symbolically preparing a guest room in your home for Christ the King. Perhaps you have a room that needs a bit of attention, a room that could be energetically cleaned from top to bottom. Rarely-used clothing, books, games, and other items could be cleared out and donated to the poor. If one of the walls has a bit of free space, you could add a religious painting or plaque — as a visible, yet gentle reminder that Christ is the King of your home.

Blessed Miguel Agustin Pro (1891-1927)

Blessed Miguel had only been a Jesuit novice for a year when revolution erupted in Mexico. As the political climate became increasingly more hostile to the Catholic Church, his superiors sent him abroad. Over an 11 year period he studied in the U.S., Spain, Nicaragua, and Belgium. He was ordained to the priesthood in 1925. Because of recurrent digestive problems, his superiors allowed him to return home to Mexico in 1926. Just three weeks after his arrival the government began enforcing a law that outlawed all public worship. Father Miguel sprang into action, distributing goods to the poor and celebrating the Mass and sacraments. When a warrant was issued for his arrest he donned disguises to continue his work. He was finally apprehended, after a car once owned by his family was used in an assassination attempt on the president. Fr. Miguel was executed by firing squad without even the pretense of a trial. He died, Rosary in hand, arms extended in the shape of the Cross, his faith in Christ issuing from his lips.

Exercise: It is fitting for the Church to remember Miguel at the end of its liturgical year, close to the Feast of Christ the King. The conviction of Jesus' sovereign rule was at the center of the martyr's life. Because Jesus is King of heaven and earth, Miguel could put up with hardship and face death unafraid, at peace in the conviction that Jesus would reverse injustice and not just restore him to life, but give Miguel a share in His own Resurrection. Knowing that Jesus was firmly planted on the Throne even gave Miguel levity in the face of darkness. Because he knew the victory was assured, persecution did not eliminate the spring in his step, his wild sense of humor, nor his practical jokes. Ask the Lord to fill your heart and mind with the grace He gave Blessed Miguel—the absolute conviction of Jesus' Lordship, even in the midst of chaos. Thank the Lord for the freedom you have to visit Him in the Eucharist whenever you desire; and, if at all possible, make a small pilgrimage to say "I love You," as you rush between appointments.

November 24

Martyrs of Vietnam (1798-1861)

And if anyone loves righteousness, her labors are virtues: for she teaches self-control and prudence, justice and courage; nothing in life is more profitable for men than these.   *Wisdom 8:7*

The common good of many is more Godlike than the good of an individual. Wherefore it is a virtuous action for a man to endanger even his own life, either for the spiritual or for the temporal common good of his country.   St. Thomas Aquinas (ST, II-II, Q 31. a.3)

On June 19, 1998, Pope John Paul II canonized a group of 117 Vietnamese martyrs beatified in groups of various sizes by his predecessors, Popes Leo XIII, St. Pius X, and Pius XII. Since the time of Dominican and Jesuit missionaries in the seventeenth century and before, there have been many groups of Vietnamese martyrs for Christ. St. Thérèse of Lisieux (Oct. 1) was so moved by the story of one that she sought to transfer to a Carmelite monastery in Hanoi, but was prevented the tuberculosis that led to her death. We know only the stories of a relative handful of these martyrs. The Vatican estimates they may number in the hundreds of thousands, most slaughtered by modern godless political regimes that did not bother to record their names or numbers. Many also suffered the most heinous and inhuman of martyrdoms by methods like amputations and disembowelments.

Exercise: Our saints for today displayed that ultimate form of the heroic virtue of fortitude. While their fortitude may not have seemed to profit them in this life, especially in the eyes of their executioners, we can only imagine the beatific vision the martyrs eyes beheld when their torture had ended in death. The image of their suffering for Christ can also inspire us to live more bravely and boldly as Christians for the benefits of those in our own nations today. Let's make sure we do not build the physical fortitude to lift heavy weights or run for miles, without developing along with it the spiritual fortitude to stand up bravely for life and for our faith.

November 25

Blessed Luigi Beltrame Quattrocchi (1880-1951) and Maria Corsini-Quattrocchi (1884-1965)

After 2,000 years of Christian history, it is unusual to hear of a "first" anymore; but that is what we have in these two Blesseds. On this date in 2001, their wedding anniversary, Luigi and Maria Quattrocchi became the first married couple to be beatified *together*. What a beautiful way for the Church to draw attention to this couple, who were able to deepen their love for each other, raise upstanding children, and become saints in the thick of the 20th century! Even before coming together, the two were quite impressive. Luigi had earned a law degree and worked for Italy's Inland Revenue Department, and Maria was of noble blood and her family was deeply involved in the cultural life of Florence. The two met during a visit of Luigi to the family home. At the time of their marriage, Luigi was a virtuous man, but it was Maria who showed him how to enter into a real friendship with the Lord. The two became incredibly generous in communicating God's love. They welcomed four children into the world; this despite the fact that during Maria's fourth pregnancy, doctors only gave her a 5% chance of survival and strongly encouraged her to have an abortion. During WWII, Luigi and Maria opened their home to refugees, and Maria volunteered as a nurse with the Red Cross. Together with their children, they reached out to children in poor neighborhoods by starting a scouting program. When three of their children heard the call to religious life, Luigi and Maria happily consented. After 20 years of marriage, they themselves felt called to a rare form of consecration, foregoing marital relations.

Exercise: Think about your family, and ask the Holy Spirit to give you a simple way to deepen its spiritual life. Could you begin leading the family in a brief prayer each morning, offering your day to the Lord and asking for His blessing? Perhaps you could read today's Gospel when your family sits down to share a meal (feeding the soul as well as the body)? Ask the Holy Spirit for inspiration and ideas!

St. Sylvester Gozzolini (1177-1267)

Abraham answered, "Behold, I have taken upon myself to speak to the Lord, I who am but dust and ashes."　　　*Genesis 18:27*

As the frailty and weakness of human nature are universally known and felt by each one in himself, no one can be ignorant of the great necessity of the Sacrament of Penance.　　*Catechism of the Council of Trent*

Sylvester was born to a noble family in Osimo, and he went to the great learning Italian learning centers of Bologna and Padua to study law, but he had a conversion of heart and "changed his major," as we might say today, to the study of theology. For this his father refused to speak to him for the next 10 years. Sylvester became a dynamic, zealous priest, and was threatened with the loss of his canonry, when he respectfully rebuked the bishop for his scandalous behavior. At age 50, he would experience a yet deeper conversion when he chanced upon an open tomb in which laid the decaying corpse of a person known for great beauty in life. He would retire to live a simple life of prayers as a hermit. Soon, others joined him, and in 1231, guided by a vision of St. Benedict, he formed the Sylvestrine Benedictines, also known as the Blue Benedictines for their distinctive blue habits. By the time of his death, Sylvester ruled 11 monasteries.

Exercise: I (Kevin) quite frequently enjoy the little "coincidences" God places in our way. Though we find ourselves reading today for November 26th, I happen to be writing this essay in the early morning hours of Ash Wednesday. And here we come across our great saint who is moved toward deeper sanctity when he sees a little proof that as for our earthly bodies, we are literally indeed, "ashes to ashes, dust to dust." Though it is right to tend to these earthly bodies of ours while alive, what a great reminder this is that our time is limited on earth, and each of us will die. Can we remember that fact about every person we see today, and treat them with the kind of loving care that might help turn their hearts to God and their souls to heaven?

St. Francesco Antonio Fasani (1681-1742)

"Padre Maestro" ("Father Master") was the title given him by his fellow Franciscans. St. Francesco was a humble priest who put his keen philosophical and theological mind to the service of his order, assisting in the formation of both novices and professed religious. Schooled in Assisi, only yards from the tomb of St. Francis, Francesco spent the next 35 years of ministry in Lucera, Italy, the city of his birth.

By all accounts, Francesco was a model of the priestly life. Each day he would distribute money and goods he had collected to the poor, visiting and praying with them as he did so. He also, on an almost daily basis, visited the imprisoned, counseling them and encouraging them to trust in merciful love for them. The bishop of Lucera also asked him to be of comfort to those awaiting execution, sharing their final moments and extending God's pardon. Francesco preached a number of retreats and missions and was known for the deft way he used Scripture to root out sin and instill a hunger for virtue in his listeners. The absolute height of Francesco's priestly duties was the Eucharist. He always celebrated Mass with great joy, and encouraged the laity to receive the Lord daily.

Exercise: Jesus told the crowd in the synagogue at Capernaum, "Do not labor for the food which perishes, but for the food which endures to eternal life . . . he who eats my flesh and drinks my blood has eternal life, and I will raise him up at the last day" (Jn. 6:27, 54). When our stomachs are full, but we still want to reach for the candy bowl or the bag of chips, what we're really doing is trying to meet an emotional need, to fill some part of our soul in which there is a void. Jesus is the only food that our spirits can live on; the rest is just empty calories. So here is my challenge both for you and for me (Shane): The next time we get the desire to snack, and our stomachs are not growling, instead of reaching for the chips, let's place one hand over the heart and the other over the stomach and invite Jesus to come in and satisfy the real need.

St. Joseph Mary Pignatelli (1737-1811)

Make yourself an ark of gopher wood...   *Genesis 6:14*

...the chief link between the Society of Jesus that had been, and the Society of Jesus that was to be.   *Pope Pius XI*

Joseph Mary Pignatelli has been called the second founder and restorer of the Society of Jesus (Jesuit) Order. For five years after his ordination as a Jesuit priest in 1762, he had worked as a prison chaplain with a special ministry to those condemned to die. Then, on April 3, 1767, his world was turned upside down, when, on the orders of King Charles III of Spain, jealous of the influence of the Jesuits in Spain and the Americas, every Jesus was expelled from Spain and its territories. St. Joseph joined 5,000 Spanish Jesuits in a flotilla of ships and they were rejected at ports in Portugal and France. After settling in Corsica for a time, St. Joseph became of student at Bologna, being unable to function as a priest. Pope Clement XIV had formally suppressed the Jesuit Order in 1773, but in 1798, Joseph encouraged the Duke of Parma to ask permission of Pope Pius VI to establish a Jesuit province in his duchy. Permission was granted and St. Joseph was named the first Italian Provincial of the Jesuit Order. He would die three years before Pope Pius VII would official restore the Society of Jesus.

Exercise: Like a second Noah, St. Joseph Mary Pignatelli kept the Jesuit Order afloat during a long period of time when it seemed as if their world could be washed away forever. And speaking of floating, let's not forget that swimming, and also "water aerobics" classes, can make a very nice addition to one's cardiovascular training regimen. Get your heart rate up for at least 12 minutes or so, and you'll reap cardiovascular awards and burn calories, with no impact trauma on your joints. As the Church is blessed with many religious orders, so too is the world of fitness blessed with "orders" of its own – Runners, Lifters, Bikers, Swimmers, etc. Join one or more today!

Our Lady of Beauraing (20th Century)

"I will convert sinners... I am the Mother of God, the Queen of Heaven. Pray always."   Our Lady of Beauraing to the visionaries

Lourdes, Fatima, and. . .*Beauraing?* Yes, in 1949, the Bishop over Beauraing, Belgium, declared that the 33 apparitions that occurred between November 1932 and January 1933 were worthy of belief. The apparitions were granted to five children, aged nine to thirteen, in the garden of a convent. The Blessed Mother appeared to them clothed in a white dress and veil, a Rosary hanging from her right arm, and her garments emitting a soft blue light. Sharp rays of golden light radiated from her face. On multiple occasions her heart was manifested to the children - gold and pouring forth golden rays of light. (Our Lady of Beauraing is also known as Our Lady of the Golden Heart.) As at Fatima two decades before, devotion to Mary's Immaculate Heart, with its recurring plea to "Pray much! Pray always!," is set before God's People as a sure means for reaching the Gospel's goal of Divine intimacy.

Exercise: Mary's heart is filled with the memory of her Son's words and actions. She meditated on them constantly during her time on earth. Begin the season of Advent by reading the first two chapters of Luke's Gospel. It will take no more than five minutes and will enrich your meditation throughout the rest of the year. Meditate on what you read as you perform today's cardio. It may be cold outside, but there are plenty of indoor alternatives: walking in the mall, a treadmill, stationary bike, Wii Fit, or swimming at the YMCA.

St. Andrew (1ˢᵗ Century)

As he walked by the Sea of Galilee, he saw two brothers, Simon who is called Peter and Andrew his brother, casting a net into the sea; for they were fishermen. And he said to them, "Follow me, and I will make you fishers of men."　　　　　　　*Matthew 4:18-19*

The cross is the unique sacrifice of Christ, the "one mediator between God and men."　　　　*Catechism of the Catholic Church, 618*

The fisherman Andrew, disciple of John the Baptist and brother of Simon Peter, was among the Apostles who were closest to Jesus. According to early Church history in the writings of Origen and Eusebius, after Jesus' death and resurrection, St. Andrew would go fishing for men in to the east in Asia Minor and as far away as Kiev in the Ukraine. Tradition holds that he initiated the see at Byzantium (after Constantine, called Constantinople, and after the Muslims, Istanbul). According to tradition, he was crucified at the city of Patras in the northern Peloponnesian Peninsula of Greece, and declaring himself unworthy to die on a cross like the one upon which Jesus was crucified, he was bound up to die on a cross in the shape of an X, which is known as "St. Andrew's Cross."

Exercise: In the exercise world, "cross-training" refers to the regular use of two or more kinds of exercise for a more complete, whole body effect. We recommend such cross-training; for example, by endorsing strength training along with one or more forms of endurance exercise. As followers of Christ however, the term "cross-training" could have a much more profound meaning. Are we truly training ourselves to bear our crosses like Christ? Is the fortitude we are building in the gym helping us face up to challenges in a spiritual life, and in fulfilling our moral duties? Today, let's think and pray about ways that the strength and endurance we are building at the gym or on the roads might cross over to other areas of our lives.

December 1

St. Eligius of Noyon (588-660)

In all toil there is profit... *Proverbs 14:13*

Everyone should be able to draw from work the means of providing for his life and that of his family, and of serving the human community. *Catechism of the Catholic Church, paragraph 2428*

St. Eligius drew favor from King Clotaire II of Paris for his excellent and honest work as a goldsmith and metalworker. When the king commissioned him to craft a throne of gold and jewels, Eligius secreted away none of the precious metal or jewels for himself, as was the norm. In fact, he crafted a second throne for the king with the materials that were left over. The king befriended him, his fame and fortune grew, and he used his wealth to ransom Christian captives and give alms to the poor. The King's successor, his son King Dagobert I, would name Eligius his first counselor. Desiring to serve God, even over king, Eligius would become a priest, and then the Bishop of Noyon and Tournai. A friend would describe him as tall, curly-headed, with "honest hands," long fingers, "the face of an angel and a prudent look." At times, he wore bejeweled clothing with a hair-shirt underneath. He built churches and monasteries and was loved by his flock for his personal kindness.

Exercise: With great patience and many repetitive strikes of the hammer does the smith ply his trade and craft his precious works. Repetitive movements are also at the heart of physical training. If you have been strength training awhile, here is a variant you might care to try. Instead of selecting a weight that allows the typical recommended 8 to 12 repetitions, select a lighter weight that will allow perhaps at least 18. Stay with that weight each workout until you achieve at least 20. This high-repetition training might be done for a month for a change, or thrown in once in a while at will, just for a workout or two.

Blessed Rafal Chylinski (1694-1741)

Blessed Rafal was beatified by Pope John Paul II, a fellow Pole, in 1991, during one of his visits home. The pope asked all those at the Mass to reflect on God's motive in having Rafal's path to canonization move forward now, instead of closer to the time of his death. The pope left it to each of us to peer into Rafal's life and, with the Holy Spirit's illumination, seek an answer. Rafal's given name was Melchior, which tradition holds to be the name of one of the three wise men who visited the Christ child. His family was of the Polish nobility, but this did not shield Rafal from difficult times. The family endured both the death of his father and the loss of the family home to fire when Rafal was in his early teens. The bishop was a great help to Rafal's mother in raising him and his brothers, even sending the children to receive a Jesuit education. Rafal went on to serve in the cavalry and was recognized as an officer within three years. Rafal later walked away from the military life, much to the disappointment of his comrades-in-arms, to join the Franciscan friars at Kracow. He was ordained in 1717, and went on to serve in the parishes of nine different cities. He was renowned for his homilies and his work as a confessor. Proficient with the mandolin, harp, and lute, Rafal put his talents to work in the communities' celebrations of the Eucharist. He also served as an exorcist.

Exercise: Rafal's life turns my (Shane's) mind to penance – the performance of a virtuous act in place of a sinful one, meant to strengthen us in our identity as disciples. Through God's grace we can perform penitential acts for our own good, but also on behalf of others. During Advent, you can offer small penitential acts to the Christ child on behalf of the times that we have failed him by our sins. You could begin today by enduring a small fast – perhaps cutting your lunch in half; or maybe later this week you could pass along the candy left by your Secret Santa to someone else. Little acts, imperceptible to anyone's eyes but God's—that was Blessed Rafal's way.

St. Francis Xavier (1506-1562)

Every athlete exercises self-control in all things. They do it to receive a perishable wreath, but we an imperishable.   *1 Corinthians 9:25*

It is not the actual physical exertion that counts towards one's progress, nor the nature of the task, but by the spirit of faith with which it is undertaken.   *St. Francis Xavier*

This refined and contented Professor of Philosophy at the University of Paris would meet a zealous former military captain who would set his soul on fire and guide him across the globe to ignite new souls for Christ in lands he had hardly heard of. On August 15, 1534, he and five companions, along with St. Ignatius Loyola, would make a holy vow that would soon lead to the establishment of the Society of Jesus, devoted to missionary work around the world. St. Francis, despite a strong tendency toward seasickness, would sail to the East Indies, land at Goa, and bring true Christian teaching and kindness to a people who had been abused by many Portuguese profiteers, Christian in name only. He lived humbly and poorly among them. He later learned of Japan and sought to bring Christ there. He adapted his methods, wearing fine clothing and bringing fine gifts to win admittance to the presence (and the hearts) of their rulers. Francis then turned his eyes toward China. On this final journey, he would die on a small island, with China in sight but never reached. Thirty years later, a group of Jesuit missionaries completed his journey.

Exercise: I (Kevin) today recommend an exercise for your eyes, your imagination, and your intellect that will be anything but painful, and that will set your heart afire. It is as simple as this: Obtain and read *Set All Afire: A Novel of St. Francis Xavier* by Louis De Wohl. Better yet, consider first this quote from St. Francis himself: "Give me the children until they are seven and anyone may have them afterwards." Consider reading this book aloud with your children. And far better yet, read all of De Wohl's novels about many great saints who appear in this book!

December 4

St. John Damascene (c. 650-749) Doctor of the Church

The Patristic Age, the Age of the Church Fathers, came to an end with the death of John. Born in Damascus, he lived his entire life under Islamic rule. His father served Caliph Abdul Malek as his counselor and chief financial officer, a position to which John succeeded upon his father's death. Both John and his adopted brother eventually left public life to seek deeper union with the Lord in the monastery of St. Sabas outside Jerusalem. Today, when we hear "summa theologica," our minds naturally fly to St. Thomas Aquinas, but John's *On the Orthodox Faith* was actually the first scholarly attempt at a theological summation of our faith. Besides over a hundred other works with which he is credited, John also wrote poems and hymns that are still used in Greek liturgies today. John is perhaps best known to history for his opposition to Iconoclasm, the belief that creating images of Jesus or the saints, or the veneration of those images, is sinful. John's orthodoxy regarding the Incarnation (that the invisible God had truly become a human being, and had become visible to His creation) allowed John to understand that Jesus' humanity and the events of His life could be represented in art the same as any other human being, and that the veneration shown to an image of Jesus or one of the saints was no more an act of idolatry than kissing the picture of a beloved relative.

Exercise: You and I are made in the image and likeness of God but it is an even greater honor to be His dwelling place, living temples. This is true of our whole person, and because of that we want to be good stewards of both body and soul. Give thanks to God today by venerating His image, His dwelling, in another – plant a kiss on the cheek of someone you love, and offer a sincere prayer for his or her well-being as you do so (Rom. 16:16; 1 Cor. 16:20; 1 Peter 5:14). Honor God through your treatment of yourself today, too: Practice temperance in eating, perseverance in exercise, chastity in expressing your sexuality, and justice in your performance of work and the taking of rest.

December 5

St. Sabbas of Jerusalem (439-532)

Behold, I am doing a new thing; now it springs forth, do you not perceive it? I will make a way in the wilderness and rivers in the desert.
                                                                    Isaiah 43:19

The most appropriate places for prayer are personal or family oratories, monasteries, places of pilgrimage, and above all the church...   *Catechism of the Catholic Church, paragraph 2696*

St. Sabbas was merely eight years old when he entered a monastery. At 18, he made a pilgrimage to Jerusalem, joined a monastery run by St. Euthymius, and upon the great abbot's death, left to live and pray in the desert. Over the years, he was joined by many others and would found a monastery of his own called the Great Lavra of Saint Sabbas the Sanctified, or Mar Saba in Arabic, overlooking the Kidron Valley. It would later be home to the great Eastern Father, St. John Damascene (see Dec. 4th), and is to this day inhabited by prayerful Eastern Orthodox monks. The monastery made the news in modern history in 1965 when Pope Paul VI, in a gesture of ecumenical charity, returned to it relics of the saint taken to Italy by twelfth century Crusaders. In the seventh century, some monks from the monastery settled in Rome and erected a church of St. Sabbas. That church is served by modern-day Jesuits.

Exercise: One miracle attributed to St. Sabbas is the production of a spring at the desert site of his great monastery, full of cells that were full of prayer. Consider the words above from the Catechism on prayer. Does your house have a "TV room," perhaps a "game room," a "study," a "family room," an "exercise room," or even perhaps a "laundry room?" Well, where, then, is the "prayer room?" No need to add on, but let's think about this. Is there a special room you can make an "oratory," literally, a room for prayer? Perhaps one of the other rooms can double up. Do you have any beautiful statues or portraits of Christ, Our Lady, or any great saints? Well, Christmas is coming! Why not make at least some part of your house literally house of prayer?

St. Nicholas (died c. 350) Bishop

Nicholas, one of the most popular saints of the Middle Ages (with over 400 churches dedicated to him in England alone) is a person we can say very little about with historical certainty. We know he was the bishop of Myra, near present-day Finike, Turkey. He was imprisoned during the reign of Emperor Diocletian's persecution of the Church, but released after Constantine's ascendency to the throne. Although his name is not listed among the council fathers at Nicaea, there is a tradition that places him there—slapping the face of the arch-heretic Arius and winding up in the dungeon for the remainder of the proceedings. There are of course a number of rich legends about the man who was eventually transformed into Santa Claus. He is reported to have been from a wealthy family and to have used his considerable inheritance to finance acts of charity. The most popular story in this vein has Nicholas saving three sisters from lives of prostitution: The girls' monetarily-strapped father was no longer able to provide for their physical needs. Unable to provide the dowries required to arrange marriages for the girls, he saw no other alternative but to sell them into prostitution. Hearing of their plight, Nicholas came by night on three separate occasions, tossing bags of gold through the windows of the home. As a result, the father was able to find suitable husbands for his daughters.

Exercise: Factual or not, Nicholas' linkage with the Council of Nicaea is fortuitous during this season of Advent. The Nicene Creed is an amazing statement of our faith in both the Trinity and the truth of the Incarnation. Use the words of the Nicene Creed to praise and thank God today for the gift of faith: "You are the one God, the Father almighty, maker of heaven and earth... I praise you Lord Jesus Christ... God from God, Light from Light... Glory be to you Holy Spirit, Lord and Giver of Life... I thank You for letting me believe here in the midst of Your one, holy, catholic, and apostolic Church..."

St. Ambrose (339-397)

I began to see that Christianity could be rational....As I listened to him, I was ashamed that I had been barking all those years, not against Christianity, but against imaginary doctrines.

St. Augustine of Hippo

Thank God today for Aurelius Ambrosius, an outstanding man, even among the company of the saints. This secular governor of northern Italy stepped in to help settle a dispute between rival factions at Milan who were unable to select a bishop. One man was so impressed at the wisdom and manner of Ambrose's approach that he began chanting for Ambrose as bishop! And indeed, the reluctant and yet unbaptized catechumen was selected. He disbursed himself of his possessions and immersed himself in the study of theology and in prayer. He would become one of the four original Latin Fathers of the Church, along with Sts. Jerome, Gregory the Great, and the man he brought into the church, St. Augustine himself. An amazingly bold and successful shepherd and leader, he rebuked the Eastern Roman Emperor Theodosis for slaughtering 7,000 people in Thessalonica in retribution for the murder of a Roman governor. The mighty emperor submitted publicly and did penance. On February 27, 380, he would declare Catholic Christianity the religion of the empire.

Exercise: In an intriguing passage, St. Augustine records his astonishment at St. Ambrose for reading silently! It had been the custom to read books aloud, even when alone. My (Kevin's) lifting partner, Mike, and I would occasionally tell the other we were "opening up the textbook," suggesting that we planned to execute our next strength exercise with perfect "textbook" form. Perhaps you have seen some at the gym who don't seem to know how to lift weights silently, emitting all sorts of wild moans and groans! When employing proper form in strength training, uninvolved muscles should be relatively relaxed, even those involved in yelling. So, take a hint from St. Ambrose, and lift, as well as read, in sacred silence!

Feast of the Immaculate Conception

"Have you been saved?" Maybe you have been asked that by one of our Protestant brothers or sisters. If our Blessed Mother had been asked, she could have given the loudest "Yes!" the world had ever heard. Her personal salvation from the stain of Original Sin is celebrated today. Mary praised God's salvation in her Magnificat and invited us to join her: "My spirit rejoices in God my Savior... henceforth all generations will call me blessed. (Lk. 1:47-48) As we all know, there are two ways to be saved from disease: once it has been contracted, a person can receive treatment, or a person can be prevented from contracting the disease in the first place! The first option is how God saves us, and the second, the way He chose to save our Blessed Mother. In both cases, the Father's sanctifying grace isn't given because of anything we have done, but because of God's unmerited Love, and in response to the actions of Jesus. Mary's salvation, too, is due to her Son—the effect of the Cross working backward in time. Mary's Immaculate Conception can even be glimpsed in Gabriel's greeting, when he called Mary "Full of Grace," *Kecharitomene* in Greek (Lk. 1:28). The term refers to a completed action—Mary *has been*, and remains, filled with God's grace, His Life. As a perfect infilling, it occurred simultaneously with her conception.

Exercise: By the physical and spiritual exercises you are engaged in, the Lord saves you in both ways. Firstly, through personal and liturgical prayer, through exercise and diet, He is repairing the damaging effects of original and personal sin. Secondly, He is using these same exercises to build virtue and shield us from even larger tragedies (Jn. 5:14); each of us already shares some portion of *Jesus' Cross*, no need to go fashioning additional ones! Today, express your heartfelt thanks to the Lord for the work of salvation He accomplished in Mary, and is completing right now in you. And there is no greater way to give thanks than by participating in the Eucharist. (*Eucharistein* is Greek for "thanksgiving.") Give thanks with your whole being.

December 9

St. Peter Fourier (1565-1640)

Do not slight the discourse of the sages, but busy yourself with their maxims...
Sirach 8:8

To harm no one and to help everyone.
Motto of St. Peter Fourier

How fitting that St. Peter Fourier selected such a motto, when St. Thomas Aquinas had written that the two fundamental principles at the heart of the virtue of justice are "Do the good," and "Do no harm." St. Peter Fourier, you see, had memorized St. Thomas's massive (over 3,000 pages in a modern edition) *Summa Theologica* by heart (and some believe St. Thomas himself had dictated it from memory!) Born in Lorraine, France, Peter Fourier would become a learned church canon, a parish priest, founder of the Congregation of Notre Dame for women religious teachers of young girls, and the founder and first Superior General of the Congregation of Our Savior for the education of young boys. In 1625, the 60 year-old was sent on a mission and won back to the Church all the "little strangers" as he called them – inhabitants of the Principality of Salm, near Nancy, who had been won over by reformers.

Exercise: Here we have another great Catholic memory master. The *Summa Theologica* that St. Peter knew so well by memory actually includes St. Thomas's advice for improving your memory (II-II, Q.49, a.1). I (Kevin) wrote the book *Memorize the Faith!* about it, and St. Albert the Great's own memory lessons are in the biography I wrote about him. Devout exercises of memory can also easily fit into your cardiovascular training. First, memorize some catechetical information of interest to you, perhaps the Stations of the Cross or the order of the books in the Old or New Testament. Next, as you walk, run, or bike, practice or rehearse what you've memorized, in both forward and backward order. For, as the ancients knew well, *"Repetitio est mater memoria,"*—repetition is the mother of memory!

Blessed Brian Lacey (c. 1550-1591)

Brian was raised in Yorkshire, England, a bastion of Catholicism throughout Queen Elizabeth I's bloody reign. He grew up not just hearing tales of martyrdom, but also actually knowing and being related to such saints. His relative, William Lacey, was a priest who lost his life for celebrating Mass. When Brian's cousin, Montford Scott, returned to England after being ordained a priest in Rome, the two set out to strengthen the underground Church. They criss-crossed England for seven years, dispensing pamphlets and sacramentals like the rosary. Fr. Scott of course celebrated the sacraments wherever they went. Their ministry came at a price, though; Fr. Scott did a seven year stretch in the Tower of London, and Brian was incarcerated twice during the same period. Once they were both free, they jumped right back into their work for the Church, only to have their whereabouts divulged to the authorities. (The government offered money to citizens reporting Catholic activities). Both men were arrested. Fr. Scott was executed immediately, but Brian was tortured for months in the hopes of obtaining the names of other practicing Catholics. He gave them nothing. In the final second before he was hung to death, his executioner informed him that he had been betrayed to the authorities by his own dear brother, Richard. He died asking God's mercy upon his brother's soul.

Exercise: Throughout Advent we look ahead to the day when Jesus will come again. We long for that day, and at the same time, have a healthy fear of standing before the Judge. You, like Brian Lacey, will probably go to meet the Judge long before His Second Coming. Pray today for the grace of *final perseverance* – the grace to finish this life firmly and unashamedly united to Jesus. Pray for this grace both for yourself and all the members of your family. The relationship between Brian Lacey and his cousin Montford Scott again reminds us of how important it is to support one another, especially within the family. Be sure to touch base with your prayer and training partners today, too.

St. Pope Damasus I (305-384)

Everyone then who hears these words of mine and does them will be like a wise man who built his house upon the rock...   Matthew 7:24

Yet, though your greatness terrifies me, your kindness attracts me.
                                        St. Jerome, in a letter to Pope Damasus

Prepare now to ponder a pious Portuguese pope. Damasus' heroic courage and devout zeal for the true faith were seen in his battling of heresies and healing of schisms within the Church as the Bishop of Rome. He employed the great St. Jerome (Sept. 30), and encouraged him in his production of the Vulgate, the Latin translation of the Bible. He called two Roman synods and gave sanctuary at Rome to Patriarch Peter II of Alexandria when driven into flight by Arian heretics. He led the Church with honor from St. Peter's chair for over 18 years until his death at near 80. St. Jerome, ever the polished scholar as well as the saint, wrote that Damasus also wrote some very fine verses and brief compositions in heroic, poetic meter.

Exercise: Recalling that strength training is the rock upon which our foundation of physical fitness is built, let's examine another advanced technique today, only for those healthy, hearty souls who have already established a firm foundation through months, if not years of steady training. We considered high repetition training as a change of pace on December 1st. Today, let's move to the opposite end of the spectrum with a system called "rest-pause" training. Using a machine like a chest press or overhead press, perform one very near maximum repetition, lowering it slowly for at least 4 seconds. Take a resting pause of about 10 seconds and try to complete one more repetition (with slight assistance from a partner if necessary.) Rest 10 seconds again. Slightly lower the weight to allow one more all-out repetition. Rest 10-15 seconds again, and with a slightly lower weight, perform your fourth and final repetition. Lower the last rep as slowly as you can, taking 10 seconds or more.

December 12

Our Lady of Guadalupe (16th Century)

"Am I not here, who is your Mother?"   *Our Lady to St. Juan Diego*

Our Lady was sent to Juan Diego at an ugly time in our continent's history. Cortez had defeated the Aztecs only ten years earlier, a civilization that practiced human sacrifice on an enormous scale. Franciscan and Dominican missionaries were able to win a hearing with only a handful of people (Juan Diego and his late wife among them) due to the horrendous treatment of the natives by the conquistadors who took control of the land. Many of the natives were treated as virtual slaves. Juan Diego was traveling to Mass on the Feast of the Immaculate Conception when Mary appeared to him on Tepeyac Hill and sent him to Bishop Zumarraga with the request for a shrine to be built so that she could show her motherly love for the people. The bishop's refusal to believe Juan Diego led to a miraculous sign: Mary's image imprinted upon his tilma, or outer garment. Mary showed herself under the imagery of Revelation 12:1, a pregnant woman, "clothed with the sun, with the moon under her feet." In Revelation 12, the woman is at war with the ancient serpent, Satan (12:9, 13), and Mary's appearance at Tepeyac was God's deathblow to paganism in the Americas. Tepeyac was where the Aztecs had worshipped Tonantzin, the mother of the gods—many who were portrayed as serpents. Mary's appearance revealed her as the exalted, yet human, mother of the *true God*. Within a decade of her appearance, nine million natives were baptized into the life of the Father, Son, and Spirit; and Juan Diego's tilma, that should have disintegrated within a matter of decades, can still be viewed in Mexico City four hundred years later!

Exercise: Beseech our Lady of Guadalupe, Patroness of the Americas, to obtain from her Son the grace of a new springtime of evangelization. We have allowed the serpent to re-entangle our continent in the darkness of sexual immorality and the human sacrifice of abortion; and only a return to Mary's Son can save us.

St. Lucy of Syracuse (died 304)

Fiat lux! (Let there be light!) *Genesis 3:3 (Latin Vulgate Edition)*

On many that were blind he bestowed sight. *Luke 7:21*

Many strange legends have accrued to the name of his early holy virgin martyr. Though devoted to Christ early in life, her family tried to arrange a marriage for her, which she delayed for several years. Her mother had been suffering from hemorrhages for years when Lucy advised her to touch the sepulcher of St. Agatha, who had been healed from a like disease when she touched the garment of Christ. Having fallen asleep in prayer, she experienced a vision of St. Agatha, which foretold of her mother's healing and of Lucy's own martyrdom for her faith in Christ. One legend has it that Lucy's jailers removed her eyes before her martyrdom by fire and stabbing, and another that God restored her sight before her death. She is often represented with her two eyes on a plate! In Scandinavia, she is honored in a yearly festival around St. Lucy's Day, the shortest day of the year, partly because her name means "light." Large grains of wheat floating in a dessert of hot chocolate are said to represent her eyes in this treat eaten only once yearly.

Exercise: Some of us are prone to dampened moods and spirits in the cold, dark months of winter, but a great antidote is a vigorous workout either out in the sun, or in a well-lit room. So, today or tomorrow, consider sending out a surge of mood-enhancing endorphins with a nice strength or cardio workout. With Christ's birthday celebration so soon upon us, 'tis the season to be jolly, after all.

St. John of the Cross (1542-1591)

So Ahab sent to all the people of Israel, and gathered the prophets together at Mount Carmel. And Elijah came near to all the people, and said, "How long will you go limping with two different opinions? If the LORD is God, follow him; but if Baal, then follow him."

1 Kings 18:20-21

Two opposite qualities cannot coexist in one person. Darkness which is passion for created things, and light, which is God, are opposites.

St. John of the Cross, Ascent of Mount Carmel

Juan de Yepes's father had been disowned by his family for marrying an orphan below their social class. He died when Juan was an infant, and Juan was raised in poverty by his mother. When the humble youth presented himself to the Carmelites as a lay brother, they recognized his capacities and trained him as a priest. Due to the presence of some corruption in the order, and his desire for austerity, he considered a life in the Carthusian Order, until, at 25, he met a kindred holy and mystical spirit in the 52-year-old St. Teresa of Avila (Oct. 15). As she would reform the Carmelite women religious through her discalced order, so too would she recruit the young saint to reform the Carmelite friars. Juan was imprisoned and tortured for several months, consoling himself by writing spiritual poetry. Though they garnered scant attention during his life, his works are now cherished classics.

Exercise: How interesting that we honor the author of *Dark Night of the Soul* the very day after St. Lucy, whose name means light. (This is also the birthday of my [Kevin's] wife Kathy, who has been my faithful companion through more than a few dark nights of the soul!) To St. John of the Cross, worshipping the things of creation and worshipping their Creator could not be more different than night and day. We are of the world. We live in it and must love its creatures, but must never lose sight of the Creator. Even as we train our bodies, we must train our hearts to love and serve the God who created and sustains both us and all that is seen and unseen.

St. Christiana (4ᵗʰ Century) Apostle of Georgia

Go into all the world and preach the gospel to the whole creation.
Mark 16:14

Go to Iberia and tell there the Good Tidings of the Gospel of Jesus Christ, and you will find favour before the Lord; and I will be for you a shield against all visible and invisible enemies. By the strength of this cross, you will erect in that land the saving banner of faith in My beloved Son and Lord. *The Blessed Virgin Mary*

Perhaps you've heard The Charlie Daniels Band's high energy, fast-fiddling "The Devil Went Down to Georgia?" Well, today we examine a high energy saint who went up to another, older Georgia (actually Iberia in those days.) As an ancient saint of many legends, St. Christiana is also known as St. Nina and St. Nino. She is believed to have come from Cappadocia, was a relative of St. George, and was directed in a vision from the Virgin Mary to spread her son's gospel to Iberia (now Georgia) in the south of Russia. She was able to heal the Queen Nana from an incurable disease, and converted her and King Mirian III to Christ.

She is venerated in the Catholic Church and highly revered in Eastern Orthodox Churches as "Enlightener of Georgia," and even "Equal to the Apostles." Her symbol is a "grape vine cross" with slightly drooping cross-arms.

Exercise: The Blessed Mother's advice to St. Christiana reminds me (Kevin) of St. Paul's wonderful imagery of putting on the armor of Christ. (Ephesians 6:13-17). A good Christian friend of a good Christian friend of mine has the habit every day in the morning of actually imagining she is donning this amour (girding the loins with truth, the breastplate of righteousness, shodding the feet with peace, the shield of faith, the helmet of salvation, and the sword of the Spirit, which is the word of God.) When you prepare to go out for your next Rosary Workout, high intensity strength session, or even a walk around the neighborhood, why not put on this armor along with the rest of your gear?

Blessed Honoratus Kozminski (1829-1916)

We think we live in interesting times? Wenceslaus Kozminski was born into a Poland under the rule of Russian invaders, and upwardly mobile Poles were abandoning the country in droves. Wenceslaus was fortunate to be born into a devout family. While attending Warsaw's School of Fine Arts, he came under the sway of "Enlightenment" thought and renounced the Catholicism of his youth. In 1846, he found himself falsely accused of an anti-Russian plot and imprisoned for a year. While there he contracted typhoid and came close to death. He survived, crediting the Blessed Mother, and experienced a return to the Faith. A new man emerged from prison. He publicly repented of his sin of apostasy, and in 1848, joined the Capuchin Franciscans, taking the name Honoratus. Within a few years, he was ordained to the priesthood. In 1863, the Russians closed the Capuchins house in Warsaw and basically outlawed participation in religious congregations. Honoratus and his comrades relocated to Zakroczym, where they were virtually under house arrest within their monastery. When a number of those who still came to him for spiritual direction expressed a desire for religious life, Honoratus made a novel recommendation: Take vows, but continue to live in the world, without wearing any outward signs of consecration. He saw this as a way to continue religious life in Poland despite the hostility of the Russians.

Exercise: Do not allow yourself to buy into deceptive thoughts such as, "I'm not called to the priesthood or a religious order; I can never achieve that kind of familiarity with God." Each and every one of us, in our current roles, is called to make Jesus present to the world. Did you realize that St. Paul supported himself by making tents? Just think of the spiritual treasures he let "slip" while talking with customers. Imagine being able to say, "The guy that made my tent? Apostle to the Gentiles." I want people 50 years from now trying to imagine what it would have been like to be one of *your* co-workers, customers, kids, etc.

St. Jose Manyanet y Vives (1833-1901)

There is no wealth better than health of body, and there is no gladness above joy of heart.
                                                            Sirach 30:16

Jesus, Mary and Joseph, may I breathe forth my soul in peace with you.
                                                        St. Jose's last words

Jose was born in Catalonia, Spain. His father died when he was but two years old, and his mother dedicated him to the Virgin Mary at five. He was raised in part by a Spanish priest and was ordained himself in 1859. He worked for a time as a seminary librarian. He came from a large family and did great works in support of the family. He later started the Congregation of the Sons of the Holy Family, the Missionary Daughters of the Holy Family of Nazareth, and The Holy Family Magazine. St. Jose never possessed the wealth of a healthy body, yet he still maintained a joyful heart. He was prone to sickness and maladies, including open wounds on his sides that never healed. He referred to them as "God's mercies." We can deduce from his last recorded words that his devotion to the Holy Family remained to the very end of his time on earth.

Exercise: Christmas is almost upon us. What gifts might you give, or what activities might you perform to enhance the physical and spiritual health and wealth of your own family? I (Kevin) picked up a tandem (two-seater) bike last Christmas and have waited patiently about three months to share in some leisurely rides with my wife and sons. Consider the possibilities to exercise with your spouse or children. If one of the parties is far more fit than the other, that's no sweat (so to speak), as the stronger party can do more of the work without losing the partner (and burning a few more calories.) It also provides time for togetherness and conversation. Consider a tandem bicycle, then, for your holy family!

St. Flannan (7ᵗʰ Century) Bishop

What would the Christmas season be without one of our Irish saints? Flannan was the son of an Irish chieftain, Turlough of Thomond. His father sent him to the monastery at Killaloe to be educated. It had only recently been founded by St. Molua, who served as abbot. Instead of returning to his father after the completion of his education, Flannan chose to remain at the monastery. His holiness and hard work were noted by St. Molua, and he eventually chose Flannan to succeed him as abbot.

While Flannan was abbot, the surrounding community, which looked to the monastery for guidance, began to thrive in every way. Flannan was noted for spending a great deal of time in nature, meditating upon the Lord as he surveyed the grandeur of His creation; and no doubt Flannan stretched his legs as he did so. During a pilgrimage to Rome, Pope John IV consecrated him as the first bishop of Killaloe. He quickly became recognized for his preaching. His father was so moved by Flannan's witness that he resigned from his position as chieftain and began to live the life of a monk along with his son.

Exercise: With the great feast of Christmas just around the corner, you want to be sure to "stretch those legs" throughout the rest of the week with some good, calorie-burning cardio. Throughout Scripture we have a pattern of work and then reward: six days of labor and then the Sabbath; fasting and then the feast. Make a point of burning extra calories now, so that you can feast and relax on Christmas day without so much as a second thought!

December 19

St. Nemesius of Alexandria (died 250)

And they crucified him with two robbers, one on his right and one on his left.
Mark 15:27

Look at the shining examples of our ancient Fathers and the Saints, in whom true perfection and religion flourished and then you will see how little we do by comparison. How can we even compare our life with theirs?
Thomas a Kempis, The Imitation of Christ

All Christians are called to imitate Christ in our lives, and some even in their deaths. As the innocent Christ suffered crucifixion between two thieves during the reign of the Emperor Tiberius, so too, during the reign of the Emperor Trajan, did Nemesius suffer crucifixion between two thieves, his only crime being that of openly following Christ. When rounded up with others by police and charged of stealing, Nemesius was found innocent. When faced then with charges of being a Christian, Nemesius admitted that "crime," and suffered heinous tortures including dislocation of limbs before he was crucified in Alexandria, as Christ had been upon the hill at Calvary.

Exercise: Have you ever read *The Imitation of Christ*? It's a riveting crash course in humility and devotion, especially crafted for those in the religious life, but rife with lessons for us all. Let's take time in our next morning prayer or during a morning walk, to ask ourselves how we can imitate Christ in every setting of our lives. How do you think Christ would behave at your gym, at your office, in your home, and heaven forbid perhaps, even in your car? Can you remind yourself that in the actions of our bodily temples, we present Christ to others wherever we may go? Are we, like the many saints we are coming to know and love, setting a shining example?

Blessed Jean-Bernard "Scubilion" Rousseau (1797-1867)

Blessed Scubilion made a complete gift of himself to Jesus, serving Him among the least respected of His brothers and sisters, the enslaved men and women of La Reunion Island. Catechesis was his passion, and he was already deeply engaged in it when he first encountered St. Jean-Baptiste de La Salle's Christian Brothers. He entered the order at age 25, and spent his first 10 years in religious life teaching in schools in France. His true calling was discovered when the Christian Brothers dispatched him from France to La Reunion Island to teach in the Brother's school there, and his heart was immediately drawn to the slave population. When plantation masters were hesitant to allow their slaves to leave the property to attend Scubilion's catechism classes, he gladly went to them. He put the Creed and other truths of the Faith into easily remembered choruses and taught his new flock about their dignity in Christ. In addition to catechism, Scubilion gave his flock an elementary education—something forbidden to slaves. The Gospel took such deep root in their lives that when their legal emancipation from slavery occurred in 1848, the people did not seek to visit retribution upon their former masters. Scubilion worked hard to help his people transition from the life of slaves to that of free men and women. He never truly retired from his work; his final years were spent taking the Gospel into the remote regions of the island and assisting local pastors in catechesis of former slaves.

Exercise: Blessed Scubilion put himself at the service of the enslaved. Would you like to set someone free today? I am willing to bet that someone wronged you in the past year, and that even though you have forgiven them, there is still uneasiness when you run into each other. Help them move past the burden of their guilt by shooting them a "Merry Christmas" email or dropping a card in the mail. Until new pleasant memories are made, we tend to dwell in the dark ones of the past.

St. Peter Canisius (1521-1597)

St. Peter Canisius was a Jesuit who at 43 was tapped to be a "secret agent" for the Vatican. The Council of Trent (which opened in 1545 and closed in 1563) had completed its main goal—to define Catholic doctrine in the face of Protestant and heretical doctrines. The definitive Catholic doctrines of the council needed to be disseminated to the European bishops. This was not an easy task because of the bulk of the work (no flashdrives, tweeting, or email available) and the hostile Protestant territories that had to be crossed to accomplish the task. Even though Canisius' predecessors failed in their attempts, Peter was able to crisscross Germany and successfully deliver the work. In addition to this feat, Peter's concern for the Catholics who were succumbing to the Protestant teachings prompted Peter to become involved in the writing of catechisms in which the Catholic teachings would not be distorted but presented in a clear and concise manner. The first catechism was so successfully received by the adults that a second, shorter catechism for middle school students was written. Peter's love and understanding of his faith became a significant obstacle to the Protestant movement that was sweeping through the population.

Exercise: Christ brought all of humanity Good News, with a capital G. In the limited, earthly realm of physical strength training, high intensity (HIT) methods bring good news with a small g – workouts that are surprisingly brief and infrequent can be very effective, if done with the proper intensity. This method produces many doubters in the weight room, who confuse the need to do *more* work to progress, with the true need to do *harder* work. In the realm of physical strength, we can indeed be guided by the results we can actually see and feel. You need not just take our word for it. In the realm of spiritual strength, though, we need to have the faith in Jesus Christ that exceeds and perfects the truths we can see with our eyes and touch with our hands. And when we believe them, we'll find ourselves perfected as well.

December 22

Blessed Jacapone de Todi (1230-1306)

You probably do not recognize the name, but if you attended the Stations of the Cross in your youth, you undoubtedly intoned his *Stabat Mater,* "Near the Cross her station keeping, stood that mournful Mother weeping. . ." Blessed Jacapone wrote it sometime in his final three years – a time of rest following a tumultuous life. Born Jacomo dei Benedetti to a noble Italian family, he seemed poised for a lucrative career in law. Even though his interests were extremely worldly, he married Vanna di Guidone, a young, extremely devout Catholic noblewoman. Unbeknownst to him, Vanna undertook arduous penances on his behalf. Her tragic death a year later proved the blow that opened Jacomo's heart to the grace of conversion. The change in his manner of life startled those around him: He sold off his earthly goods and distributed the money to the poor, and then spent the next ten years going through his city in penitential rags. The city began making a play on his name, calling him *Jacapone,* "Crazy Jim." In his great humility, he embraced the name. In time he joined the Franciscans as a lay brother.

Exercise: When Jacapone and two cardinals took umbrage with a elected pope, Boniface VIII, and began seeking his resignation, Jacapone was excommunicated and jailed. He acknowledged his wrongdoing and accepted his imprisonment in a true spirit of penance.

Did you receive the Sacrament of Reconciliation this Advent? If not, perhaps you can still make arrangements. If you are free of mortal sin, then at least perform a thorough examination of conscience in preparation for Christmas. Ask for perseverance in avoiding your venial sins throughout the new liturgical year. Zero in on the venial sin you most struggle with, and after you have asked the Holy Spirit to guide your thoughts, spend five minutes thinking of concrete steps you can take to achieve victory over that sin.

St. Servulus (died 590)

I will bless the Lord at all times; his praise shall continually be in my mouth. My soul makes its boast in the LORD; let the afflicted hear and be glad. O magnify the LORD with me, and let us exalt his name together!
Psalms 34:1-3

While we would see the ancient adage "a sound mind in a sound body" become even more generally realized in the present generation, it is the duty of everybody to look with particular compassion on those whose lot it is not to enjoy such well-being.
Pope Pius XII

St. Pope Gregory the Great (see Sept. 3rd) would sing the praises in a famous sermon of this great, though unlikely, saint of his personal acquaintance. Born quadriplegic, Servulus was unable to sit or stand, to roll from side to side, or to bring food to his own mouth. His brother and mother would carry him to the steps of the Church of St. Clement, where he would beg for the alms to sustain him. Servulus, however, gave others more than they could give him. He loved to be read to from the Scriptures and would memorize verse after verse. He loved as well to sing songs of praise and thanksgiving to God, enjoining those near him to join right in. He was also quick to share his alms with other poor beggars around him.

Exercise: St. Servulus reminds us of some very important caveats. In tending our temples, we are not preaching a cult of the body beautiful. We are to be the best possible stewards of whatever kind of earthly body we've been blessed with. We must share our possessions and our love with the sickly, diseased, and the aged if we are to live lives like Christ. Pope Pius XII has stated with great wisdom and compassion that those unable to engage in sport or exercise due to physical frailty have a "special title to nobility and greatness of spirit" when they can share without envy in the joy of their physically robust neighbors. Christ is in you and your neighbor whether you or your neighbor bristles with muscles or is confined to a bed or a wheelchair. Let's learn from St. Servulus, then, to share Christ's love with all and gladly sing praises to God's name.

December 24

Christmas Eve – St. Charbel Makhlouf (1828-1898)

St. Charbel is an ideal saint for the Church to remember on Christmas Eve. He was of this earth, at home in the harshest of conditions; and yet, there was an otherworldly character about him. He was born in the highlands of Lebanon, the youngest of five children. Blessed with two devout parents, his father died when he was only two years old. His uncles helped his mother raise all of the children; two of these uncles were monks of the Lebanese Maronite Order. Our young saint served Mass each morning before going off to shepherd the family flocks – an occupation that gave him an abundance of time to pray and meditate on God amidst the beauty of creation. St. Charbel entered the monastic life without a word to his family. He simply slipped away one morning before anyone else arose. He went Annaya Abbey and took the name Charbel (his given name was Youssef). After eight years of preparation, he was ordained a priest. He lived at the abbey for another six years before moving to one of the nearby hermitages where his only companionship was the Lord Jesus and the Communion of Saints. Charbel endured the coldest of mountain winters in nothing but his robe, spending every night on his knees before the altar, after which time he would celebrate Mass. During his seventieth year, while celebrating Mass just a week before Christmas, he suffered a stroke while elevating the consecrated Host. He passed from this world on Christmas Eve.

Exercise: St. Charbel made his whole life a sacrificial gift to the One Whose birth we commence celebrating at midnight. Make your life a gift to Jesus by quietly doing whatever you can to assist in preparing for your family's celebration of Christmas. The stress of last-minute errands and getting the house ready for guests can make for frayed nerves. Ignore the hurried tones and harsh words; make your only response an understanding smile and two helping hands. This is the kind of sacrifice, the kind of Christmas gift, the Lord Jesus truly desires. St. Charbel, on this anniversary of your entrance into glory, pray for us.

December 25

The Nativity of Jesus Christ

And she gave birth to her first-born son and wrapped him in swaddling clothes, and laid him in a manger, because there was no place at the inn.
Luke 2:7

No pagan legend or philosophical anecdote or historical event, does in fact affect any of us with that peculiar and even poignant impression produced on us by the word Bethlehem.
G. K. Chesterton, The Everlasting Man

We know that our flesh is a good thing, since God chose to clothe Himself in it in the person of His Son through the great miracle of the *incarnation*, a literal "enfleshment." G.K. Chesterton has waxed eloquently about how a God so limitlessly big and powerful chose to become so tiny and weak for a time, for our benefit of eternal salvation. St. Albert the Great (Nov. 15), would marvel at the incarnational mystery foretold in Jeremiah 31:22: "For the Lord has created a new thing on the earth: a woman protects a man." In the Latin Vulgate translation "protects" reads *"circumdabit,"* to encircle or enclose. It would be nothing new for the womb of a woman to enclose an ordinary child, but for the womb of a virginal woman to enclose within its confines the very Lord of the universe, that indeed was a "new thing!"

Exercise: Christmas has arrived and truly this is a day for celebration with our loved ones and with our fellow parishioners. What can we do on this very special day commemorating Christ's birth, to show to God and man just how appreciative we are of this incomparable gift of Himself? Let's share our gifts gladly with nothing but appreciation. Let's go to Mass (if we haven't already participated at midnight!) and spread joy at our Christmas meal. Eat heartily, though without gluttony. Be sure to try a bite of Aunt Rita's famous Texas cake, and don't forget Marjorie's frozen pink marshmallow salad. (I [Kevin] can't remember what mom called it.) In our family tradition, on this special day, even the kids get a little taste of sweet concord wine as well. Let's make this day a day of sweet memories for all the generations.

St. Stephen (1ˢᵗ Century) Deacon and Martyr

What is the Church thinking, following Christmas with the feast of its first martyr? She is doing exactly what the Lord Jesus did – shocking us with the paradox of the Gospel: "For whoever would save his life will lose it; and whoever loses his life for my sake, he will save it. (Lk. 9:24). The joy of the incarnation always exists side-by-side with the sobriety of the Cross – and thanks be to God, side-by-side with the glory of the Resurrection too! In St. Stephen we see how this reality took flesh in someone exactly like us, a sinner regenerated and continually strengthened by the Sacraments. St. Stephen was in the Church's first class of deacons, ordained to see to the material needs of neglected community members. The Spirit moved him to also speak eloquently of the Lord Jesus, infuriating those opposed to the infant Church. His bold public witness eventually led to him being brought before the Sanhedrin and being accused by false witnesses. Just before his being stoned to death, he was granted a vision of the glory that awaited him at the Father's throne, alongside his resurrected Lord. Acts of the Apostles then reveals that Stephen's stoning as a participation in Jesus' Cross; Stephen made Jesus' dying prayer his own, "receive my spirit." (Acts 7:59-60). We see one of the effects of Stephen's prayer later in Acts, when the man who watched the cloaks of Stephen's executioners received the grace to become the Apostle Paul.

Exercise: Yesterday we heard of how Jesus was laid in a manger, a feeding trough for animals, at his birth. He came into the world to make a gift of Himself, both to God and man. He was a gift who would be "chewed up" – in anger by the world, and in humble awe by those of us who receive Him in Holy Communion. Both are connected to the Cross, Jesus' pain – one leading to it, and the other flowing from it. You and I must make a complete gift of ourselves too. Make an offering of soul and body to the Lord today by returning to your regular schedule of prayer and exercise; and make a gift of yourself to your family by straightening up the house.

St. John the Evangelist (1ˢᵗ Century)

Each had the face of a man in front; the four had the face of a lion on the right side, the four had the face of an ox on the left side, and the four had the face of an eagle at the back...　　　*Ezekiel 1:10*

But there are also many other things which Jesus did; were every one of them to be written, I suppose that the world itself could not contain the books that would be written.　　　*John 21:25*

As a young child, I (Kevin) recall with fascination the images of the four evangelists painted high between the inside arches of the old St. Agnes Church. Based on traditions of the Church Fathers drawing on Scriptural passages from Ezekiel and Revelation, Matthew was symbolized as a man with wings, Mark as a winged lion, Luke a winged bull, and John as an eagle (of course, with wings!) who could stare into the face of the Son. St. John was the youngest of the Apostles, and was beloved by Christ. He was there leaning at Christ's breast at the Last Supper, at the Transfiguration, at the agony in Gethsemane, with the Blessed Mother at the foot of the cross. He was the first Apostle to believe in the resurrection and the first to recognize the resurrected Christ when He appeared by the Sea of Tiberias. He would live to an old age, and while exiled on the island of Patmos write the book of Revelation.

Exercise: What can *we* do to be "beloved of Christ,"—to live in the hope of seeing Him face to face in the bliss of the beatific vision? Like St. John, we need to let our thoughts soar to the heights like an eagle and not become mired down low in the things of the earth. St. Thomas Aquinas said that with the Holy Spirit's gift of understanding, we "penetrate deep into to the heart of things." St. John rested his head on the very heart of Jesus and looked Him in the eyes. Christ Himself, in his famous mountain sermon, told us what we need to purify our hearts to see Him: "Blessed are the pure in heart, for they shall see God." (Matthew 5:8).

December 28

Holy Innocents (1st Century)

It is one of the ghastliest episodes in the gospels – Herod's slaughter of innocent children in the vain attempt to harm Jesus. Secular histories do not even mention of it; the deaths of twenty or so children in a hamlet like Bethlehem appeared insignificant, and especially so when compared with Herod's other crimes, like murdering three of his own sons. Our society today recoils at such actions, or do we? At the time of this writing, the United States is in furious disbelief at a Florida jury's inability to convict Casey Anthony in the murder of her two year-old, Caylee. Night after night, the country hears commentators such as Nancy Grace decry the lack of justice for little Caylee whose body was disposed of along the highway like "trash." Never have I heard one of these reporters ask why our country reacts with such horror to this case, but can continue to tolerate legalized abortion, where aborted fetuses have literally been disposed of in dumpsters behind clinics? How can the country hate a woman such as Casey Anthony that, no matter what a jury says, it will always consider guilty of murdering her two year-old, and yet refuse to overturn laws that allow any mother to end the life of her two month-old?

Exercise: Have you ever stood in prayer outside of an abortion clinic? I (Shane) have not. I pray for an end to abortion. I share my opposition to it in conversations with friends, and I refuse to vote for any politician who supports it. But I have never stood in front of a clinic, shoulder-to-shoulder with other believers, praying and publicly witnessing to the value of unborn life. So here is a challenge, for me personally, and for you if you feel so inclined: Contact your diocese's pro-life office and find out when people will next gather for prayer outside of an abortion clinic. I need to stop just shaking my head at the world's callousness and allow my legs to take me where I need to be, so I can pray: *"Holy Innocents, who lost your lives because of your nearness to our Lord, and Mary and Joseph – who saved Jesus from death – please intercede for the lives of our unborn children. Jesus, save our nation and world, from this cancerous sin. Our Lady of Guadalupe, Patroness of the Unborn, pray for us!"*

St. Thomas Becket (1118-1170)

No man can serve two masters...   *Matthew 6:24*

I served our Theobald well when I was with him: I served King Henry well as Chancellor: I am his no more, and I must serve the Church.
Lord Alfred Tennyson, Becket

Thomas Becket was King Henry II of England's royal chancellor. In a time of fierce struggle between powers of Church and state, this Henry (sixth in line before the Henry who would rent asunder England's affiliation with Rome), sought to consolidate his power by appointing his good friend, Thomas, to the highest Episcopal seat in England, the Archbishopric of Canterbury, in addition to his role as chancellor. Thomas hesitated to assume this role, but it was put upon him. Surprisingly, though, a true and holy change took place. He was made a priest and through study, prayer, sacrifice, and sacraments, became a true man of God and son of the Church. He resigned his chancellorship and defended the Church against King Henry's encroachments on its possessions, rightful powers, and moral laws. When King Henry voiced his irritation at such mistreatment "from a low-born clerk," certain nobles interrupted this as an order for the archbishop's murder. On December 29, 1170, four knights and a band of armed men slew the unyielding archbishop with sword strikes through his skull in the transept of the church. The public was moved and outraged. King Henry himself responded with fasting and public repentance. Within two years after his death, St. Thomas Becket was a canonized saint.

Exercise: As we near the year's end, we see yet another example of the saintly, heroic fortitude of the martyr. Thankfully, in the modern Western world, Christian martyrdom is rare, and will hopefully stay that way. It is our job to muster a much less heroic, but still virtuous, fortitude to do hard things for God, like enduring the strength and cardiovascular training that will perfect the temples that we are.

Blessed Eugenia Ravasco (1845-1900)

Blessed Eugenia was what we call "well-grounded." She had her priorities straight – a good example as we approach the start of a new calendar year. This isn't to say that Eugenia's life started smoothly. By age 10, she had lost both parents and had relocated three times. She and her five siblings were raised by their uncle Luigi Ravasco in Genoa, Italy. He provided them, as well as his own ten children, with a noble example of charity to the poor and a sound formation in the truths of the Faith. The Eucharist and devotion to the hearts of Jesus and Mary became the hallmarks of Eugenia's spirituality. By her late teens she felt called to religious life. She started volunteering in her own parish instead of applying immediately to a religious order. She taught catechism classes to girls who were being raised more by the streets than their parents. At first Eugenia appeared quite naïve and sheltered to the girls, but her sincere interest in them allowed the girls to look past the differences in circumstance and recognize her as an older sister. At age 23, she founded a new religious congregation, the Sisters of the Sacred Hearts of Jesus and Mary. Ten years later the order was able to open its first school for girls. Its mission was to form future Christian teachers. Under Mother Eugenia's leadership the congregation opened new houses in Switzerland and France. Today her congregation is found in South and Central America, Africa, and the Philippines.

Exercise: Live your priorities today. Begin by re-consecrating yourself and all of your activities to Jesus, through the Sacred Heart of Mary. Invoke the Church's saints and blessed to pray for you. Put in your minutes of cardio or perform your HIT session. Give an honest day's work at your job. Make sure to give your family the attention they deserve; mute the television and really listen to what they have to say. Laugh. Laugh some more. And make sure to put a smile on your Mother' face before your head hits the pillow by praying the Rosary.

St. Catherine Laboure (1806-1876)

I have fought the good fight, I have finished the race, I have kept the faith.
2 Timothy 4:6-7

O Marie conque sans peche priez pour nous que avons recours a vous. (O Mary, conceived without sin, pray for us who have recourse to thee.)
Text of the Miraculous Medal

When I first saw a photo of this great saint, I was rather surprised that Peggy, our pilot, let me (Kevin) write this one, since her habit's winged headpiece reminded me of the beloved "Flying Nun" television show that I watched as a kid! St. Catherine was a humble, loving woman graced with visions of the Blessed Mother. It is said that when her own mother died when she was very young, she kissed a statue of Mother Mary and said that she would be her mother now. In the summer of 1870, Mary appeared to her in visions and displayed herself bearing colorful rings, standing inside an oval frame that rotated on the back and was surrounded by stars, featuring a capital M surmounting a cross, with an image of the Sacred Heart of Jesus encircled by thorns and an image of the Immaculate Heart of Mary pierced by a sword. Mary told her to report her vision to her confessor and have the image cast into medallions that would be worn to obtain her graces. This was indeed done, and today millions wear the "Miraculous Medal" and pray for Mary's graces.

Exercise: As we come to the end of the year, two parting thoughts come to mind. First, hopefully you feel now like you are indeed fighting the good fight in developing the habits to glorify God through a properly tended temple. But remember, too, that virtuous habits are the oars on our ships, but God is the wind in our sails. The Blessed Mother (whose Immaculate Conception had not yet been pronounced as dogma at the time of the casting Miraculous Medal) told St. Catherine that some of the colorful rings on her fingers did not emit light because people had not asked for those graces. We need to do our part to live our lives in Christ, but we must never forget to ask for some help, especially from his Mother!